PRAISE FOR *A COMMON STRUGGLE*

"A stunningly unvarnished portrait of one of America's most private public families."   —*People*

"In his book, Patrick breaks what he calls the Kennedy code of silence."
—Lesley Stahl, *60 Minutes*

"[A] raw and honest book."   —*Star Tribune* (Minneapolis)

"Searching and fearless."   —Kevin Cullen, *The Boston Globe*

"I am personally really proud of Patrick. I think what he's doing is consistent with everything that my family has stood for. . . . He needed to start that journey by telling his own story of mental illness. I think it's noble, and it's heroic, and I have nothing but admiration for him."
—Robert F. Kennedy Jr. on *Ring of Fire*

"[Patrick Kennedy] has undeniably turned his fame toward a good cause—of raising understanding about the prevalence of mental illness and addiction in our society, and the need to help our brothers and sisters who cannot help themselves. There are easier ways to make money than speaking out honestly about one's own life, and we admire the courage Mr. Kennedy has shown in discussing these difficult issues."
—*Providence Journal*

"Fascinating. . . . This book is a must-read, not only for those suffering from mental health and substance-use disorders but also for the professionals who treat them and for those who pay for that treatment."
—Dr. George Koob, Director of the National Institute on Alcohol Abuse and Alcoholism, *Clinical Psychiatry News*

"Kennedy's eye-opening book is a public call for action. *A Common Struggle* also is a call for understanding, not only for those with mental illness but for all those affected by the mostly misunderstood, and often devastating, illness. As Kennedy points out, no one is immune from mental illness."
                                                                    —*Wichita Times*

"His new memoir, which recounts the troubles he and his famous family experienced, will help move the needle when it comes to public policy regarding mental health and substance abuse. . . . It shine[s] a needed light on a serious problem."

                                                                    —*The Oklahoman*

"If your readers do nothing else today, they should buy or order this remarkable book. . . . I always admired Kennedy's passion and willingness to fight not only on mental illness issues but also such topics as gay rights and gun control. This book should enhance your understanding and appreciation of the work he did in Congress and the ambitious mental health initiatives he is leading now. And for the happiness of his marriage and fatherhood. . . ."

                                                —M. Charles Bakst, on WPRI TV blog

"I think Patrick Kennedy is quite courageous for bringing this book out. . . . What he is doing is really the equivalent of what Betty Ford did when she exposed her own alcoholism."
            —Dr. Thomas McLellan, former deputy director of the White
                House Office of National Drug Control Policy, on MSNBC

"Patrick Kennedy should receive a Profile in Courage Award for his book, *A Common Struggle*. . . ."   —Dan Rea, CBS-TV Boston

A COMMON
STRUGGLE

A COMMON STRUGGLE

*A Personal Journey
Through the Past and Future of
Mental Illness and Addiction*

PATRICK J. KENNEDY
& STEPHEN FRIED

BLUE RIDER PRESS
New York

blue
rider
press

An imprint of Penguin Random House LLC
375 Hudson Street
New York, New York 10014

Library of Congress Cataloging-in-Publication Data
Kennedy, Patrick J. (Patrick Joseph).
A common struggle : a personal journey through the past and future of mental illness and
addiction / Patrick J. Kennedy & Stephen Fried.
p.   cm.
ISBN 978-0-399-17332-5 (hardcover)
1. Kennedy, Patrick J. (Patrick Joseph), 1967—Mental health.   2. Legislators—United States—
Biography.   3. United States. Congress. House—Biography.   4. Manic-depressive persons—United
States—Biography.   5. Drug addicts—United States—Biography.   6. Patient advocacy—United
States.   7. Mental illness—Social aspects—United States.   8. Drug abuse—Social aspects—
United States.   9. Mental illness—Treatment—United States.   10. Drug abuse—Treatment—
United States.   I. Fried, Stephen, 1958–   II. Title.
E840.8.K358A3   2015   2015025738
616.890092—dc23
[B]

Blue Rider Press hardcover: October 2015
Blue Rider Press paperback: September 2016
Blue Rider Press paperback ISBN: 9780399185717

Printed in the United States of America

Book design by Meighan Cavanaugh

PROLOGUE

I'm never going to remember what actually happened that night in early May of 2006 when I slammed my green Mustang into the police barrier in front of the US Capitol. I retain a faint memory of flashing lights and people in uniforms knocking at my car window. That's about it. No idea how I got there. No idea how I got home.

But I will never forget what happened the next day. I got up late, walked from my apartment building to Capitol Hill (because I had no idea where my car was), and then sat in my congressional office waiting in terror for the phone to ring.

I was waiting for someone to call and say: "You finally did it, you killed somebody. This is it."

When the call didn't come, I drank a couple Red Bulls to try to clear my head and took a meeting with the leaders of the Campaign for Mental Health Reform, which was lobbying on behalf of patient, provider, and clinician groups. They immediately noticed I didn't appear mentally healthy myself: I was having trouble following the conversation and my hands were shaking. We were all saved from further embarrassment when I was called away to the House floor to vote on a lot of amendments for a port safety bill.

As the voting ended, the phone call finally came. I was summoned off the House floor into the cloakroom, where there were booths that allowed private conversations. It was my chief of staff.

"Patrick," he said, "we have a problem."

Apparently I had half woken up at around two thirty in the morning, several hours after mixing medications to get to sleep—Ambien and Phenergan, both recently prescribed, along with all the other asthma and mental health meds I was taking. Convinced I was late for a vote, I threw on a suit and tie, stumbled to my car, and drove, headlights off, several blocks down Third Street until I barely managed the left onto C Street. Then I barreled straight toward the security station for the House of Representatives. I swerved into oncoming traffic, nearly hitting a US Capitol Police vehicle, which somehow dodged me and then made a quick U-turn to chase me. I slowed down but didn't stop until my car slammed into the security barrier.

Luckily, my chief of staff explained, only my car was damaged, because nobody was on the streets or the sidewalks where I was driving in the middle of the night.

After making sure I wasn't hurt, the Capitol Police quietly took me home and moved my car into the congressional parking lot. But word spread and someone from the media had noticed the banged-up car in the lot.

"You've got to get back here, right now," my chief of staff said.

I made a beeline back to my office and barricaded myself in. The next hours were a blur of phone calls of support and tough questions for which there were no easy answers. But the call I remember best came from my dad.

The first thing he said was, "I saw a picture of the car, and I don't know why they're making such a big deal of this. It looked to me like it was only a little fendah bendah."

Very old-school. No "How are you doing?" Just "a little fendah bendah" (or, for those not raised in New England, "fender bender").

In fact, that's pretty much how he suggested I play it with the press and the public.

I wanted him to understand that I was sick, and that untreated mental illness and addiction was not about little fendah bendahs. It was about multicar pileups where people were injured and killed.

His insistence that this was a fendah bendah was a key to our issues as father and son. I worshipped my dad. He was the North Star by which I navigated my life. My dad loved and supported me as best he could, but he didn't always respect me, and he didn't understand the chronic medical condition I struggled with. He often said that all I needed was a "good swift kick in the ass."

Did I say any of this to him? Of course not. I grew up among people who were geniuses at not talking about things. When I was a teenager going for therapy during my parents' divorce, I wouldn't tell my psychiatrist the truth because I wasn't sure I could trust him to keep things private. Then one day I walked into a bookstore and browsed the "Kennedy section" and saw that many of the books included the "family secrets" I had refused to discuss. But I still wouldn't talk about them.

So my father was stunned when, several hours later, I admitted everything that happened to the press and then very publicly left for an extended rehab at the Mayo Clinic. He was also pretty concerned when I tried to demand jail time in my plea agreement so it wouldn't look like I was getting preferential treatment.

And my dad was *really* not thrilled when, after returning from rehab, I started being much more public about my private struggles with bipolar disorder and addiction. I promised myself I would have the most transparent recovery and treatment ever, all but donating my brain and its diseases to science while I was still living. I wanted to aggressively tie my personal story to my ongoing legislative fight for mental health parity—an effort to outlaw the rampant discrimination in medical insurance coverage for mental illness and addiction treatment. And winning the parity fight would be the first step to overcoming all discrimination against people with these diseases, their families, and those who treated them.

So I decided to go public exclusively to the *New York Times*. I did this with my Republican House colleague Jim Ramstad from Minnesota. Before my crash I had known him, although not well, as one of the only members of Congress who was openly in recovery. But after my arrest and hospitalization he was the first one to come visit me at the Mayo Clinic. I asked if he would be my sponsor in recovery—I had never had a real sponsor before—and he invited me into his network of friends in recovery on Capitol Hill.

While we thought this could have an impact, there was no way we could have predicted that the resulting story would run huge on the front page of the *Times*—or that it would run on September 19, 2006, two days after the death of my father's sister Patricia Kennedy Lawford and the day before her funeral in New York City. There was also no way to predict that the reporter would quote me talking about the veil of secrecy in my family regarding depression and substance use, and then call my dad for comment about his own drinking habits at such a sensitive time.

So, of course, he was livid. When the family gathered after the funeral service at my Aunt Pat's house in New York, he cornered me. He called the article a "disaster"—the word he always used to describe the most extreme situations. How *dare* I talk about the family this way? How *dare* I discuss "these things" in public?

I stood there on the verge of disintegration. I was early in my sobriety and still pretty vulnerable. And I watched my father circulate around the room, talking about the article.

Then my cousin Anthony Shriver came up to tell me what his sister, Maria, had just done. When my dad got to her to complain about the *Times* story, she apparently challenged him.

"I think what Patrick did was *fantastic*," Maria said. "That's what we need in our family, someone to talk about this."

And, in that moment, I knew what I had to do.

THIS ISSUE OF not talking openly about "these things" is hardly just a Kennedy issue. It is a problem in most American families. Most of the challenges of mental illness and addiction feel incredibly unique and private when, in fact, they are remarkably common: nearly 25 percent of all Americans are personally affected by mental illness and addiction every day, one-third of all U.S. hospital stays involve these diseases, and they have a huge impact on everyone else.

But, in this situation, there was a very specific, very personal and political way for me to address this on Capitol Hill. It was a bill called the Mental Health Parity Act.

Ten years earlier, a mental health equity act had been signed into law. It was supposed to finally end prejudice against mental illness by making it illegal to treat diseases of the brain any differently than those of any other part of the body.

The act had failed. And now it was up for renewal. I was lead Democratic sponsor of the House version, my father was lead Democratic sponsor of the Senate version, and the two bills couldn't have been more different.

The Senate bill was much the same one that had failed to make much impact ten years ago—in part because, as a matter of political expediency, it only covered what are called the most "serious" mental illnesses (such as schizophrenia) and ignored more common mental illnesses and substance use disorders.

My bill included *all* the brain diseases. House Resolution (HR) 1424 was meant to be a kind of medical civil rights act, which once and for all would end—or at least make illegal—any discrimination in coverage for these illnesses.

Basically, in my dad's Senate bill, what was wrong with me—bipolar disorder, addiction—would *not* be fully covered, would not be medically equal. In my bill, they would be.

But, of course, it was all much more complicated than that.

ALMOST SIX YEARS after that front-page *New York Times* story about my recovery, I slipped very quietly into the Mayo Clinic in Minnesota. Again.

I ended up in the Generose Building. That's where they do psychiatric care, and drug and alcohol rehab. After checking in at the front desk, I was brought to see the same doctors who had treated me there before, along with my favorite counselor, John Holland. He runs the infamous "process groups," which are like AA meetings on steroids— very intense—with your peers just smashing down your denial.

John and I caught up. Since the last time we had seen each other, a lot had happened. My father had died, I had left Congress, I had fallen in love, I had truly committed to sobriety, I had gotten married for the first time at age forty-four, and I had moved from New England to the Jersey Shore, where my wife, Amy, and her family lived. We had just had a son and were also raising her daughter from a previous marriage.

I also shared with him a recent devastating loss: my older sister, Kara. John knew Kara but hadn't known about her sudden, unexpected death at fifty-one.

He said that he had recently lost his older sister. Drug overdose.

It was a relief to be able to tell him that I wasn't there to be admitted. I was there to see a friend and colleague who had been texting me from rehab, asking for my help.

I was led through several doors, each one locked behind us, into the corridors of the Generose Building, where I had walked so many times before. I was finally brought to a patient room where the door was opened to reveal my longtime fellow Congressman Jesse Jackson Jr., sitting on the edge of a hospital bed.

I was stunned by how dejected he was—what a grip depression had on him. I had served with Jesse for sixteen years and saw him all the time because we were on a lot of the same subcommittees together. And he always had this kind of bravado about him—a proud guy with an incredible physical bearing and this power personality. Now he was really frightened by the depth of his own despair.

He said he had put on his nice shirt because I was coming. He was now measuring things differently in life—the simplest act, of putting on a clean dress shirt, had become a big gesture. It was hard.

Jesse had been secretly suffering from bipolar disorder. Although his family was insisting he was being treated for, you know, "exhaustion," he realized it was time to come clean. But he wasn't in any condition to do that yet. Nobody close to him really understood. So he wanted me to be the messenger.

I sat down next to him and we talked. He spoke achingly about his kids and what kind of father he was, how he felt he had let everybody down. He said he couldn't imagine not being there to walk his daughter down the aisle. When I thought about what that meant—that he wasn't sure he would live through this—it left me speechless.

I figured the best way to encourage him was to tell him about how it was when I was in his situation. He knew I had been treated at Generose in May 2006 after the car crash. But what he didn't know, because nobody did, was that part of the reason I wrecked my life was because I failed to take my treatment seriously enough when I was at Mayo five months *before* the crash, during Congress's Christmas break in 2005.

During that previous hospitalization, I tried to game the situation, refusing to be treated in Generose because of the stigma. I didn't want anyone to think I was "crazy." So I forced them to keep me at the medical facility at Mayo, where I could detox from opiates but still, technically, not be in rehab. I got treated physically but not mentally and spiritually. And after that treatment, I only stopped using opiates— not the other drugs I used, which didn't have such a pejorative label. When you're good at self-medicating, you can abuse just about anything.

I told Jesse I was glad he wasn't making the same mistake and was committed to doing the treatment right. Everyone finding out wasn't such a bad thing. In fact, everyone finding out was probably the only reason I was still here. But, at the time, I hadn't known what was going to happen; I felt my life was over and I had let everyone down. I was a loser and a failure.

"I know, I know," he said, nodding his head. "But I don't know who I'm supposed to *be* anymore. My father is this great man and I've been trying to be a great man, but I don't know if I can be."

I told him he was a great man and this was going to make him an even *greater* man. And, frankly, in the political world we live in, his openness on mental health would advance the cause of civil rights as much as anything he had ever done. Because it's all about overcoming stereotypes, prejudice, and marginalization.

He asked if I'd be willing to tell his father that. As quickly as I said yes, he was speed-dialing the number on his cell phone. I thought it was funny when he handed it to me and said, "Here's the reverend."

I explained what Jesse Jr. and I had been discussing, and he declared, as if he were in the middle of a sermon, "The cross is a lot easier to bear if you're not bearing it alone." I actually had to stop myself from saying "Amen."

I told the reverend that I wasn't sure which was a heavier cross to bear, being Ted Kennedy's son or being *his* son—at which point Jesse, sitting next to me, started to smile for the first time, and actually laughed.

After we wrapped up the call, Jesse was talking about the sense of persecution he felt, and his confusion about whether to resign from Congress—because of the ethics investigation he was in the middle of and because of his illness. It turned out he was in the same healthcare dilemma as so many other Americans.

"I can't resign," he said. "I need to finish my treatment, and I won't get any care if I resign. All these years I never needed healthcare. Now when I need it, how am I going to get it?" This was also making him wonder how his constituents got mental healthcare. I told him that was a good sign—if he was still thinking about other people, he would be all right.

We took some pictures, we hugged, and then I left.

As I walked down the hall to the exit, I thought about all of the "aha" moments there are in the world of these diseases. So many people hiding and pretending, so many people who just want to be able to say out loud what's wrong with them and get proper treatment, so many people all over the country who are facing the same problem but rarely find each other—and if they do, it's often too late.

We need to better engage those who think these illnesses don't affect them, to help them move from prejudice—which they often don't realize they have—to at least an enlightened curiosity.

Several hours later, I fulfilled my role as Jesse's messenger, speaking to NBC News about my meeting with him. "No one wants to admit that they suffer from a mental illness, because of the stigma," I said. "Both of us suffer from major depression. He knows that I've been through a lot of the same things that he's going through now."

I made it clear that while Jesse was ill and I was, at the moment, doing pretty well, I knew there would likely come a day when our roles were reversed, and he would have to be there for me. These are chronic illnesses. So far, we have no cures. Only medical treatments, meetings, research, spirituality, hope, and belief in a common struggle.

I LEFT CONGRESS at the end of 2010 to change and, hopefully, to save my life. Since then, I have been crisscrossing the country on a sort of Lewis and Clark expedition into the new frontiers of medicine, politics, economics, and human emotion in mental healthcare and brain research.

I speak to groups who want to hear about my personal challenges and my political challenges, and about the future of healthcare—especially healthcare from the neck up. I meet with top scientists in their labs and see the cutting edge of research. I hold public hearings for patients and families denied their mental health benefits. And I'm constantly pulled aside for private and incredibly revealing conversations with an amazingly broad cross-section of people.

They often just need someone to talk to about their own challenging experiences with brain diseases, someone who "gets it." But they also appreciate having that conversation with someone who is deeply involved in the worlds of mental health policy, medicine, science, law, and economics—so when they ask what they can do to help, or what the future looks like, they can get a useful answer. Or at least an informed opinion on what isn't yet known.

For the past twenty years, including my time in the House, I have been immersed in the big science and big business of mental health, as well as the small steps of progress in many people's care. I interact with everyone from heads of state and international business leaders who privately suffer with mental illness to the local family we know, whose mentally ill son was shot to death by an untrained police officer.

I also get deeply involved in the politics of the brain, which are fascinating and inspiring but also sometimes bruising. The fight to save "beautiful minds" can get pretty ugly.

I've had a chance to see these frictions from a unique perspective. While sitting on a House committee being asked to fund all these competing approaches and perspectives, I was also suffering from, and not always taking very good care of, the mental illnesses of bipolar and anxiety disorders, and the substance use disorders of binge drinking and opiate dependence. I have watched debates by top scientists, policy analysts, treatment professionals, drug manufacturers, and insurers and then, just weeks later, sat in group therapy commiserating with fellow inpatients about the same problems from a wholly different vantage point.

It takes a while to understand and navigate these worlds as a patient or family member. And a shocking number of people walk away from treatment that works after reading something inflammatory about the politics and economics of care—or they game the failures of integration in the system, hide between the cracks, and make themselves sicker. I have, in my "career" as a patient, seen and done both. But, working in the politics of medicine, I also understand that everyone in the world of brain diseases has attitudes formed in an environment of discrimination and prejudice.

Most of the varied approaches to care began getting traction before there were actually any medicines that worked. And the business of those medicines now often competes with the business of behavioral therapies and supports, as well as the housing and employment assistance usually required to keep people in any kind of treatment and healthy lifestyle. Each sector treating mental illness or addiction is challenged, underfunded, and discriminated against in its own way. But it's still hard to watch people who care deeply about brain diseases and have devoted their lives to their treatment competing on medical, legal, or financial issues—as if certain diagnoses or therapeutic approaches are supposed to *win*.

It is sometimes hard to remind all these people—who, by the way, work incredibly hard in their own worlds—that they are all treating the same organ, the brain. And, just like for every other organ, we need to support, research, and reimburse a menu of evidence-based approaches. We need to build bridges between all the disparate researchers and clinicians in neurology, psychiatry, psychology, developmental disabilities, and cognitive impairments—as well as the people they treat and their families. We need to help inspire an increasingly "one-minded" approach to not only mental illness and addiction but brain diseases from autism to Alzheimer's, bipolar disorder to traumatic brain injury, seizures to PTSD.

We need to constantly remind people that this is a common struggle.

People have been lamenting the stigma of mental illness and addiction for centuries. So why do I think anything is going to change now?

Simple. Until very recently it was completely legal to discriminate in treatment and insurance coverage against those with mental illness and addictions. We have referred to this phenomenon as "stigma," as if there were some justification and shared responsibility for the questioning and blaming and undermining of those with certain types of illnesses, describing their traumas and challenges as "little fendah bendahs."

But it's time to stop asking to be destigmatized and instead start demanding an end to discrimination.

Because what many still don't realize is that this discrimination is now a federal crime.

Mental health parity is finally the law of the land. Based on the guarantees of the Mental Health Parity and Addiction Equity Act—which my father and I helped pass together in 2008 but has only recently started being implemented—and the Obama Patient Protection and Affordable Care Act, it is finally illegal to cover mental illness, addiction, and intellectual disabilities any differently than other medical conditions, and preexisting conditions can never again be used to restrict access to coverage. While these laws were signed several years ago, because of court challenges and the seemingly endless process of government rule-making, they couldn't begin to be fully enforced until July 1, 2014. And they are still barely being enforced today.

The Mental Health Parity Act is the equivalent of a medical civil rights act, a brain disease equal rights amendment—the legal end of the discrimination that is at the heart of the stigma of brain diseases. As a politician, as a patient, and as a member of a family haunted by mental illness and addiction, I have waited my entire life for this moment.

But I also know that since we weren't sure this moment would ever come, we are largely unprepared for it. We're still struggling to figure out how the promise of mental health parity will be put into practice.

Fifty years ago, when "civil rights" became the law of the land, nobody was really sure how to outlaw racial discrimination. It was up to people like my Uncle Bobby, as Attorney General and later as a Senator, along with many others to figure out how to operationalize and enforce such a societal change. And we will have to figure out how to do the same for this "parity" by outlawing medical discrimination, stigma, and inadequate care.

It is a daunting, exciting challenge. We have all lived our entire lives, as did our parents, our doctors, and our leaders, making decisions about mental illness and addiction under the assumption there would always be prejudice, there would always be institutionalized, legal stigma and discrimination. We have to start adjusting to the unfolding realities of a post-parity world, and help change that world.

We must do it now, together, and in the open.

OUR SECRETS ARE our most formidable adversaries. The older I get, the more I see secrecy as "the enemy within," which blocks recovery not only for individuals but for society itself.

That phrase has a special meaning to me. Not long before he died, my father gave me his copy of his brother Bobby's 1960 book about union corruption, *The Enemy Within*.

It is autographed: "To Teddy, who has his own enemy within."

Giving me that book was the closest my father ever came to acknowledging *anything* to me about his own struggles. Which is probably why I have been so invested in exposing the secrecy around mental illness.

Since I first "came out" about my treatment for bipolar disorder and addiction, I have found myself talking incredibly frankly to an enormous number of people who feel it isn't safe to share the secrets of their illnesses. I've had these intimate and moving conversations with an astonishing number of people, from the powerful to those who feel utterly powerless, in all kinds of settings.

Sometimes the conversations become a huge step in their ability to acknowledge the common struggle. Other times they reinforce the hypocrisy and pain of our stigmatizing society.

You would not believe how many times a Congressman or other public official has pulled me aside for advice and counsel because they, or a loved one, suffer from a mood disorder or an addiction, and they need a recommendation for treatment.

And I still have a hard time believing how many of these same public officials have failed to support funding for mental illness or addiction research, and even voted against parity for their treatment.

Recently, I have found myself being more open in my advocacy, perhaps because the national tragedies involving mental illness have made the cost of remaining quiet more clear. I have also been reaching out to the doctors who treated me over the years, to discuss my own care and the state of mental healthcare. These conversations have been fascinating, especially now that I have the perspective of today's science and my own personal perspective from the longest period of continuous sobriety I've experienced since the age of thirteen.

That sobriety has not been very long, and I don't kid myself that it will ever get any easier to maintain. I began counting it several months *after* my last days in Congress, on February 22, 2011—what would have been my father's seventy-ninth birthday.

And the main reason I am able to stay sober is because of a stroke of luck and coincidence that I am more than happy to attribute to divine intervention: the spring before I left Congress, I met and fell in love with my wife, Amy, a middle-school teacher in coastal South Jersey, where I now live. Amy has saved my life in so many ways but, more important, has provided the love and support I needed to commit to the daily work—and joy—of saving my *own* life.

Amy and our young children are what keep me on my spiritual journey of recovery and hope. In fact, they are probably the only reason I am still alive. They remind me every day of our most underappreciated treatments for these illnesses: *love and faith*.

They also remind me of the biggest reason to fight for mental health parity. My own children are at considerable genetic risk, just as I was, of developing mental illness and addiction. Which means that they can, and *must*, be part of the first generation in American history to have their brain diseases treated like every other disease.

Our children *must* be part of the first generation for which routine doctor visits include a "checkup from the neck up."

When you have heart disease or cancer, nobody questions your diagnosis—even if it changes or your treatment changes direction. And nobody uses setbacks in treatment as an excuse to question whether or not cancer or heart disease really exist, or if they are all "in your head."

My goal is to change the way we talk about mental illness and addiction in this country, move the conversation from a painful existential debate to a more useful and forward-looking discussion about proper diagnosis and care. The sad truth is that while we still have so much to learn about the brain, most patients don't even benefit from what we already know. More than half the people who have been diagnosed with any mental illness do not get treatment at all. It is time for this to change.

My hope is that by writing about and exposing the worlds I get to visit—as a politician, advocate, patient, and family member—I might be able to make your journey less isolated. These struggles are much more common than most people realize, but too many of us still face them alone, if we face them at all. That isn't necessary, it isn't healthy, and it isn't how any of us want to live our lives.

I believe more than ever that we have the power to help change the world for people who have mental illnesses and addictions, and for all of those whose lives are touched by these brain diseases—which is to say, *all of us*.

In fact, I have bet my life on it.

Chapter 1

During the winter of my sophomore year at Providence College, in early 1988, my back started hurting. First it was just occasional pain, then spasms would wake me in the middle of the night, and then I noticed I was stubbing my toe all the time, because I wasn't lifting my leg normally when I walked. I went to several doctors, who told me they couldn't find anything wrong. One night I decided to drive to the hospital but had to put the seat way down to even get into the car. At the ER, they weren't sure whether or not to give me pain-killers, since they thought I might be faking to get drugs.

After all, I was not considered the most reliable patient at that time. I had already been in rehab for cocaine, after a binge during spring break of my senior year in prep school. Then I had bailed out of my first semester at Georgetown, before ending up at Providence.

I had suffered with severe asthma since childhood, which was considered as much a pain in the neck as a disease. My asthma was set off by a lot of things—animal hair, smoke—and besides my inhalers, I sometimes needed oxygen. Yet "He's asthmatic" had, over the years, taken on meanings far beyond my breathing problems. And while I clearly suffered from depression and anxiety, they were not really viewed medically—they were seen, mostly, as symptoms of my parents' divorce.

Because I was living away from home—my mom was in Boston, my dad in DC—the ER staff decided to call my local doctor to see if it was okay to give me medication. That was my psychiatrist, a young guy named Peter Kramer, who five years later would become famous for writing *Listening to Prozac*, but at the time was just a rising psychotherapist who actually used medication pretty sparingly, if at all, the way it was supposed to be used: to help treat symptoms and enhance talk therapy, not to replace it.

Peter vouched for me—he considered it part of my work with him that he and I figure this out without calling my father. And they sent me home with the pain meds. But I had to agree to see him the next morning and then also get an evaluation from an internist he knew.

Of course, the painkillers knocked me out so much I slept through the appointment. So Peter decided to devote the therapeutic hour of my missed session to driving down the street to my apartment and banging on my front door until I woke up and he could make sure I got to the doctor's appointment. The internist took me a little more seriously than the ER docs had and did a full-body scan.

And that's when they found it. There was a tumor on the vertebrae of my neck. A pretty big one, actually, nearly an inch around. While it was likely benign, it was wrapped around a nerve root in a way that made removing it—or not removing it—very risky for possible paralysis.

When I got this news I was, in some strange way, thrilled. While I now find this hard to believe, I remember that, at the time, I actually welcomed this diagnosis. Because, for the first time in my life, there was something wrong with me that everyone agreed was "real." For the first time in my life, people acted like they had a legitimate reason to worry about me and what I was going through. No more of that "Oh, poor Patrick"—but, instead, a solid "Oh my God."

If you are lucky, you have no idea what it's like to have a disease that society questions because people can't "see" it and aren't sure they "believe in" it. I have a couple of those illnesses, which are easy to deny or downplay. While people always tried to be sympathetic—I was, after all, a scrawny, good-natured, redheaded kid who sometimes couldn't breathe—I also felt dismissed as weak, as if I could control these illnesses but simply chose not to.

But, suddenly, a *tumor on my spinal cord*! Top surgeons at Mass General going through all the X-rays and pointing to the tumor and talking about how complicated the surgery would be and even if it wasn't malignant I *could end up being paralyzed*. The tumor was *growing* and *tangled around my spinal cord* and all this great medical stuff that sounded terrifying to everybody else but actually gave me this strange kind of peace. There was something wrong, there was something they could do, but, more important, I had something that I wasn't ashamed of.

I recall actually saying to my twenty-year-old self: "Thank God I have cancer."

My parents were terribly worried, and everyone was calling them to say, "How awful, another son with a devastating illness." And all the time I was thinking, *This is great*.

This is something I wish for everyone who has a mental illness or addiction disorder.

Not to have a tumor, obviously, but to have your illness taken as seriously and sympathetically as cancer. (Luckily, the surgeons had my tumor biopsied and it was benign.)

And just to show how overwhelming and empowering that feeling was, I hobbled out of Mass General after three weeks in a hospital bed—walking with a cane and sporting a massive neck brace—on

May 7, 1988. And in less than a month I was making plans to run for the Rhode Island state legislature, in the district where I was heading into my sophomore year of college.

It was a part-time political job, paying $300 a year—and the incumbent, a five-term Democrat and Deputy Majority Leader, was a local funeral home director. But I was so high off the feeling of my health being taken seriously—and, in retrospect, while I hadn't yet been diagnosed with bipolar disorder, I suspect this was somewhat manic behavior—that it all seemed quite logical. My older brother, Teddy, had decided he would not seek public office. So this was a way for me to do something that would really connect me with my dad— who I revered, and who I desperately wanted to respect me instead of just feeling sorry for me.

There were 4,700 registered voters in the district where I went to college. My opponent and I each spent about $30,000 in campaign funds to woo them, and even after I put in close to $50,000 of my own money, I won by only 315 votes, 1,324 to 1,009.

But it didn't matter. I had joined the family business.

Chapter 2

When I was seventeen and a junior in high school, I got a letter around Thanksgiving from my father's older sister Eunice Kennedy Shriver—as did every member of my generation of the family. The letter described the work of the Joseph P. Kennedy Jr. Foundation, which had been started in the 1940s to memorialize my father's oldest brother, Joe Jr., who was lost in aerial combat in World War II. The foundation was about to celebrate its fortieth anniversary and Aunt Eunice basically suggested it was time that we young people start taking some interest in it. Not only did she want us to learn more about the foundation and its work, but she wanted to know what each of us thought about it—so her friend Lou Harris, creator of the Harris Poll, had volunteered to individually question each one of us young Kennedys, Shrivers, Smiths, and Lawfords about our "own policy concerns."

I'm not sure just how many policy concerns I had at seventeen. But as I look through all the stuff I still have from my teens, this letter—and the fact that I saved it—is probably the earliest inkling of where I would end up professionally. I have no recollection of what I told Lou

Harris then, but I now have a much better understanding of the importance of the questions my aunt was posing to us.

When the Joseph P. Kennedy Jr. Foundation was started in 1946, it was not specifically meant to fund work in healthcare. Joe Jr. had died in what now might be seen as one of the first military drone accidents. He and another pilot were flying a plane outfitted to be used as a radio-controlled unmanned dive bomber; on the way to its target in occupied northern France they were to arm the bombs, and then parachute to safety. Instead the bombs went off right after they were activated, and both pilots were killed instantly.

The foundation memorializing him served several philanthropic roles during its first years before Eunice took control of its mission in the midfifties and began using its funds more systematically to help advocate for pediatric medicine, especially in improving the lives of children with intellectual disabilities—who were then referred to as "retarded" and, mostly, sent away to institutions. She was moved to do this because she could see how the care of pregnant women and infants needed dramatic improvement. But she was also inspired by the experience of her oldest sister, Rosemary—even though, at the time, much of that experience was a family secret and something of a medical mystery.

Rosemary Kennedy was born during World War I with some form of developmental disability—it will never be completely clear which, because even the known facts about her case were gathered at a much more unsophisticated time in our understanding of the diagnosis and treatment of these conditions. Unlike most people with developmental disabilities, she was raised mostly at home with her family, just with a lot of extra help. But in her late teens and early twenties, her behavior changed and became more extreme—which was baffling to doctors of the day, who did not know, as we now do, that people born with developmental disabilities can still develop psychiatric disease at the same age everyone else normally does.

In 1941, Rosemary's father, my grandfather Joseph P. Kennedy Sr., made one of the most regrettable—and most resonantly regretted—decisions in the history of diagnosing, treating, and researching diseases of the brain and mind. He chose to have her treated with a terribly extreme new psychiatric procedure, a lobotomy. Instead of improving her life, this ill-conceived procedure dramatically worsened the brain damage she had experienced at birth, and she was never the same. She was cared for in a convent school in Wisconsin and, by my guilt-ridden grandfather's edict, wasn't seen at family events for years.

In the mid-fifties, Aunt Eunice decided to use the Kennedy Foundation to explore what could be done to help those born with developmental disabilities, as well as improve prenatal and postnatal care in the hope of preventing brain damage. Her goal, to a large degree, was to wrestle the care of those with developmental disabilities away from psychiatrists.

Psychiatry represented to her both the unresponsive medical establishment and the eugenics movement of the not-so-distant past. The psychiatrists also didn't do a good enough job differentiating the needs of those born with developmental disabilities from those who developed psychiatric illness later in life—usually starting in their teens, when mood disorders and psychotic disorders normally first manifest themselves. (In their defense, there was a lot we didn't know then about either area of medicine—and those who treated both of these deeply stigmatized groups were also, in the medical community, pretty stigmatized themselves.)

Psychiatrists generally oversaw the large state institutions where both people with untreatable mental illnesses and those with developmental disabilities were warehoused if their families couldn't afford a private institution. While many in these overcrowded, underfunded institutions didn't belong there, it was for different reasons. Those with intellectual disabilities primarily needed care because their challenges came at birth and were not believed to be treatable or improvable; many of them could have already been living at home, but their families were too stigmatized. Those with mental illness had diseases that generally began manifesting during their teen years, sometimes responding to treatment, sometimes not, and sometimes improving on their own in natural (if unpredictable) cycles—as long as the patients didn't harm themselves while sickest. The available treatments were the same kind we have today, but just much more rudimentary, and often given at much higher doses than we now realize is necessary. There was talk therapy and there were medical treatments, including the earliest psychoactive medications (mostly tranquilizers but also the very earliest antidepressants and antipsychotics) and the earliest types of direct brain stimulation (electroconvulsive therapy and insulin shock therapy). And there was watchful waiting.

The federal government was already paying attention to mental illness, having passed a law in 1955—cosponsored by young Senator John F. Kennedy—establishing the Joint Commission on Mental Illness and Mental Health. But, as Aunt Eunice often pointed out, there was "nothing" for people with intellectual disabilities. She would have to create something herself.

The first action of the Kennedy Foundation was to offer grants that would seed the creation of separate offices—state by state, because that's how healthcare is largely delivered—to improve the care and treatment of children who grew up like Rosemary. Eunice worked on this state strategy for a number of years before her brother Jack was elected President in 1960, and she began encouraging him to create federal legislation to help people with intellectual disabilities. A year later, just before Christmas of 1961, my grandfather had a debilitating stroke, which, among its other impacts, freed his wife, Rose, my grandmother, and her children to begin interacting more overtly with Rosemary and talking more openly about her. It is no coincidence that in the summer of 1962, Eunice created a small summer camp for children with disabilities in her backyard in Potomac, Maryland—which is what eventually grew into the Special Olympics.

That same summer, she wrote an article for the *Saturday Evening Post* revealing for the first time that her sister Rosemary, who was about to turn forty-four, was "mentally retarded." She then began using her position with the Kennedy Foundation even more aggressively to fund such summer camps all over the country, in schools, parks, and other recreation facilities. And she used what turned out to be the last year of her brother's presidency to lobby him to make bold legislation to help all the "special" children and adults who, largely, were living in institutions.

That article Aunt Eunice wrote about Aunt Rosemary also represented the beginning of a tradition of which I am now a part: the Kennedy family sharing its own health concerns to encourage and personalize medical advocacy. That tradition continued the next summer when Jackie Kennedy gave birth to a son who was five and a half weeks premature and died after only thirty-nine hours. The White House was quite open about the challenges of that son, Patrick Bouvier Kennedy, and those of the First Lady after the loss, calling international attention to the challenges of premature births, infant respiratory issues, and postpartum health for mothers.

In 1963, President Kennedy finally decided it was time to reverse "our approach to mental affliction." His goal was to respond to all the lobbying from his sister Eunice by creating new institutions and funding for the care of the "retarded," and also to reform existing mental healthcare, largely in response to a sweeping study and book-length report from the Joint Commission on Mental Illness and Health, which had taken over five years and was published just after he took office. Both efforts were deeply important and long overdue. In retrospect, combining them may not have been ideal.

In February of 1963, JFK delivered his landmark "Special Message to the Congress on Mental Illness and Mental Retardation," which represented the first time that either of these medical challenges ever had been discussed in public by a world leader. He called for "a new approach to mental illness and mental retardation" and said when that approach was "carried out, reliance on the cold mercy of custodial isolation will be supplanted by the open warmth of community concern and capability. . . . We cannot afford to postpone any longer a reversal in our approach to mental affliction." Mental illnesses were covered first in the speech, in part because there were three times as many patients institutionalized for those diseases, and a much larger treatment bureaucracy already in place and desperately in need of reform.

The resulting legislation, however, was more focused on addressing the smaller, but overall needier, group of children born with brain-related birth defects. On October 24, the President signed the Maternal and Child Health and Mental Retardation Planning Amendment to the Social Security Act, which focused on improving maternity and infant care, and preventing developmental disabilities.

And on October 31, he signed what was now called the Bill for the Construction of Mental Retardation Facilities and Community Mental Health Centers.

His rhetoric on signing the second bill was amazingly powerful and still resounds today:

It was said, in an earlier age, that the mind of a man is a far country which can neither be approached nor explored. But, today, under present conditions of scientific achievement, it will be possible for a nation as rich in human and material resources as ours to make the remote reaches of the mind accessible. The mentally ill and the mentally retarded need no longer be alien to our affections or beyond the help of our communities.

Three weeks after that speech, my uncle, President Kennedy, was assassinated.

While we now call that second bill the Community Mental Health Act, you can see it really wasn't that at all. It was primarily a well-thought-out plan to change the lives of those with intellectual disabilities, to which was added a small but significant number of changes culled from a much larger, more ambitious mental health reform plan. In the President's defense, at that time it was harder to know the difference between intellectual disability and severe mental illness, and people with one or the other (or both) were all being warehoused in the same shamefully run institutions.

My Uncle Bobby loudly referred to them as "snake pits," which certainly fit in with the rhetoric of the day. Ken Kesey's *One Flew Over the Cuckoo's Nest*—which showed how a sane man pretending to be crazy to avoid jail was harshly treated and, eventually, lobotomized—had just recently been published, and two weeks after the Community Mental Health Act was signed, a theatrical version of the book opened on Broadway with Kirk Douglas starring as Randle McMurphy.

The main strategy of the bill was to move those stuck in large, often outdated and cruel facilities into smaller, more community-based centers (and, in some cases, back home) while dramatically increasing research into prevention, treatment, and cures. This impacted the two groups of patients quite differently. Many people with intellectual disabilities were able to live at home and they were all fully covered for their care and their needs for the rest of their lives—especially after

Medicare and Medicaid were established in 1965. They were viewed as not being responsible for their disabilities and there was a government-supported process in place to try to care for them, destigmatize their situation, and prevent the injury, disease, or problem in the brain that caused their disabilities.

For those suffering from mental illness and/or addiction, however, something different happened. The act led to the closing of many of the large institutions where these illnesses were treated but did not provide the funding for them to ever be replaced with smaller community health centers. In fact, we actually *still* can't build modern psychiatric facilities today because of a clause in the 1965 Medicaid law: the dreaded "IMD exclusion." The exclusion was established to help hasten the emptying of outdated facilities by prohibiting hospitals where more than 51 percent of the patients are mentally ill from getting the new Medicaid reimbursements. Today this outdated law just makes modern inpatient facilities all but economically unfeasible, leaving the nation with a serious shortage of hospital beds for patients with mental illness. (This is also a big part of the reason why so many Americans with mental illness are now housed in prisons.)

The new laws also helped lead to the creation of a separate but unequal reimbursement system for care. Not only were these illnesses not viewed as disabilities, they weren't even viewed as "real" illnesses. This helped create a situation where even though the science of the treatment and genetics of mental illness improved, the way it was viewed by society and covered by insurance did not keep up.

Now, this bill certainly did not *invent* these problems. The prejudice against mental illness and addiction is as old as medical care itself. But while JFK's act made major progress in stopping the stigma against those with intellectual disabilities, it did little to stop the stigma against mental illness and substance use disorders. By separating out those with intellectual disabilities, people with mental illness and addictions were actually *more* easily labeled as mostly responsible for their own problems and willfully going out of their way to not solve them.

My aunt changed the world, and she showed us all how to employ laser focus and relentlessness—and the Kennedy name—to herd cats and convene the unconvenable. But she also taught us that even the most well-meaning and powerful advocacy can later turn out to have unpredictable results.

Chapter 3

I grew up in a household where both of my parents had mental health issues. My mother inherited her own mother's dark disabling alcoholism. And my father . . . well, I can now see my father suffered from PTSD, and because he denied himself treatment—and had chronic pain from the back injury he received in a small plane crash in 1964 when he was a very young Senator—he sometimes self-medicated in other ways.

My father would have been President of the United States if there had been progressive mental health treatment for him—someone saying, "Since two of your brothers were shot and killed, maybe you need to get support and services, because you suffered trauma." But no one could say that to my father, who had lost two siblings when he was a child and then had to survive the unthinkable: having not just one brother murdered in front of his eyes, and having it repeated over and over on television, but then having a second brother murdered, watching that repeated over and over, and wondering if he was next. That is psychological trauma beyond comprehension.

The difference between my parents was that my dad was much

more highly functional with his illnesses. My mom was just the opposite. She spent much of my childhood in her room, doing little but drinking and surviving, as her mother did before her. Occasionally she would come out and try her best to be attentive, like driving us somewhere. And when she swerved slowly down the street, my brother, sister, and I would just giggle because we didn't know what else to do. Sometimes she would disappear to go back to rehab, for weeks or months at a time. We didn't know much about it except for the obligatory family counseling session we had to go to. She did have a sustained period of wonderful sobriety during the late seventies and early eighties—during which I got to know a very different woman and mother than the one I grew up with, and we were able to travel together to the Holy Land, to London, and to Rome. But my mother has spent too much of her life harshly impaired by the cycles of disease.

I WAS BORN IN JULY OF 1967; before me, my mother had my sister, Kara, in early 1960; my brother, Ted Jr., in the fall of 1961; and then two miscarriages. I was at the tail end of the kids born to my father's generation of Kennedys—just as he was the youngest of his siblings. My birth was the reason my parents decided to leave their house in Georgetown and build a larger one on a six-acre tract along the Potomac River in McLean, Virginia, not far from where my Uncle Bobby's family lived at Hickory Hill. The house had wonderful views and a separate wing for my brother, sister, and me, and the governess who helped take care of us. The new house was seen as a fresh start for the family.

In Kennedy history, I was born several months after my uncle, then a Senator from New York, came out against the war in Vietnam, and eight months before he declared his candidacy for President. He was assassinated in June of 1968, just weeks before my first birthday. In the aftermath, during our regular summer family time in Hyannis, my mother says my father, then in his mid-thirties, would often privately burst into tears. He needed help but didn't get it.

That fall and winter in McLean, and then the next spring at Cape Cod, the family had a new dynamic. Instead of he and his brother Bobby trying to be father figures to Jack and Jackie's two kids, my father was now on his own trying to be a father figure not only to Caroline and John Jr. but also to Bobby and Ethel's eleven children—which he had to balance with taking care of Kara, Teddy, and me.

By the summer of 1969, my mom was also pregnant again and on strict bed rest because of her previous miscarriages. Four days after my second birthday that July, my father attended the annual summer reunion in Martha's Vineyard of the "Boiler Room Girls," who helped run my Uncle Bobby's campaign. That was the night my father accidentally drove off a bridge on Chappaquiddick Island, killing his passenger, a young woman named Mary Jo Kopechne. Her funeral was four days later. Even though my mother was terrified to lose another baby by leaving her bed, she joined my father at the funeral, because it was felt it would look bad if she wasn't at his side. She miscarried not long after that.

And then, just a few months later, my father lost his own father.

It has taken me a long time to even begin to understand how we were affected by all of this. I knew there was huge suffering going on in my family. But it was never spoken of when I was growing up. My mom discussed it some much later, during her periods of sobriety. But my father went on in silent desperation for much of his life, self-medicating and unwittingly passing his unprocessed trauma on to my sister, brother, and me. My dad never stopped working for others who were suffering, and he experienced a great many moments of joy and triumph. But his own anguish was palpable and unspoken.

And since he was the more emotionally available of my parents, I derived most of my emotional foundation from his strength and his turmoil.

I knew I was born a fragile person. I wasn't strong, I had severe asthma. I remember feeling awkward, anxious, separate, like a loser. In my family, however, "asthmatic" became a catchall phrase for all the other aspects of my emotional fragility, because there wasn't any other way to put your finger on it.

Oh, he's *asthmatic*. Oh, okay, sure.

Not only did my asthma reflect my emotional turbulence, but my asthma attacks were the one time I could get the nurturing and undivided attention I craved from the person who was most important to me: my dad. Asthma attacks were my safe zone, because the only thing that would make him drop everything—and he had a lot of everything—was if one of us was sick. And the very minute we were no longer sick, he was sucked back into being a senator.

I later came to understand my asthma as an illness that was exacerbated by stress, and there were also mood swings because I was taking large amounts of prednisone, the steroid people were prescribed back then. But, at the time, I just thought of myself as scrawny, scared of my own shadow. And nobody said anything about it because, in my family, that's how we were taught to cope.

THERE WERE, OF COURSE, many wonderful things about growing up in my family. When I was very little, I would hang around my father's dressing room in the morning as he got ready to go to the Senate, and we'd argue over what to watch on TV, the *Today* show or my favorite morning cartoons, especially *Deputy Dawg*—which is why he gave me the nickname "Dippity Dog." Many evenings after dinner he would invite me up on his lap and I would lay my head on his chest while he held me tight. And then, with me still there—I seemed to fit perfectly—he would finish his dessert and his Sanka.

Like most people, my childhood memories revolve around summer vacations and winter holidays. Summers were spent in and around Hyannis Port, where many family members had homes close to what I always called "Gramma's house." Having a summer birthday was especially great, because so many family members would be around in July, and everyone would head to Gramma's house, tanned and windswept, walking down side streets and through openings in the trees and shrubs between the houses, gathering for any celebration. For my birthday parties, though, my dad sometimes arranged for a professional fireworks display that lit up Hyannis Harbor.

The family summers were all organized around sailing, swimming, and fishing, which began on weekends as early in the spring as possible and continued as deep into the fall as was reasonable. (My wife, who grew up at the Jersey Shore, is constantly amazed that I'm still swimming in the cold ocean in October, since she grew up rarely going into the ocean after Labor Day.) There were still football games on the big lawn that Americans had grown up watching in the sixties, but that wasn't my best event. I tried playing in those games, but I was not only the smallest in my family but the one most likely to have to stop early in the game and catch his breath.

For a skinny kid with severe asthma, family football on the lawn was primarily a spectator sport. The ocean, however, was something quite different. I was on and in the ocean as early as I can remember. On a wall in my study, I have one of the framed pictures of my dad on his boat that he signed to me when I was still a baby, saying that he couldn't wait to go sailing with me. For many of the regattas he sailed in with family members, the rule was four to a boat. But, just as he often did in the Senate, he studied the rules until he found a loophole that allowed me to join in as a fifth because I was under twelve. He refused to leave me behind. When we raced in foul weather, there was lots of salt water and salty language. Those experiences not only broadened my vocabulary, but they also built my self-confidence.

Although I didn't realize it then, he was teaching me a lot of his political philosophy in those boat races. On a boat, as in a country, there was a role for everybody, a way for everyone to contribute, and no place for those who didn't try their best. And in a regatta, as in life, it didn't matter how strong the forces against you were. As long as you kept driving forward, there was nothing to lose—and it was also the only chance you had of coming out a winner.

Dad bought me a little Boston Whaler fishing boat with an outboard when I was sixteen, but my real joy was to be out with him on his big sailboat, along with as few other people as possible. And since this was all before cell phones, sailing was actually the only real escape for my father—and for us—from the rest of the world.

Besides the group sailing, when I was eight, my dad started taking me on his boat the *Victura* for three-or-four-day adventures, just the two of us. We'd leave with nothing but a bag of Kingsford charcoal and a little lighter fluid, a cooler full of steaks and cold cuts and condiments and soft drinks, sleeping bags, and a couple fishing poles to sail around the islands near Martha's Vineyard and Nantucket. Those were magical times.

All the Kennedys, Shrivers, Smiths, and Lawfords were together in the summer—my Aunt Ethel's house was next door to Gramma's; our house and Aunt Eunice and Uncle Sarge's house were down the street. And during the school year, I went to the same school, the Potomac School, with a lot of my Robert Kennedy and Shriver cousins, who lived close by and also gathered for each other's birthdays. We generally did Thanksgiving just at our house with my parents and siblings, but then during the winter holiday break we would often take skiing trips together as one big family. And during spring breaks we would take turns visiting Gramma's Palm Beach house.

While some of our trips were the height of personal, private time, I look back on some of the bigger, more involved family trips now with a little more of an eye for everything that was going on. These were joyous journeys for our family, but some of them were also being shared with the public. My childhood photo albums are crammed with the blurry, rounded-edged snapshots everyone has, along with gorgeous, sharp images done by the late photographer Ken Regan of Camera 5. He was close to the family, a very good guy, and had been given "exclusive" access to us. Which is why I have wonderful professional shots of us at the bottom of the Grand Canyon, on an amazing rafting trip my dad organized for the family.

Whenever the family was together, in groups large or small, there was usually singing. We sang wherever there was a piano and a bench full of old sheet music, belting out "When Irish Eyes Are Smiling" and "You Are My Sunshine" and many beloved show tunes. At Gramma's house, the room between the dining room and the sunroom was called "the piano room" and we often sang there. But there were also pianos in our living room in McLean and on Squaw Island. When my mother was well, she would play the piano. She would accompany us or, since she was classically trained, would play pieces by Chopin or Mozart.

On summer evenings, the family sometimes watched movies together. My grandfather had, during his years in film production, outfitted his basement with a full professional projection room and several rows of movie-theater seats. There was a decent-sized stage, which could accommodate a screen that lowered from the ceiling—and we watched a lot of movies there. It was also a great place to put on skits and play charades.

To get down to the basement theater, we had to walk through a narrow hallway where my grandmother's international doll collection was stored—all those glass or button, unblinking eyes staring out at us from floor-to-ceiling cases. I would never tell my Gramma how many nightmares I had about those dolls or how, when I was in uncomfortable social settings and felt disconnected or judged, I was reminded of their stares.

UNDER THE SURFACE, I grew up with a lot of tension and unprocessed trauma. And while I felt judged and stared at, the truth was I was capable of being as judgmental and unsympathetic as everyone else. I saw my mom's alcoholism and depression through the lens of my father's old-school attitude that she just couldn't keep it together. I can still hear him: "Here she goes again . . . oh my God . . . I can't believe it!"

I got the message early on: I didn't want people saying, "Oh, we need to take care of Patrick," the way they dismissed my mom: "Oh, we need to take care of Joan." I realized pretty young that this was less about anyone actually needing help than it was about making sure we avoided a public relations crisis.

I'm not proud of how I viewed my mom then. But I didn't know any better.

It's ironic that the politician who, from the early 1970s on, was probably the nation's leading voice on healthcare reform and its loudest advocate for universal national health insurance had blind spots on some mental health and addiction issues. My dad wrote in his memoir, "I grew up in a family of people who didn't want to hear you complain and, quite frankly, I don't have a lot of respect for people who whine or go around feeling sorry for themselves." But I doubt he was out of step with most of his voters. I suspect his "snap out of it" attitude was how most people viewed these illnesses then. And too many still do.

Interestingly, during these years, my Aunt Rosemary was back with the family more often and I recall seeing her at many Kennedy events.

I recall her acting in a way that today we might describe as a form of Tourette's, where she would sometimes say a bunch of random words or yell them. As a kid, this scared me a little, mostly because nobody explained anything about it. No one said, "Hey, your Aunt Rosemary's coming, and you know she suffers from a disability, and don't worry when she yells these things, it's just part of her condition." I really would have appreciated a conversation like that.

Yet I did perceive through the silence that my family embraced Rosemary much more than my mom, even though they both had what Uncle Jack had called a "mental affliction."

In June 1972, in a cover story in *Good Housekeeping* magazine, my mom became the first family member—and, honestly, one of the first Americans—to speak openly about her "long emotional struggle that led her to turn to psychiatry." Alcoholism was never directly mentioned in the long story, which was otherwise surprisingly revealing—especially considering that it was based on an interview arranged through my father's office. While it discussed psychiatry, there wasn't a word in the piece that made it sound like she had a medical illness—it mostly said that she was unable to handle the pressure of all the traumas, and of course "the other Kennedy women" to whom she was supposedly comparing herself constantly, "inwardly certain that she didn't measure up." So the piece seemed completely judgmental, unlikely to encourage anyone else to get help.

When I talked to my mom about this story recently, she said she viewed her being open as something she did for my father. But she was proud if it made a difference to destigmatize mental health and addiction care.

In fact, within weeks of the cover story's coming out, it was clear just how bad the stigma still was.

A new Kennedy book was published, timed for the upcoming Democratic convention—for which my father was considered a possible presidential or VP candidate—and it included bold and painfully un-sympathetic assertions about my mother's alcoholism. And then, later in July, Senator Thomas Eagleton, just selected as Democratic candidate for Vice President, was hounded off the national ticket by cruel coverage of his previous psychiatric treatment.

After all that, my mom's challenges were hardly a secret. It was fair game in the media to make light of her drinking and psychiatric care—just as it was to question my dad's faithfulness to his marriage, especially every year at the Chappaquiddick anniversary.

I sometimes learned more about my family from the press coverage of Kennedy books than I did from any Kennedys. The books were often riddled with inaccuracies, but also riddled with facts that probably would have been much easier to hear first from close family members, and perhaps with some context.

For example, the only time my father ever talked to me about Chappaquiddick was when he said he wanted me to come take a walk with him on the beach one July when the anniversary was approaching. I remember wanting the conversation to end before it even started because it was obviously so painful for him. His face was just pure anguish.

And all he said was, "You're going to be hearing a lot of people talking about what happened at Chappaquiddick, and I just want you to know how bad I feel about everything, and I'm really sorry you have to hear about it." That was it. Then we just walked in silence.

But, with my dad, silence was never silent. He had a way of gazing slightly away and I could see from the expression on his face how much he was still saying to himself—loudly.

IN THE FALL OF 1973, when I was six, my brother, Ted, who was twelve, said he felt a strange pain in his right leg. It developed into a welt and then one day he was taken to the hospital. When my parents came back, my father called Kara and me to their bedroom. It was the longest walk *ever* down that hallway, past Dad's bathroom and changing room, then Mom's, both on the right, until we got to their room. My father did all the talking. He said, "Your brother is going to need an operation, he has cancer and we're going to have to remove his leg." And Kara and I were just standing there, silent, with no real way to comprehend what was going on or how to react.

Looking back, I think it's significant how important it was for him to talk, very straightforwardly, about my brother's rare malignant bone cancer, about "physical" health. But we never said a word about Aunt Rosemary, and we never talked about the fact that my mom was walking through the house like a shadow in the middle of the day. Those things were never discussed.

A few days after we were told about this, Teddy's right leg was amputated just above the knee. It was a scary and surreal experience, during which we received an outpouring of support and love, all partisanship put aside. While we were accustomed to notable adults coming in and out of our house and lives, I can still vividly remember Muhammad Ali sitting on my brother's bed telling him he would fight through this.

Given the age difference between me and my brother and sister, I had always looked up to them. After my brother's brave recovery from the amputation the feeling was just that much stronger.

His illness, treatment, and recovery put amazing pressure on my parents. They disagreed about how Teddy should be treated: my father wanted a lot of celebrated, encouraging people around him all the time pumping him up, and my mom thought things should be quieter, more private. Every few weeks for a year and a half, Teddy flew back to Boston so he could get an experimental chemotherapy, after which he got violently ill.

When Teddy did recover, he was fitted with a prosthesis, and my father quickly pushed for him to become active again. He was outfitted with outriggers so he could ski on one leg. Dad also had the idea that riding go-karts was something Teddy could do competitively— and something I could do with him without much threat of an asthma attack. So he had a special go-kart made to accommodate Teddy's leg. The two of us became so obsessed with go-karts that we even started attending some of the pro racing events for which go-karts were the opening act. These creative accommodations raised my brother's consciousness of the needs of others with disabilities, which became a big part of his life's work (and Dad's, leading to the landmark protections of the Americans with Disabilities Act).

But as Teddy improved and the emergency passed, my mom's symptoms grew progressively worse. Several months after Teddy's surgery, in May of 1974, she checked herself into Silver Hill in Connecticut for a three-week rehab. The statement from my dad's office said she had gone for "emotional problems"—but since Silver Hill was best known for its treatment of alcoholism, it was clear why she was there. Several weeks after being discharged, she went back, for what my dad's office called the "second phase" of her treatment for emotional strain.

TEDDY'S CANCER AND Mom's treatment were covered not only in the regular press and the supermarket tabloids, but in a new medium somewhere in between them: *People* magazine. It had grown out of *Time* magazine's "People" column as interest rose in "personality" journalism—initiated by the success in the late sixties of several city magazines and then the *Washington Post* "Style" section—and debuted the week of March 4, 1974. In its first several months of publication, my family was the cover story in two of the initial seventeen issues: one covered our family skiing trip to Vail and featured my dad and brother on the cover (noting that my mom, "who was not feeling well, stayed at home in Virginia") and the other was a big piece on my mother.

By creating and presenting a whole new level of "respectable" personality journalism—previously seen as "soft" news for the "ladies' section"—*People* magazine changed the role of public figures in America. It also presented a new forum for mental illness and addiction to be discussed more openly. This was good, in theory, because it did help expand the dialogue about illness and treatment—it was the very beginning of Americans realizing this was a common struggle. There was something powerful in seeing, say, Martha Mitchell—the divorcing wife of Richard Nixon's Attorney General who was caught up in Watergate—talking about her problems with prescription drugs and alcohol. But there were also plenty of half-truths and myths perpetuated in some of those stories.

The story about my mother, for example, featured an interview with my maternal grandmother, Virginia Stead Bennett—though every other quote in the story was from an anonymous source. She denied my mother had any problem with alcohol dependence and insisted she had gone to Silver Hill because "she needed a rest." The article later noted that my grandmother had once been at Silver Hill herself, but only because it was where she "retreated during her divorce" from my grandfather.

Nobody in the family, and none of her friends, wanted to say out loud that my mom suffered from alcoholism. In 1975 her father, Harry Bennett, finally admitted it in an interview, as my mom's side of the family started getting more involved in offering a different spin than my father's press office. While my grandfather was more open about my mother's drinking, he did offer the same explanation for it that everyone else had: not the disease of alcoholism, but the unique pressures of being a Kennedy.

In reality, my mother's father knew full well that she had inherited this illness, which affected every member of her family, regardless of whether they had married a Kennedy. My grandfather had issues with alcohol. My mother's younger sister struggled with alcohol and would later become active in the recovery movement.

But my mother's mother was the most ill. She was, by that time, living by herself in an oceanside apartment in Cocoa Beach, Florida, incredibly isolated because she had burned every single bridge with her family, her friends, and her community. On April 8, 1976, my grandmother was found dead in her shower. Apparently she had been that way for several days, before her body was discovered.

She was only sixty-five. When we got the news, it was the first time I ever saw my mother cry.

Chapter 4

My parents informally separated in 1977, when I was ten years old. We had been living in McLean, Virginia, and my mom, an accomplished pianist and musician, announced she wanted to spend more time in our Boston apartment so she could pursue an advanced degree and study more music. This was, like many statements my family issued about personal stuff that probably wasn't anyone else's business, technically true. In reality, she was leaving to try to save her own life, and finally get her alcoholism under control, by doing what an increasing number of Americans were doing—joining the free, all-peer-supported twelve-step programs of Alcoholics Anonymous. It was a brave thing to do.

Her care had, up until that point, been controlled by medical experts my father brought in—often the absolute leading people in their fields, but not people who could help my mom create any real care community she could rely on every day. She got intensive treatment at inpatient facilities, which always included a few sessions for us kids, sessions we viewed as so silly, famous therapists looking at us in horror that we weren't heartbroken and crying ("families usually do that, you know," they would tell us). We had lived in turmoil our whole lives, so the notion that this was especially traumatic was almost absurd to us.

So she would have these intensive inpatient experiences, and then she was back in the real world of one-on-one psychiatry a couple times a week.

After many cycles of this approach proved unsuccessful, my mother wanted to try something different: a twelve-step program with daily meetings. This was a big risk because, at that time, twelve-step programs were very separate from, and often critical of, most of the medical rehab facilities that had been her lifeline.

AA had sprung to life in the thirties and forties and was popularized in the early sixties when the main character of the Oscar-winning film *Days of Wine and Roses* (played by Jack Lemmon) was in the program. By the early seventies—when its founder, Bill W., died, not long after partially breaking his famous anonymity by testifying before Congress with no photos allowed—the organization reportedly had more than 300,000 active members worldwide (today that number is more than two million). But the mainstream mental health establishment viewed it as something of a cult and a threat. This was largely because AA was peer-run without professionals, and was based on daily free meetings, which competed with paid individual or group outpatient sessions offered by medical rehab centers. AA also had a spiritual basis for recovery, and mental healthcare at that time prided itself on being secular, because in the distant past of mental disease, patients had been accused of being "possessed." And AA adhered to a model of alcoholism as a "disease," which was, frankly, ahead of its time but also without much scientific evidence, just a lot of quietly satisfied customers.

Besides the conceptual debates, there was also the matter of privacy. Much of rehab—medical or in AA—was based on group sessions during which people were expected to be honest and supportive. Most people in these groups were trustworthy, but in both the closed medical rehab groups and more open AA groups, there was a fear that intensely personal things shared in meetings might not remain secret. This was especially worrisome for a very public family like ours, and when my mom first tried a twelve-step program, everyone's fears were justified.

In early 1976, she had checked herself into a place in New York City called the Smithers Rehabilitation Center, which was private and medical but also employed the AA model, which a few other places around the country also did, following the example of Hazelden in Minnesota. She was very open during her twelve-step meetings at Smithers. And then she had to endure the violation of trust when two of her fellow patients, including one who had clearly been targeting her to talk to during treatment, sold stories about her to the *National Enquirer*.

Presumably, it would be a little safer for Mom to attend twelve-step meetings in our hometown, where people might be a little more respectful of her challenge and the process.

She took to AA very aggressively. Since I was living with my dad full-time in Washington, I remember being a little taken aback the first time I visited her and saw how she had redecorated her Beacon Street apartment with AA slogans: "One day at a time," "Live and let live," "Serenity is not peace from the storm, but peace amid the storm." There were framed posters, bumper stickers, pillows, oh my God, the pillows—it was like walking into a recovery gift shop. We'd kid each other about how sappy all this stuff was, but she was truly into it. I didn't really understand then how important the fellowship and community of recovery could be in combating the isolation of these illnesses.

It was like she was in another world. But then, we were all in another world, because of the separation.

With my sister and brother heading to college, I felt increasingly lonely living in a big house outside of DC, being raised by my dad and a nanny, seeing my whole family together only at holidays. When the Senate was in session, I saw my dad mostly between evening meetings—although sometimes he would bring me into the sessions to lighten the mood and, occasionally, even ask for my opinion. He did, however, always drop everything when I was having a medical emergency with my asthma, which I too often did. The problem was, I was trying so hard to be normal, to be well, to be one of the guys, that I hated to tell anybody I was starting to wheeze, because I knew it meant we would have to go home early from wherever we were, and it was just a real pain; it would ruin everything. So I would wait and wait and wait, until I was really in trouble.

Asthma was harder to control then, and all the treatments weren't as easy as they are today: I have this image of my dad, whose back never really healed properly from the plane crash he was in during the early sixties, lugging my twenty-five-pound Maxi-Mist nebulizer everywhere we went, always looking for a three-pronged plug for it. And the meds back then weren't what they are today, so they were a bigger deal to take and the standard dose was probably a lot more than I needed. We didn't know as much about prednisone as we do now, didn't realize how much taking it could affect moods. Considering my genetic predispositions, these steroids, while the standard of care at the time, probably weren't helping my youthful mental health.

IT WAS DURING THIS TIME, as my mom was starting to make some progress with her alcoholism, that I first tried drinking. It honestly never occurred to me that what I was doing had anything in common with my mother's illness. I was more interested in drinking and trying pot to try to impress my older brother and sister and their friends, who were, like all kids in the seventies, "experimenting." I wanted to be wild like some of my cousins, who to me didn't seem to be *depressively* into drugs and alcohol; they just did it for fun.

In AA, it's not uncommon to talk about the first time you ever drank. My story is a little atypical for most meetings: I got drunk during my father's first diplomatic trip to China, in the winter of 1977. I was ten years old.

My mom came on the trip, along with my Aunts Eunice, Pat, and Jean, and my Uncle Steve Smith, with whom my dad was very close, as well as my cousins Caroline and Michael, who were college-age, and my brother and sister. I recall we visited Japan during the trip and spent one night in a place called the Three Sisters Inn—where my dad and Uncle Steve spent a long time jokingly speculating what an inn would be like if it were run by Jean, Pat, and Eunice.

I also remember—well, I sort of remember—drinking a lot of rice wine in the Forbidden City during one state dinner. Then–vice premier Teng Hsiao-p'ing hadn't attended the dinner, saying he had a cold, and there was some question of whether he was slighting the US. But, apparently, he actually did have a cold, and ended up meeting with my family the next day. He even mentioned to the press that I had lost a tooth during the visit (completely unrelated to the rice wine) and said, "You have left a part of you behind. You must come back."

It was a couple years before I really tried drinking or drugs, but I was still pretty early in my teens for that—and I am still amazed that, given how irritating any kind of smoke was for my asthma, I still insisted on smoking pot to keep up with the older kids. This was, after all, the late seventies, and young people were moving from pot and hallucinogens to more drugs people snorted. I was getting some psychotherapy during this time. But it didn't seem to be geared toward treating any symptoms I was displaying, but rather toward trying to psychologically immunize me against my parents' impending separation. In retrospect, I'd say I was probably already suffering from some anxiety and situational depression by my early teens. And I was certainly self-medicating. But the therapy wasn't about any of that: the therapist just wanted to discuss how I felt about my parents.

I do worry that by explaining my depression and anxiety this way, it is easier to minimize. This is one of the basic challenges of all mental healthcare, that somehow a person is less sick, less disabled—temporarily or permanently—by illness, because some of the external stressors involved are somehow not extreme enough, not overtly "traumatic" enough. It is really difficult to make people who don't have these illnesses, or don't treat these illnesses, understand that it doesn't matter if your particular combination of genetics and life experiences seems destructive enough to an outsider to lead to a crippling depression or anxiety attack. The question is only whether your symptoms—however you got them—have reached the point where they are preventing you from living a normal life.

Some people find themselves able to emotionally surf across the biggest waves of family trauma and dysfunction, the harshest circumstances of business or war. Other people can't.

The notion that mental illness and addiction are directly "caused" by bad parenting was rejected years and years ago—but the news just doesn't seem to have reached enough people yet. Up through the early 1960s, mental health professionals were still being taught that even treatment-resistant schizophrenia was caused by "bad mothering"—and could only be prevented by good mothering. We now know that people genetically predisposed to schizophrenia get it regardless of how they were raised. We also know that some people drink and take drugs and get addicted to them, and others drink the same things and take the same drugs and don't.

This is not to suggest that childhood traumas do not have impact in many areas of health. The Adverse Childhood Experiences (ACE) study done by the CDC and Kaiser Permanente, which has followed a group since they enrolled as young people in the mid-1990s, found dramatic correlations between childhood maltreatment and compromised adult health. But that doesn't change the fact that the strongest predictors of mental illness and addiction are clearly genetic in nature, and bad parenting can't "turn" someone schizophrenic or bipolar.

Someday we will truly understand why. But the biggest challenge facing us today is to get people to realize that what they think they understand about this is incorrect, and there is finally some good science to prove that.

Are there some aspects of my childhood that look especially challenging and unique? Sure. And I'm sure that's true of your childhood, too. But don't you know people who had similarly challenging childhoods and do *not* suffer from debilitating mental illness and addiction? Of course you do.

Chapter 5

Although I didn't see her as much during the next couple years, my mom did make great progress getting control of her illness in AA. In the summer of 1978, not long after former First Lady Betty Ford made the very first public revelation of her struggle with alcohol and painkillers, my mom gleefully announced to *McCall's* magazine that she had finished her first year of sobriety. Unfortunately, by the time the issue came out, there was talk that she had "slipped" or had a "relapse." (In recovery, a "slip" is a one-time or brief substance use that interrupts but doesn't completely compromise treatment and sobriety; a "relapse" is more sustained use, after which you generally have to start again. When people casually use the word "relapse" I think they forget that for addicts their natural state is to be using substances.)

Some of her slips we didn't know about at the time, but only discovered later when my mom's personal assistant—and fellow AA member—decided to violate all confidence and decency to write a tell-all book to cash in on the experience. She actually had the audacity to suggest she was doing this for my mom's own good, and to help AA. My dad's driver during this time period also later wrote a tell-all memoir. It's no wonder we were always taught to keep everything a secret, even things that didn't need to be secret. (That's how shame grows in children who are too young to even know what shame is.)

In the middle of all this, my father was urged to run against incumbent Jimmy Carter, whose presidency was floundering. This required a number of family meetings. He met privately with me and my brother and sister to get our blessing—not only for the public appearances we would be doing but for the heightened risk on my father's life. We told him, however reluctantly, that we were on board. Although, really, what else were we going to say?

And then there was a meeting of the grown-ups, to discuss whether or not my mom was well enough to handle this. With my mother's permission, my dad ordered an exhaustive retrieval of all my mother's medical records going back to childhood, and a survey of the leading research in addiction care. And then he convened a team of physicians—his own healthcare adviser, my mom's regular psychiatrist, and leading experts from Yale, the Mayo Clinic, and elsewhere, along with my aunts Jean, Ethel, and Eunice, to discuss with my parents what risks a campaign would pose to my mother's health.

One of the surprises of the research, at least to my father, was that my mother apparently had documented problems with alcohol as far back as college in the 1950s—undermining the popular notion that her health problems were nothing more than a reaction to the Kennedy tragedies of the 1960s. Aunt Eunice—with whom my mom was closest in the family—was apparently the most concerned about whether a national campaign would be safe for her. They ultimately decided it would be.

Now, I suppose you can be cynical about this and say that my father was doing due diligence mostly on my mom's stamina, not her feelings, and that if she relapsed and he was blamed it would hurt the campaign. And, given how her illness played out, I can only imagine how the pressures of the White House might have aggravated her alcoholism and depression. But I will note that there is something about this discussion they had—the kind of thing that almost never happened back then—that seems sort of progressive. It was in no way judgmental; nobody was asking how and why my mother had reached this point in her life and her treatment, only what the status of her illness was and what she thought her capacity might be. They wanted her to make the most informed decision possible about her own health, with all angles considered.

As a twelve-year-old, I'm sure I rolled my eyes over this at the time. Now it strikes me as kind of enlightened—not emotionally, because my mom was putting her health at risk in hopes of saving her marriage and advancing my father's career, but simply as cutting-edge disease management. If she had heart disease and they were talking about going mountain climbing, it would make sense to consult expert cardiologists beforehand. Why not have such frank discussions about alcoholism and mental illness?

THIS DISEASE DUE DILIGENCE is especially interesting if you consider what was going on at that very moment in the politics of brain health. When Jimmy Carter took office in 1977, one of his first acts was to create the President's Commission on Mental Health, the main legislative priority of his wife, Rosalynn, who was named honorary chair.

At the beginning of the Carter administration, there were high hopes for President and Mrs. Carter's ambitions in all of healthcare reform. My father was optimistic—this was, after all, the first Democratic president since Lyndon Johnson. And I recall a White House family picnic during his first summer in office, during which President Carter noted that I was the only member of my immediate family with red hair and freckles. He said I looked "more like one of [his]" than a Kennedy.

Mrs. Carter always had been passionate about advocacy for people with mental illnesses and developmental disabilities, and when her husband became governor of Georgia in 1971, it became the primary focus of her public life. She got to know my family first through my Aunt Eunice, because as First Lady of Georgia she was very active in the state's Special Olympics and sat on the state commission to improve services for what they called "the Mentally and Emotionally Retarded." But she was equally if not more interested in mental illness—medically and socially—in part because people with mental illnesses had not received the same funding and protections as those with developmental disabilities. Her main focus was on "serious mental illness"—whose victims either don't respond to treatments or are unable to stay on them, and therefore often end up disabled, homeless, or in prison. But her goal was to hold hearings leading to a broad bill that would help everyone suffering from a brain disorder.

The hearings addressed many of the problems identified in JFK's Community Mental Health Act that had remained unsolved—or in some cases had actually worsened—since that historic legislation. The commission's deliberations went on for more than a year and drew an incredibly broad cast of characters, most of whom agreed on almost nothing. This was partly because, in an attempt to be broadly "inclusive" at a time before a true medical understanding of mental illnesses had emerged, every social, ethnic, and gender issue that might produce psychological stressors was included in their discussions.

At the same time this was going on, a quiet revolution was beginning in mental healthcare—the first major rethinking of the diagnosis, treatment, and underlying causes of mental illness in decades, perhaps since Freud at the turn of the twentieth century. It came in the form of a landmark revision of the primary manual of psychiatric diagnosis in the US—the *Diagnostic and Statistical Manual of Mental Disorders*, published by the American Psychiatric Association. The *DSM*, as it's called, began in the 1950s as little more than a slightly expanded and Americanized version of the mental health section of the World Health Organization's standardized listing of the name, description, and code number of every known illness, the International Classification of Diseases, or ICD. (The ICD's history goes all the way back to 1893, when it was the "International List of Causes of Death," issued by the International Statistical Institute.)

Some people still refer to the *DSM* as "the bible of mental health," though it's actually more of an encyclopedia; in the late 1970s it wasn't culturally powerful enough to be widely known as either. It was known mostly because in 1973 homosexuality was removed as a mental illness and replaced by the category of Sexual Orientation Disturbance for those seeking therapy about gender issues. The codes and descriptions in the *DSM* only became hugely important later in the eighties and nineties during the rise of managed care, when the treatment of mental illness—like the treatment of all illness—became more mechanized, medicalized, centralized, and capitated by the influx of more corporate-run HMOs.

In the late seventies, the revision that became the *DSM-III*—led by Columbia psychiatrist Dr. Robert Spitzer—was more of a medical and intellectual endeavor. Its main goal—besides producing a much longer and in-depth *DSM*—was to help psychiatric diagnosis move on from blaming everything on "neurosis," largely the reaction to faulty parenting. The hope was to develop diagnoses based more on the idea of brain illnesses that are partly genetic and partly triggered by any number of possible causes, but needed to be more accurately described and categorized.

This work was driven, in part, by the research Spitzer and others did to prove the current, simplified, neurotic diagnoses were being used differently by different doctors. ("Schizophrenia," for example, meant different things to different clinicians around the US and in the UK.) But also, the first generation of useful psychiatric drugs—Haldol to sedate and address the hallucinations and thought disorders of psychotic disease, imipramine to help pull patients out of unipolar depression, lithium to help balance the mood swings of manic depression—were already showing that certain symptoms could be lessened just by the right medication. While they weren't cures, they allowed for the possibility that patients could see psychiatric symptoms for what they were—symptoms—and develop insight into their diseases and the value of sticking with the treatments, however imperfect. And the rise of directed, short-term "cognitive" psychotherapies—which focused not on your past, but on reinforcing your ability to function in the present and see the future—was suggesting a new role for diagnosis and the different forms of treatment.

The new *DSM-III* was meant to offer a road map to all that. It was also meant to be written in such a way that nonphysicians might use and understand it.

With all this going on in mental healthcare, and the Carters and the Kennedys working together to forward JFK's historic agenda, it was an odd time for the First Family and my family to pair off against each other. But that's what we did.

On May 15, 1979, President Carter submitted the Mental Health Systems Act to Congress, and my dad and his colleagues began marking it up. Three months later, my father decided he was going to run against President Carter for the Democratic nomination.

I WAS TWELVE YEARS OLD when my father's presidential campaign began, but I have strong memories of it, because he often brought me along to keep him company. That began before the race even started, since I was the only other family member present for the infamous interview my dad gave Roger Mudd of CBS in Cape Cod, which forever changed the level of media scrutiny of my family.

It was the last weekend in September of 1979, and the first day of filming for what was going to be a one-hour CBS Reports prime-time news special about my father and his presumed presidential run—scheduled to run during November sweeps against the network premiere of *Jaws* and raise the curtain for his official announcement. The CBS camera crew was invited to Hyannis Port to cover a typical family weekend at the Cape. But, at the last minute, my eighty-nine-year-old grandmother became ill and left. Then my mom begged off, saying she didn't feel well, so she didn't drive down from Boston. My sister and brother bowed out. So it was just Dad and me. He expected to do a pretty easy, benign interview with his friend Roger Mudd, and then he and I were going to sail.

My father, Mudd, and the CBS crew decided to do a sit-down interview in the backyard of my parents' house on Squaw Island, which is just a five-minute drive from Gramma's house in Hyannis Port, but a little more secluded. Dad and Mudd were dressed casually, sitting in captain's chairs on the lawn, which overlooks the ocean. While the cameras rolled, I peeked from the side of the house to see what was going on.

My dad sat and gave stock answers to stock family questions. He was not really comfortable talking freely about personal things, in public or in private. But this wasn't enough for the CBS producers, who had come all this way on a weekend to get good Kennedy family scenes for their prime-time special. Nobody, however, mentioned this problem to my dad.

After forty minutes of filmed conversation, the cameras stopped and we thought we were done. Dad told me to go start getting the boat ready, and he would catch up with me in a moment. Then Roger Mudd asked my dad to sit down again for just a few more minutes.

This time, Mudd went right for the tough questions. This should not have completely surprised my father, but somehow it still did. Mudd asked about my parents' marriage, he asked about Chappaquiddick, and he asked why my dad wanted to be president. My father mumbled, backpedaled, completely choked—he was always better on offense than defense in public speaking. The moment it was over he knew it had been a disaster.

The CBS crew left, and we went sailing. Out on the water, he tried to pretend everything was fine. But he just kept shaking his head, looking out to sea, and muttering to himself. He was replaying the interview over and over in his head. It was painful to watch. I had never seen him so upset with himself.

ALTHOUGH THE CAMPAIGN had a rocky start, it turned out to be great fun for me. I had a lot of time with my dad on campaign planes and in hotels. We'd play crazy eights when he had breaks. And he would always have an extra set of index cards made up for his speeches, so I could have one of my own and follow along, drawing stars next to the lines I thought worked best.

I kept a handwritten journal of the adventure in a school composition book, where I described everything from the campaign events ("our motorcade was really neat") to family escapades ("Anthony Shriver and I . . . met up with my mom at a Ramada Inn. There we played ding, dong, ditch, till 2:00 am") and campaign strategy ("mom's speeches are a little different than dads her speeches talk about ERA instead of inflation, Education instead of economy").

When he traveled without me, I was often worried about his safety. He called me every night just to chat and catch up, but he and I both knew that the real reason for the phone call was accomplished the moment I heard his voice: he was calling to assure me that he was okay.

He never let on that he was worried anything would happen to him. But after he died I was given something that showed me one way he dealt with the risks. It was a letter my father had written to me at the start of his presidential campaign in case he was assassinated. In it, he talked about how much he loved me and how I had given him so much love. He said he would never forget the times we went fishing and sailing. He advised that I should follow the example of my brother and sister and do what they suggested.

It was amazing and chilling to get this letter recently—especially since it was handed to me by Dr. Larry Horowitz, a physician and political adviser who had been one of my father's closest confidants, first as staff director for him on the Senate Health Committee, and later as his chief of staff. Larry was also my father's family healthcare consigliere, and he played a crucial role in my relationship with my parents. Without ever breaking the rules of confidentiality, he had been a healthy sounding board and reality check for me with my parents from my earliest diagnosis with asthma. When my parents couldn't handle my emergency calls—and even when they could but didn't know what to do—Larry was usually the next call. Later, when I was a Congressman and my staff was concerned about my mental health, they would reach out quietly to Larry for help. He knew a lot of things my father never knew about me. So I was deeply moved when he gave me this old letter—because, he said, he felt I finally was well enough, and had been sober long enough, to handle it.

Actually, one of Larry's earliest medical interventions on my behalf came during the latter part of my father's presidential campaign. By this point, the race wasn't going well and we were stuck on smaller and smaller propeller planes. We were flying across the Midwest one day when I experienced a really sudden and severe asthma attack. While some wanted to keep going, Larry insisted to my father that we needed to put down as soon as possible at the nearest airport, which turned out to be in St. Louis, so I could get emergency medical care.

MY FATHER'S PRESIDENTIAL BID ended on the evening of August 12, 1980, on a stage at the Democratic National Convention in New York's Madison Square Garden. My mom stood with him on the stage during his speech—pretty much the last time I was going to see my parents together looking like husband and wife. And my sister, brother, and I watched from the wings.

We were called to the stage near the end of the speech, to be with him before he delivered the famous finale. He actually sounded a little more nervous than people remember, but still captivating, as he declared, "For me, a few hours ago, this campaign came to an end. For all those whose cares have been our concern, the work goes on, the cause endures, the hope still lives, and the dream shall never die."

While I admit I'm a little biased, I feel in some ways that last line is more inspiring than many of the quotes of my uncle's presidency. JFK's words speak to great American youthful hope, but my dad's words speak more to the reality of what is required to get back up and continue after life fails to cooperate, loved ones are taken, hopes are dashed, all appears lost.

The older I get, the more "the work goes on, the cause endures" resonates in my day-to-day life.

ON OCTOBER 7, 1980—four weeks before the election—President Carter held a big signing ceremony for the Mental Health Systems Act in the White House. It was a fascinating day in the politics of brain health, because it was clear that during even the most frictional parts of the campaign the Carters and the Kennedys still had somehow figured out a way to keep working together on this historic, if flawed, legislation, which created a new federal/state partnership and new funding to treat and prevent mental illness, addictions, and developmental disability. My Aunt Eunice was introduced during the ceremony; my father was asked to give remarks directly after Mrs. Carter. And after the President signed the bill, he couldn't resist the temptation to make one more point about the personal politics of mental healthcare.

"You might be interested in knowing," President Carter said with a grin, "that all during the spring campaign, when Senator Kennedy and I were communicating, um, through the media"—which got a laugh—"quite often I would come in and find Rosalynn and him communicating very intimately about the Mental Health Systems Act. So, it kind of bridged the gap . . . and I'm very grateful that all of us have been able to share in this delightful and exhilarating and gratifying experience."

The delightful experience lasted just a few more weeks. Not only did President Carter lose convincingly in the general election to Ronald Reagan, but the Republicans gained control of the Senate for the first time in over two decades and made substantial gains in the House.

And one of the first things Reagan and the Republican leadership did was throw out almost every single aspect of the Mental Health

Systems Act, passing on all mental healthcare to the states through block grants at lower levels of funding than ever before: seventy-five cents for every dollar that would have been spent under the Carter bill. What had been meant as the federal government's largest foray *ever* into improving care of mental illness and researching new treatments, prevention methods, and cures actually turned into its single largest and most resonant setback. The National Institute of Mental Health (NIMH), which had been founded in 1949 as one of the original National Institutes of Health, was defunded from any direct centralized involvement in mental health services and policy, and became just an adviser to the states. The massive deinstitutionalization that was feared during the sixties appeared to be instigated on purpose by the Reagan administration in the eighties.

When it came to addiction treatment, the Reagans appropriated the title of President Nixon's original "War on Drugs" from the 1970s but ignored the most important part of Nixon's effort. Just as he had done for his War on Cancer, Nixon had poured money into improving research, prevention, education, and, most important, *treatment* for drug addiction—the only multipronged approach with any chance of success. The Reagans instead decided to slash funding for addiction treatment and addiction education, and attempted to solve the growing problem by spending massively to quash supply—in the US and, militarily, abroad. They addressed the complex issue of demand with Nancy Reagan's reductive "Just Say No" campaign. While presumably well-meaning, the campaign also spent millions trying to reinforce the idea that addiction was a character flaw—something you could stop by "just saying no"—and not a disease.

This became, inadvertently, one of the most destructive and stigmatizing efforts ever undertaken by the federal government in the area of addiction or mental health. It reinforced, to an entire generation, that not being addicted, not being mentally ill, was as easy as "just saying no" if you only had the moral strength to do it. We have been trying to undo its damage ever since.

While I suppose you could argue that "Just Say No" had one message consistent with the abstinence called for in twelve-step programs, it offered no funding for the supports that would help someone struggling to keep saying no. It also laid the groundwork for the problem we still experience today: we now have a handful of medications that can be successful in helping treat addiction, but some people are refusing to use them because they think you're supposed to "just say no" to them, too.

All this "Just Say No" moralizing pervaded the culture just as some major breakthroughs were happening in mental health that could really have helped reduce stigma. In diagnosis, the *DSM-III* went from being an obscure technical manual for a small number of clinicians to a bestselling book used by teachers, lawyers, and judges to make sense of the growing field of psychiatric diagnosis. For the first time, when clinicians all over the country used the terms "schizophrenia" and "depression," most of them now meant the same thing. The book did not suggest how to treat the illnesses—just how to identify and describe them more accurately. But there were also advances going on in new medications and forms of shorter, more directed therapies.

This should have been a time when treatment began dramatically improving and discrimination against brain disease actually began retreating. Instead, this period in mental health is mostly significant because the situation became so terrible that consumers had no choice but to, out of sheer frustration, create the modern consumer medical advocacy movement as we now know it. The only good thing about the years to come in mental health is that they were so bad they encouraged much of the consumer advocacy we take for granted today.

AFTER MY FATHER'S PRESIDENTIAL CAMPAIGN, I felt lonely. Over the previous year, my whole nuclear family had spent more time together than they had since I was very young. And now it was over. Dad was back at work in the Senate, my mom was back in Boston, Teddy and Kara were away at college, and suddenly the house in McLean seemed very big and empty.

My father really did try his best to make sure we had private father-son adventures during holiday breaks. We went to Latin America together, just the two of us. We took this wild fishing trip to Alaska, which ended with our almost being arrested in the Anchorage airport because we tried to bring home a petrified twenty-four-inch walrus tusk we found on Round Island in Bristol Bay. ("The youth returned the tusk," said the Associated Press story on our vacation gone awry.) Looking back, I can see how hard he tried to compensate for how I was feeling about the impending end of my parents' marriage.

But he couldn't really make up for the isolation of my daily life with him in McLean. Especially the evenings, after I went to bed. My bedroom was the one closest to the main driveway, so I would always hear if someone came to visit my dad at night. He and my mom were separated by then, so, in theory, he was free to do what he wanted. But it was still very weird for me to realize what was going on behind his closed door.

I developed a way of expressing my feelings without actually saying anything. There was a phone intercom system in the house and my parents' bedroom was button number one. When I realized he wasn't alone, I would often push button number one, and hold it down as long as it took for my dad to pick up the phone. Then I would hang up and pretend I was asleep.

After all those nights pressing the intercom, I decided to ask for a change of scenery. So I actually told my father I wanted to be sent away to boarding school, preferably somewhere closer to my mother. I went to Fessenden—my dad's alma mater—which is in West Newton, near Boston, as a full boarding student for eighth grade. Of course, I wasn't at boarding school long before I started missing my dad.

I recently discovered a letter sent to my dad during this time, apparently written by a clergy member who knew our family pretty well, which offered a really harsh and insensitive portrayal of my mom and her illness and how it could affect his ongoing personal and political life. It chilled me to read it. The writer referred to my mother's "use of liquor and all too frequent recourse to psychiatry" and expressed a "deep-seated worry" about my mother's custody of me. While acknowledging that "you have both lived through tragedy," the writer went so far as to suggest that unless my mother made "contact with God as he is (not as she wants him to be)" the result could be "the loss of a mighty good president for the U.S.A." Whoever wrote this unsigned letter has not made contact with the compassionate God I worship.

With my parents' formal divorce approaching, they decided I should have weekly therapy with a top adolescent psychiatrist with an office at McLean Hospital. Mom would pick me up from school one day a week, drop me off at the doctor's office, wait for me for an hour, and then drive me back to Fessenden.

I don't remember much about the therapy—I felt I was doing it for my parents, not for me. But one thing does stick out. The psychiatrist would often ask me to be more specific about my experiences in my family. I was unsure if I could trust him to keep things private, so I would edit things out.

Some of that burden of ultra-secrecy was finally dropped the next year, when my father announced that he would not run for president against incumbent Ronald Reagan—and basically said that his children were the deciding vote against another campaign. While he did

talk to Teddy, Kara, and me a lot about whether or not to run, in retrospect I think the press was encouraged to overplay this—almost as if
we were making the decision and not my father. Since I had already
learned quite a bit about politics, I vaguely understood then—and better understand now—what was really going on.

The whole idea of asking us what we thought has really been misinterpreted by people who don't understand politics. In my view, you
don't run for office because you weigh this and weigh that. You run
because you have the fire in the belly for it. You either have that or you
don't—there's nothing deliberative about the decision at all, it's totally
intestinal. It's about motivation, not calculation.

My dad had a lot of expectations on him, people always wanting
him to run. Remember, a lot of people staked their careers on his running, people working for him to create public policy and churning out
amendments and markups and speeches. He had all the smartest people working for him, the cream of the crop. You couldn't attract such a
high-powered group and not understand they had higher expectations. After 1980, when he knew it wasn't in the cards for him, he also
understood that he had the biggest campaign infrastructure in the
country of any Democrat. He had to back down in a very methodical
way; he couldn't roll it back abruptly. He had to do a lot of listening
sessions, follow a calculated process—all of which was a way for him
to internalize a decision he had already made. He wasn't going to run
and he was going to commit to being a senator, but he couldn't just say
that. And nothing works better than "the kids are worried about my
safety." You say that, and everybody will back off.

Personally, by that time, I didn't really think as much about the
safety issues. Both of my uncles were killed before I was old enough to
be conscious of what was happening, so this trauma was not embed-
ded in me as it was for my siblings and cousins. I grew up and honored
the anniversaries; I saw my dad wear a bulletproof jacket and be pro-

tected by Secret Service. But I also really liked it when my dad had run for president. I consistently spent more time with him that year than during almost any period I can remember in my entire childhood and adolescence. I was like the son who wanted every day to be "take your kid to work day."

So I wasn't the only reason my dad didn't run against Ronald Reagan. I was just part of the way that he and my family could let that dream die, so all the work could go on and the causes could endure.

Chapter 6

By the time I was fifteen and at high school at Andover, I was ill. It would be years and years before anyone suggested I had bipolar disorder. And it's one of the only times in my life when I wasn't getting much of any mental healthcare. But as I look back now, a lot of the behavior that was blamed on my asthma during the week—and easily correlated with my drinking and drug-taking on the weekends—was pretty textbook bipolar disorder.

Actually, at that time, the textbook—the *DSM*—only described one basic kind of bipolar disorder with a few variations. But research had already begun to tease out two distinct types of the illness. In traditional manic-depressive illness—one of the first psychiatric diseases ever categorized, by German psychiatrist Emil Kraepelin in the late 1800s, and now called bipolar I—patients generally swing between long periods of full-blown depression, and the increasingly out-of-control racing thoughts and hyperactivity of full-blown mania, with periods of wellness in between.

In what is now called bipolar II, patients go all the way to the depths of depression but are less prone to experience full-blown mania where they completely lose control and become "psychotic," or thought-disordered. They are more likely to swing only to the less intense—and often sometimes hyperproductive—state of "hypomania," but are also more likely to "rapid cycle" between depression and hypomania, and have very agitated "mixed states." That's me.

Bipolar II is in some ways a more unpredictable illness than bipolar I, and often harder to diagnose and treat. And my symptoms got more significant when I was fifteen and sixteen.

My dad used to joke that I logged more time in the infirmary than any student in Andover history. But I just don't think he understood what was going on. There was always some other reason—I had mono, had recurring asthma. But mostly what I had was depression. And because I did have asthma, it was an easy thing for the nurses to say I "needed to rest."

I was seriously impaired by depression. And I really did not want to feel that way. So on the weekends I'd go out to nightclubs. Early on, my sister was at Tufts and sometimes she and her boyfriend would take me out with them, sneak me in. I just went right for the kamikazes (vodka, triple sec, lime juice); I didn't want anything but to get obliterated. No drinking beer for me. I just wanted the strongest drink they had so I could feel better—or at least different—right away. Or sometimes I would go myself. From Andover I used to sneak out of my dorm and take the bus into Boston, and come back early in the morning, violating all the rules. I would just introduce myself to the bouncer, and nobody ever kicked me out. They all knew who I was.

Also, well, it was the eighties. Besides kamikazes, there was cocaine everywhere in the clubs. I *really* liked cocaine. It made me feel good, so I just tried to get more.

I DON'T REMEMBER any of this behavior feeling particularly risky, just fun. I was, in many ways, happy for the relief that self-medicating brought, along with the sense that I could now fit in with the older kids. In early 1984, however, the party turned scary.

My cousin David, who was twelve years older than me, had a serious drug addiction that had many in my family worried. During Easter break of 1984, we were together in Palm Beach because my grandmother was very ill after a series of strokes, and they weren't sure she would make it.

David was, by this time, suffering from what we would now call a "stage-four addiction." (Substance use disorders are generally viewed as having four stages: experimentation, steady use, dependence, and addiction.) He had reached the point where it wasn't comfortable for him to stay with us at the Palm Beach house. So he got a room at a hotel nearby and would periodically visit the house but not stay very long.

I was into Hacky Sack at the time, and I remember being behind the house, showing David how to play. It was just my teenage way of trying to connect with him a little bit. I never knew what to say, what to talk about with the older kids, especially him, because he was brilliant and sensitive and in seemingly constant turmoil. At the same time I really appreciated that he would take the time to play with me.

So we were all waiting to hear if my grandmother was going to make it. And then I remember the doctor saying she was going to pull through, so I should go back to school, there wasn't any sense in waiting around. So I went back. The next day, my dorm master at Andover pulled me aside and said, "Your brother is calling," and I thought, *Oh my God, my grandmother.* He took me down to his apartment on the first floor of the dorm, and since kids weren't ever allowed to use the housemaster's phone, I was really bracing myself.

My brother said, "I've got some really bad news." And when I asked, "Oh, Gramma died?" he replied, "No, *David* died."

It was very difficult to reconcile this with the very clear image I had of David from just the other day: he was wearing his shirttail out and his collar kind of open with his long hair hanging over it, and he was young and thin and we were playing Hacky Sack. And now he was dead from a drug overdose.

I remember driving to the wake at my aunt's house, Hickory Hill, with my father. He didn't say a whole lot.

The house was full of family and friends and I remember just the two of us went into the room where David's casket was. I sat down with my dad and he started talking about his brother, my Uncle Bobby. He remembered Bobby telling him that, as a father, he needed to spend more time with David.

He also recounted a story Uncle Bobby had told him just before his own death. On the day before the California primary, the Robert Kennedys had gone swimming in Malibu, to relax together. David had been knocked over by a wave and got caught in the undertow, and his father had come to his rescue. When Uncle Bobby told my father this story, he talked about "the undertow" in broader terms, how there was an undertow in life and David, who was then only thirteen, already seemed vulnerable to it. And then, just hours later, Uncle Bobby was murdered as David watched the TV coverage in their hotel room upstairs.

It was unbelievably poignant to hear my father tell this story. David was in the casket next to us. And I wasn't that much older than David was when his father worried whether he could survive the undertow.

After David died, the family started paying much more attention to what all of us were doing. Especially because, just days after the funeral, a controversial new book about the family came out—*The Kennedys: An American Drama*. It was written by two magazine journalists, one from *Rolling Stone*, and it included some interviews with several of my cousins, including David and Chris Lawford.

Among many other things, the book revealed some of the controversies surrounding Aunt Rosemary's lobotomy, which had been previously reported but never publicly acknowledged by anyone in the family. The book quoted David—who was likely under the influence when he gave some of these interviews—suggesting he was the Rosemary of his generation.

The book also included a scene of David hanging out with gonzo journalist Hunter Thompson. Afterward, Thompson reportedly said of David, "This kid's going to the edge, all right. But I don't know if he'll make it back."

It never occurred to me that, just a few years later, people would be saying the same thing about me.

LATER THAT SUMMER, something scary did happen to me. I was riding with my dad in Hyannis Port, a couple blocks from the house, in his beloved blue 1972 Pontiac GTO convertible—one of a pair that he and his close friend, California Senator John Tunney, had bought together. We were heading up a slight hill when a pickup truck pulled right in front of us and we collided.

Dad wasn't hurt badly. But I was—in a way that was minimized when it happened, as most head injuries were, but now may help explain a number of things. At the time, it was announced to the press that I had a "mild concussion." In fact, according to the documents from a series of neurological tests I had beginning later that year, I suffered a fairly substantial head injury: a small skull fracture in the left

frontal area and a laceration over my left eye that required stitches. I
was unconscious for nearly a half hour and had amnesia of events before and after the crash.

In the months after my head injury, my parents and my school noticed some changes in my sleeping habits—I could sleep twelve or
more hours a day unless forced to wake up—and the attention deficit
I had long experienced in school seemed to be getting worse. My
mother also thought I had had a slight personality change, that I had
become less inhibited. And they noticed I was having trouble with
memory and with calculation. When my parents sent me to get tested
during winter break, the first thing the doctor recorded was that I
came into the office very concerned that I had undertipped the cab-
driver because of difficulty figuring out what I owed him.

Today, I would be seen as someone still recovering from a relatively
serious head trauma—a neurological patient. Back then, the recommendation for my treatment after all this observing and testing was
"Patrick should continue in psychotherapy so that he can develop a
greater ability to recognize and accept his feelings and expend less energy in avoiding them."

In reality, some of these things they were suddenly noticing about
me now appear to be clear signs of a mood disorder worsening at the
age when many of these illnesses commonly start to become clinically
significant. And, while the head trauma didn't help, I had been suffering from cycles of deep depression and then little bursts of mania for
a while (to the point where I was figuring out how to trigger hypomania to quickly finish all the work I had ignored while depressed). It
may have been because the family was being more vigilant after David's death that anyone noticed any change in me. But more likely it
was the head injury, because now there was a "reason," an "excuse," for
my mood swings.

With all the medical attention I received as a child and an adolescent, it still astonishes me that nobody talked to me about the possibility of depression when I was so obviously depressed.

IF DAVID'S DEATH and my head injury were supposed to be a wakeup call, I slept through them. Over the next year and a half, I struggled in school and in life.

In school, I was really impaired by depression. I could sleep seventeen hours a day. The only reason I made it through, actually, was a great teacher named Robin Crawford, who taught early American history and really helped me emotionally. The irony is that he was known as the toughest teacher on campus—he never smiled, and he had this grimace, just a stone-faced, miserable-looking guy, like a drill sergeant in the marines. He was also in charge of college counseling, and he was notorious for taking all these smart, preppy, Ivy League–bound kids from privileged backgrounds into his office and leaving them crying by the time they left. He almost relished giving them a dose of the real world. I remember all the smart kids would raise their hands in class, and he would just eviscerate them. So he was the most unlikely person to take me under his wing.

He gave essay tests, and I didn't do well on them. During one of our final essay exams—which was worth like a third of the overall grade— I just blanked on it. I was sitting there falling apart, in this big exam hall. After most of the kids had finished the test and left, I was still sitting there, with pretty much nothing. Finally he said we had to turn in our papers and I brought mine up. My eyes were filled with tears and I was heartbroken that I couldn't get it together. I felt I really had let him down.

He said not to worry. And that kindness meant everything to me. (So did passing his class.)

Today, we have a much better idea of the role teachers can play in the early recognition, diagnosis, and treatment of mental illnesses. They can be much better trained on warning signs and emergency care and suicide prevention, through programs like Mental Health First Aid, and they can be given more tools than just sending kids to the nurse or detention. They also need more training on the finer points of what is called "social and emotional learning," an idea my cousin Tim Shriver helped spearhead over twenty years ago. In 1994, he co-founded CASEL, the Collaborative for Academic, Social, and Emotional Learning, which promotes student self-awareness, social awareness, and responsible decision-making skills.

But this all has to start with teachers who go the extra distance for those students who need extra care. I was one of those students, and thank goodness Robin Crawford was one of those teachers.

IN THE SUMMER OF 1985, I stayed with my brother, Teddy, in the house he bought in Somerville, Massachusetts, to establish residency there. He was twenty-three, and my father really wanted him to run for Congress. Speaker of the House "Tip" O'Neill had just announced he wouldn't run again for that seat—the very same one where President Kennedy had begun his career in elected office. From a timing and publicity perspective, you couldn't have asked for a better narrative, and everyone knew it. Dad recently had taken Teddy with him to South Africa on a trip hosted by Bishop Desmond Tutu. And NBC had just agreed to make a TV movie called *The Teddy Kennedy Story*, detailing his heroic recovery from cancer and scheduled to be shown during the fall of the election.

We were both getting more attention from Dad than we were used to, Teddy because of the congressional seat—which he still wasn't sure he really wanted to run for—and me because Dad was constantly calling me asking, "What's going on with your brother, what's he thinking?"

I remember one afternoon my brother and I were sitting together in the bleachers at an empty baseball field in a park in Somerville. Teddy was very emotional, and he said, "I don't think I'm ready for this. Dad wants me to do it, but I'm not up for it." He was active in disability advocacy and other medical causes, and was thinking about law school.

I remember being proud of him for announcing, that July, that he wasn't going to run, clearing the way for our thirty-three-year-old cousin Joe Kennedy Jr. to successfully seek the seat. It took incredible courage for him to say he wouldn't run.

BACK AT SCHOOL THAT FALL, I was increasingly out of control: lots of lost weekends on cocaine, many weekday nights calmed down to sleep by Xanax, lots of weekday mornings too depressed to get up, my own bipolar cycles just made more vicious by chemicals. Then on Sunday, March 16, 1986—just three months before I was supposed to graduate from Andover—I flew down to Palm Beach for a week with a couple of my high school friends and a chaperone.

We were staying at my grandmother's house down there, and I thought we had enough drugs to make it through the whole vacation. But what was supposed to last a week was gone by the third day, and I started realizing I couldn't go on. I was doing a lot of drunk-dialing when I was high. So I called my dad, called my mom. I don't recall much of what I said, but I know I just kept telling them over and over and over how much I loved them—a cry for help.

My dad had a sort of tough-love response, and then he turned me over to Larry Horowitz, who as a physician had a much clearer understanding of what was going on and what to do. Larry arranged for someone to come get me and fly me home. I left my friends down there on vacation and was taken immediately to the rehab he had arranged.

By Friday, I was checking into Spofford Hall, a rehab facility in New Hampshire, as "Patrick K." And soon I found myself filling a kelly green college notebook with all the AA sayings from the pillows I had been making fun of in my mom's living room.

The first things I wrote were "One day at a time," "Obsessed with possessing," "No more mind altering," "Live and let live," "There are no degrees to addiction," "I'll get sober if it doesn't interfere with the rest of my life," and what later became my life's motto—in good and bad ways—"Fake it until you make it."

I DID NOT TAKE REHAB as seriously as I should have. In my first group meeting, I was asked what I would do instead of drugs.

"Hunting and scuba diving," I shot back, getting a laugh. Afterward I scribbled to myself that "it was sick" my glib answer had come so easily and definitively.

On my self-reporting forms, I wrote I used marijuana and alcohol infrequently; hallucinogens, narcotics, amphetamines, barbiturates, inhalants, and PCP never; and tranquilizers like Xanax and Librium daily. Next to "cocaine" I checked the box for using one or two times per week, but then wrote in "would be" and an arrow toward the box for "every day."

After ten days, I was checked out of Spofford Hall early, against medical advice, because my family had other ideas for my treatment. They wanted me to return to Andover, but under constant live-in supervision. They hired this guy Don Juhl, who ran a concierge recovery service for people who didn't want to stay in rehab. He was the same guy who had "supervised" my cousin David, back when the family thought that might help him overcome his addiction.

I felt like my dad wrote me off at that point; I was just an enormous disappointment, like my mom. Just the idea that I had the same guy with me who had taken care of David made me feel shunned. At the time, I was told that my father had convened a meeting of the best and brightest about me and my health—just as he had when Teddy got his bone cancer, and on numerous occasions concerning my mother. There was also an assessment from my Spofford caregivers. I was told that the prognosis offered about my future was simple: I was never going to get well. I was a child of an alcoholic and showed all these indications of such trouble at a young age. My prospects of living a healthy, productive life were pretty bleak. I was apparently defective long-term, the curse of the illness.

I was eighteen and knew I was already considered hopeless.

I can understand how, at the time, this wasn't such a hard vision to subscribe to. My mom was already totally incapacitated by this illness. But nobody should ever put a teenager in that kind of box.

YEARS LATER, I had a revelation about this time period with my dad. He admitted that before I went to rehab, "I knew you were in trouble." When I asked how, he said, "I used to get all of the receipts from your ATM bank withdrawals, three o'clock in the morning when you're blowing hundreds of dollars."

I thought to myself, *Why didn't you do anything?* But, of course, I didn't *say* that.

I was moved out of the dorms and into an apartment where there was room for Don; when he needed a break, his wife and partner,

Patty, would be with me. His job was to make sure I finished high school. It was actually pretty great to have someone's total attention all the time. I had never realized how much I wanted that. Don dropped me off for classes and picked me up afterward. We played basketball together, talked about life together.

At the beginning, I was supposed to go to twelve-step meetings pretty much every day—on discharge from Spofford they require "ninety in ninety," which means ninety meetings in the first ninety days. There was also an aftercare support group at Spofford twice a month.

But Don Juhl, who was overseeing my care, was not a strict AA guy. He subscribed to what was referred to as the "Malibu Model," which grew out of a rehab in Malibu, California, and was based on the idea that perhaps alcoholism wasn't a disease, and perhaps complete abstinence was not necessary to remain functional and well. This is, of course, part of a very large, emotional, and never-ending debate in the world of addiction. Since its inception in the 1930s, AA has always been completely unwavering on this issue: there is only one definition of sobriety—complete abstinence.

There has been some liberalization over recent years concerning the use of psychiatric medication for patients with comorbid alcoholism and mental illnesses. (More debatable in AA are the medications prescribed to help wean people off drugs or alcohol, some of which are themselves addictive but not disabling.) But the general goal is to treat the addiction with abstinence, spirituality, and meetings, and nothing else. But from the moment that AA and the twelve steps became popularized, there were programs that wanted to retrofit the twelve steps into something more forgiving.

When I was in my teens and twenties, this seemed logical to me. This was especially true since I had two parents who abused alcohol but who functioned—or failed to function—pretty differently. My mom was the classic poster child for the AA approach, since she could only function if she was completely abstinent, going to meetings, working the twelve steps. My dad had a drinking problem and was deeply in denial about it, but, well, he did still function as a US Senator, and a powerful one. So it is unsurprising that he didn't believe in abstinence. And even after I had been in rehab at eighteen, he didn't seem concerned about my drinking, or even drinking too much. He seemed mostly concerned that I not get into trouble or attract any negative attention to the family.

For example, less than three months after I left rehab, I got a letter from him, on Senate stationery, in which he attempted to lay down some rules about my use of his house in McLean, Virginia, and the family house at the Cape. He was mostly concerned that I alert him and the staff several days in advance if I was going to have any guests. He did note that the liquor bill my friends and I had run up the previous summer was "still vivid in my mind." But rather than suggest or reinforce that I shouldn't be drinking, he explained, "The rule that I want you to understand for this summer is that any time you are with me, picnic lunches, cocktails, or dinner, I am glad to entertain our guests . . . but, what I don't want this summer are the last minute drifters returning to the house and then feeling free to help themselves to the bar and the icebox. I think if we follow these guidelines, we'll avoid some of the problems we've had in the past. Love, Dad."

At the time, I thought this letter was fine. Now it seems pretty surprising. At the time, I also thought the Malibu Model made sense. Now, I have to say, I know it could never work for me.

DON HELPED ME get through high school, although I ended up not graduating with my class—which my parents weren't happy about—and finishing one term paper over the summer. And then, after several years of living near Boston, and near my mom, I moved back to DC to go to Georgetown. I was surprised I got in at all, especially to the School of Foreign Service. But Robin Crawford, the college counselor who helped me at Andover, knew someone there and my father was, well, my father.

In reality, whatever strings may have been pulled, nobody really did anyone any favors. I was in no way prepared to be at Georgetown, especially the highly competitive foreign service program, either academically or psychologically. I went to DC for a summer class at Georgetown to get a head start on it, and to work as a page for Senator Bill Bradley. But without supervision, I started drinking—binge drinking.

I did maintain my cocaine sobriety. But since I needed stimulants to help push me out of depression and into hypomania, I was using more and more caffeine—in coffee and over-the-counter pills. I would also exploit some of the euphoric effects of the prednisone prescribed for my asthma.

I lasted at Georgetown only a few weeks. I was in way over my head, and out of my head. In disgrace, I quietly moved out of my dorm and back in with my dad, feeling like a complete failure.

Our house in McLean had a tennis court, and sometimes early in the morning, my dad's good friend Connecticut Senator Chris Dodd would come over to play. Chris's father had been a powerful senator, so he knew all about generational issues, especially in Irish political families.

One morning after a tennis match, Chris told me he thought it might be mentally healthy for me to get a fresh start in a smaller fishbowl, somewhere away from the glare of DC or Boston. He had gone undergrad to Providence College, and he thought his alma mater and the town of Providence, Rhode Island, would be a great place for me to begin again.

My dad agreed, but for a different reason. "Yes, Rhode Island is great politically," I recall him saying. "If you ever want to think of running for office, it's a great place."

I was utterly blown away to hear him say this. The fact that he even mentioned the possibility that I could have a political career meant that even though I had been in rehab and had blown everything at Georgetown, I might have a second chance. Or at least my dad thought so—which was, to me, actually more important than if it were true.

Saying this was like throwing a lit match on a fuel depot. I just exploded—I knew exactly what I was going to do. I would move to Providence, get back on track academically, and show my father I might be worthy of his confidence.

Chapter 7

It was in Providence as a second-try college student that I first became aware of the larger world of mental healthcare. I volunteered to work on a local suicide hotline—where my code name was "Patrick 507"—and I had to learn not only how to talk to people who were floridly mentally ill, but how to connect them to emergency healthcare. It was the very beginning of my education in the mental health system—besides, of course, being a consumer—and it came at a time when the field considered itself deeply under siege. This was largely because of cutbacks from the Reagan administration—which decided to get the federal government out of the mental health business but didn't really fund or empower the states to do the job. But the cutbacks were exacerbated by the rise, during the 1980s, of the first generation of managed care—which made mental health and addiction care, already stepchildren to all other medical care, even less well funded and more aggressively capped. For many people, mental illness and substance use disorder care were becoming increasingly do-it-yourself.

This was still the early days of suicide hotlines, and the technology that helps them work. We didn't have cell phones and caller ID and reverse directories available to us so we could quickly identify where the person was calling from and send someone to revive them. There were a lot of calls where the person passed out on the line, or the line went dead, and you just didn't know what happened. It was very frustrating. We couldn't send police to them; we were generally trying to get them to go to emergency rooms.

While I suppose, deep inside, I did understand that the people I was talking to and trying to help were like me in some way, I mostly did this to get out of myself and as an educational adventure. I wanted to have this window into suffering that I couldn't make sense of myself. I felt a great sense of satisfaction doing it. I never left that room without feeling like I had in some way helped someone.

At the same time, I had taken on an honorary position for Aunt Eunice at Let's Play to Grow, one of the spin-off organizations from Special Olympics. The group focused on helping parents connect with their babies and infants with intellectual disabilities by breaking down their fear of playing with their children, and also being involved in local clubs—there were several hundred around the country—with other parents facing similar challenges.

As for taking care of myself, my parents helped me find a psychiatrist in Providence who I could consider my own doctor. It was a smart thing to do and, at the time, something pretty uncommon. We now know better that the beginning of college is one of the most vulnerable times for anyone with any predisposition to mental illness or addiction. It is when many of the major mental illnesses begin to express themselves in earnest, with symptoms that simply can't be blamed on anything else (although they still too often are). It is the first time that most young people have complete freedom to use drugs and alcohol. It is also the exact time when most young people have outgrown their pediatricians and really need to start taking control of their own health.

Back then, student healthcare was often grossly inadequate. (For mental health it still is at many schools, and organizations like the Jed Foundation—the nation's leading nonprofit for campus mental health and suicide prevention—would be even more effective if the colleges and universities were more proactive.) So it wasn't uncommon that nobody noticed there wasn't a real safety net until you (or your kid) fell through it. I'm sure in 1987, the idea of seeing a private psychiatrist off campus seemed like an indulgence. It's now much more common, and student health plans offer many more options for on-campus care. But one thing is still the same—at eighteen or nineteen, it is incredibly important for young people to take some control of their healthcare, especially their mental healthcare.

My parents got a recommendation for a psychiatrist in Providence, Dr. Peter Kramer, who had worked previously in Washington for what was then called the Alcohol, Drug Abuse, and Mental Health Administration (ADAMHA)—the federal entity that, since 1973, had overseen the National Institute of Mental Health, the National Institute on Alcohol Abuse and Alcoholism, and the National Institute on Drug Abuse. Among his responsibilities during that time was to help refute damaging testimony to the Senate Finance Committee about the efficacy of psychotherapy that claimed there was little proof it was anything more than "rent-a-friend." (This has been an ongoing issue in mental healthcare. At the time, in the 1980s, there were few actual studies to prove the efficacy of psychotherapy. There are now many studies proving the effectiveness of several types of psychotherapy—especially cognitive behavioral therapy—either paired with medication or by itself.)

Kramer was now teaching at Brown, had a small private practice, and had just begun writing a regular column for the *Psychiatric Times*. He was a youthful forty and seemed closer to my age than any therapist I'd seen.

This was long before Dr. Kramer wrote *Listening to Prozac*. In fact

Prozac—fluoxetine—hadn't even been approved by the FDA yet. (That happened in December of 1987, almost a year after I had started seeing him.) Mostly, Kramer was listening to me. Since I was depressed, he did try me on the drug that was, at the time, the gold standard of treatment, imipramine. That landmark antidepressant had first come on the market in the late 1950s and was—with lithium and Haldol—the beginning of truly effective psychiatric medications for the major mental illnesses. Each, of course, had its side effects, as all medications do, and some had dietary restrictions: imipramine was easier to take than the other popular antidepressant of the day, Nardil, which had some annoying food interactions.

As with all psychiatric medications, there were also risks that grew out of the challenging process of diagnosis. Antidepressants are created to yank the brain out of a depression, which means pushing it in the other direction. Mood stabilizers for bipolar disorder are created to balance swaying moods. Mood stabilizers won't bother patients who primarily suffer from depression (although antidepressants will work better). But antidepressants can make bipolar patients manic, sometimes dangerously so. This is a predictably unpredictable response—a patient and clinician often only know it when it happens.

The problem can be quickly identified and corrected, which is why it's so important for patients on new meds to be closely monitored. But until we learn enough about the brain to have reliable tests to clearly see the difference between unipolar depression and bipolar disorder, some patients will only learn which illness they have because of a bad reaction to medication. (There are now some early stage genetic tests to help inform psychiatric drug choices; they hold out promise that there can be "personalized medicine" for brain diseases just as we are coming to expect from the rest of healthcare.)

I actually tolerated imipramine pretty well, for someone who would later be diagnosed with a bipolar disorder. But my drug situation was complicated by all the meds I took for my asthma. Dr. Kramer believed that any psychiatric medication I took would mostly be useful to control my symptoms enough so I could work on what he considered my more pressing problem, which was growing up, taking more responsibility for my actions and my life, and moving past my childhood and my parents—who were, for me, both distant and dominating. Mostly, the treatment was about process, about ways to try to control symptoms and control actions.

UNDER DR. KRAMER'S CARE, I tried my best to make a new life for myself in Providence while struggling with symptoms of depression and anxiety. Getting up for classes was a huge challenge; picking up my mail at the student center sometimes caused me total panic. But I did my best to muddle through. Even as a freshman I lived off campus, alone, so I wouldn't risk anyone knowing what was really going on with me.

In addition to school, I interned at the State House, acting as a page for legislators and doing research for the Legislative Council. In the fall of 1987, I worked for the Lieutenant Governor in his attempt to unseat US Senator John Chafee. I revived the Young Democrats group at Providence and decided to run as a delegate for the 1988 Democratic National Convention, pledged to Michael Dukakis. In early March of 1988, I was elected as a delegate.

And this probably would have been what my life looked like for the foreseeable future—school, political and mental health volunteerism, therapy, drinking sprees, and oversleeping—if I hadn't developed that tumor on my spine. Instead, I entered Mass General on April 18 for back surgery and got caught up in receiving the same family and media attention that had greeted Teddy when he faced his amputation.

I was still in my hospital bed recovering when I first told my dad that I planned to run for office, immediately. He was not, initially, very supportive of the idea, said he was worried about my health and whether I was jumping in too soon. But then, like he always did, my dad started thinking politically. He shifted his queries to more practical matters, like whether I really knew enough about the district I would run in. I convinced him I had been studying all the players and the dynamics of the district and really did know what I was doing. Also, the state legislature in Rhode Island was part-time, sitting only six months of the year, so it would be possible to stay in school and be a state rep.

By the time I was discharged from the hospital on May 7, we were already using my coming-home party to announce my campaign. We had four months until the election, and I spent the first weeks going door-to-door, still wearing my full neck brace and walking with a cane. It was an unusual way to meet a twenty-year-old candidate. But, given the percentage of elderly people in the district, my condition—and my ability to make jokes about it—made it easier for me to strike up conversations and connect with voters of all ages.

Early in the campaign, I was fortunate to get the support of the state's current Democratic Senator, Claiborne Pell, who had been elected the same year John Kennedy became president and had many legislative triumphs—the best known of which was the Pell Grants for college students. He came to a kickoff breakfast we had but, perhaps because I was challenging a five-time Democratic incumbent he had known for many years, he didn't immediately rise to speak like some of the other politicians there.

As people were just starting to leave, I got up the courage to go over to him and ask if he might say something. He didn't speak loudly—he never did—but I never forgot his words.

"I want to say why I'm here to support Patrick Kennedy," he said. "I believe that he shares the values of President Kennedy. And every night

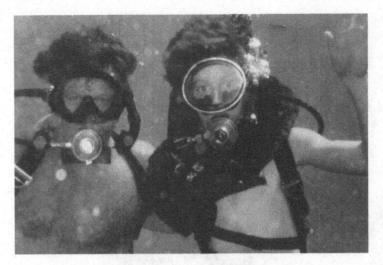

Scuba diving with my father.

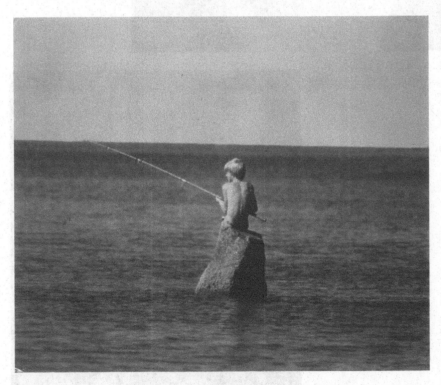

Fishing at the end of Squaw Island.

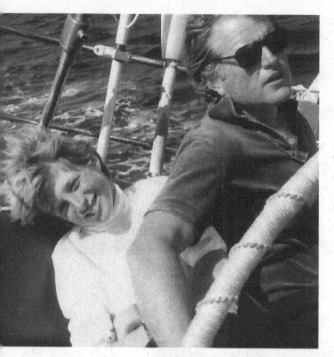

On the water with my dad, September 1979, in his boat, the *Curragh*.

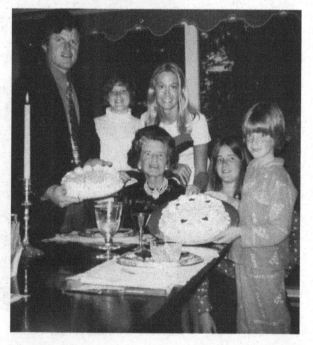

Gramma's birthday.

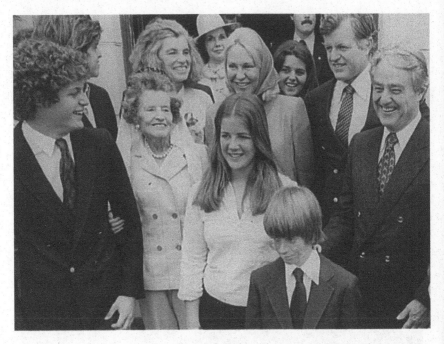

Kennedys and Shrivers. Back row, from left: Bobby Shriver, Aunt Eunice Shriver, Mom, Maria Shriver, Dad. Front row: my brother Ted, Gramma, my sister Kara, me, Uncle Sarge Shriver.

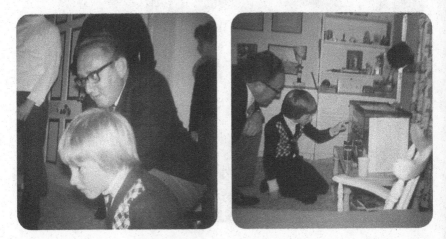

In my bedroom at the McLean, Virginia, house, showing Henry Kissinger my aquarium.

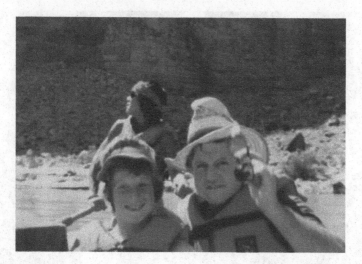

My father and me during the big family rafting trip he organized
down the Colorado River into the Grand Canyon.

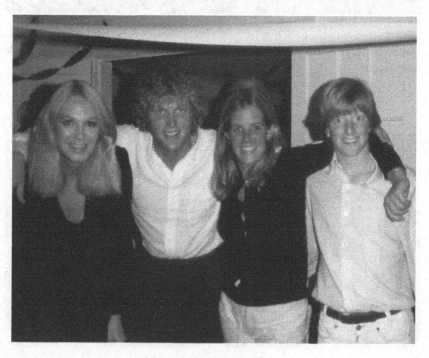

My mom, Ted, Kara, and me.

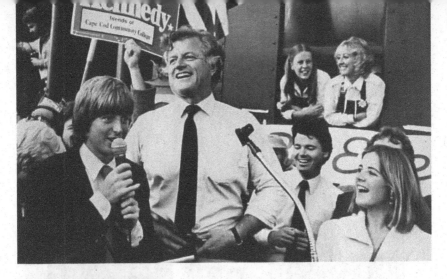

ABOVE: My father, me, and Kara (far right) at a campaign appearance during his 1982 Senate race.

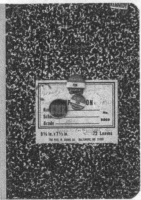

LEFT: My campaign diary from my father's 1980 presidential campaign.

BELOW: What my father's car looked like after the car crash in Hyannis Port in 1984, in which I received a head injury that was minimized at the time, but was more serious than anyone let on.

The Boston Herald, Saturday, August 18, 1984

TEDDY AND SON IN CAR CRASH SCARE ON CAPE

By SHELLEY MURPHY
AND STEVE
CONNOLLY

HYANNIS PORT — Sen. Edward M. Kennedy and his youngest son Patrick suffered cuts and bruises yesterday when their convertible collided head-on with a plumber's pick-up truck that veered suddenly into their lane, police said.

Kennedy, 51, 17-year-old Patrick, and plumber Leonard J. "Jack" Bell, 63, of Hyannis, were treated for facial cuts and bruises at Cape Cod Hospital after the 1:50 p.m. accident, hospital officials said.

Thomas Gargan, 13, a Kennedy cousin and a passenger in the senator's car, was not injured and Edward Martin, a spokesman in the senator's Boston office.

Hyannis Police Sgt. Frank J. McKenna said Bell was cited for driving to endanger. He added that "there was no indication of liquor involved in the accident."

Kennedy, who reportedly was treated for cuts on the head and knee, left the hospital and returned to the family compound. Later, last night, he and his son Teddy went swimming.

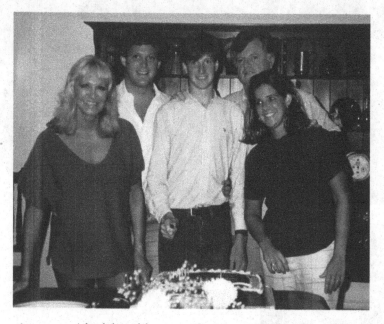

A birthday celebration at the Squaw Island house.

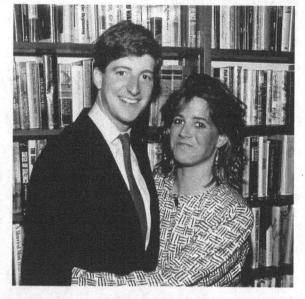

My favorite picture of Kara and me, taken at the Mount Pleasant Public Library in my district when I was a Rhode Island state representative.

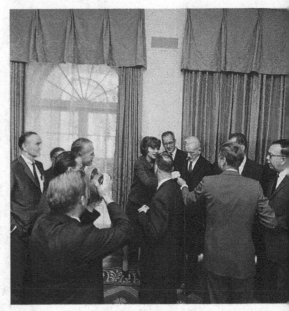

My Uncle Jack (back to the camera) handing my Aunt Eunice one of the pens used to sign the landmark Mental Retardation Facilities and Community Mental Health Centers Act of 1963, or what we now call the Community Mental Health Act. The signing ceremony, on October 31, 1963, was his last. (Courtesy JFK Library)

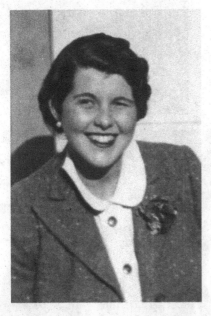

My Aunt Rosemary at age twenty-one, in April 1940. It was her life and the challenge of her medical conditions— a developmental disability from birth, the onset of mental illness in her early twenties, and then a tragic mistake in her treatment in the 1940s—that inspired my family's commitment to changing the world for people with developmental disabilities and brain diseases. When I was seventeen, my Aunt Eunice invited me and others of my generation to get more involved. (Courtesy JFK Library Foundation)

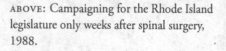

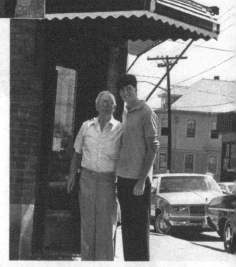

ABOVE: Campaigning for the Rhode Island legislature only weeks after spinal surgery, 1988.

RIGHT: With my Providence political mentor and friend, Frank DiPaolo, in front of his beloved diner, Castle Spa, where I ate almost every day. (Courtesy *Providence Journal*)

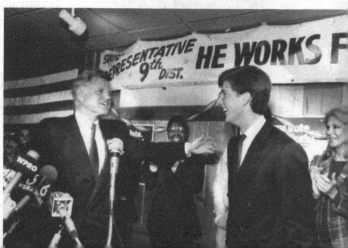

Election night, 1988, in Providence with my parents. (Courtesy *Providence Journal*)

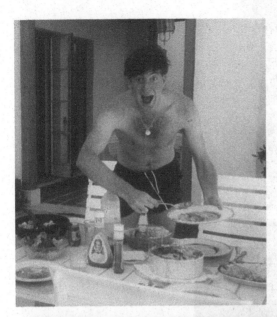

In Palm Beach during a break from Providence College and the Rhode Island State House.

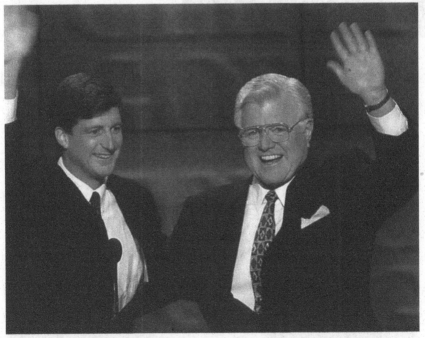

My father and me onstage at the Democratic National Convention in Chicago, 1996.

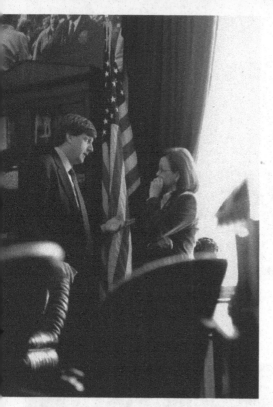

In my congressional office with my executive assistant and protector, Terri Alford.

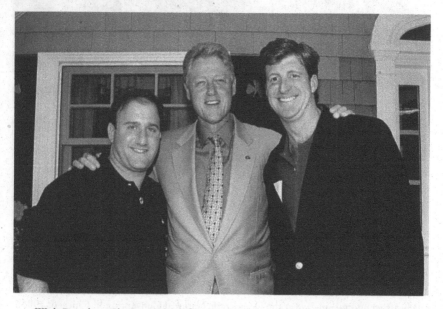

With President Clinton and my first congressional chief of staff, Tony Marcella.

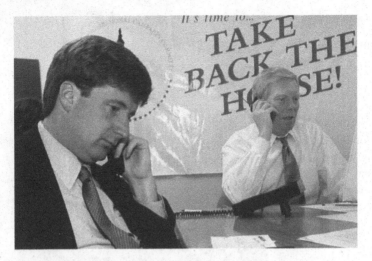

Fund-raising call with my first House political mentor, then Minority Leader Dick Gephardt. (Photograph by Bill O'Leary/*The Washington Post*/Getty Images)

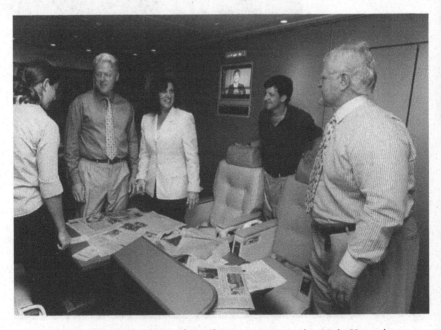

On *Air Force One* with President Clinton, my stepmother Vicki Kennedy, and my father, during the 2000 campaign. (Courtesy The White House)

With Hillary Clinton outside Gramma's house during a Rhode Island political action committee event.

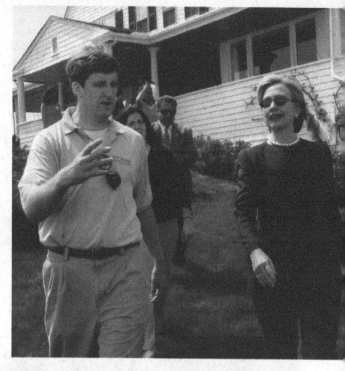

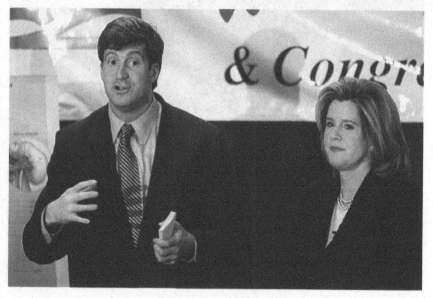

With Tipper Gore at the Woonsocket, Rhode Island, senior citizens event in February 2000, where I first publicly admitted I suffered from a mental illness and was being treated with medication and therapy. (Courtesy *Providence Journal*)

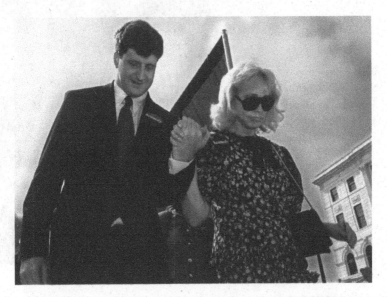

With my mom after announcing my bid for reelection to Congress, in front of the Rhode Island State House. (Courtesy *Providence Journal*)

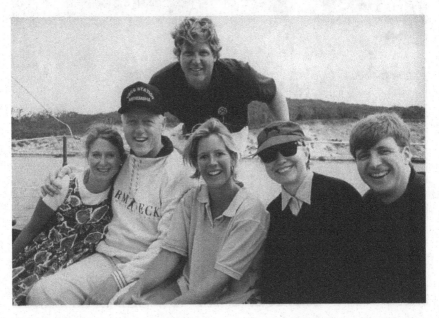

Sailing with the Clintons. From left: my sister-in-law Dr. Kiki Gershman Kennedy, the President, my sister Kara, Hillary Clinton, and me, with my brother Teddy behind us.

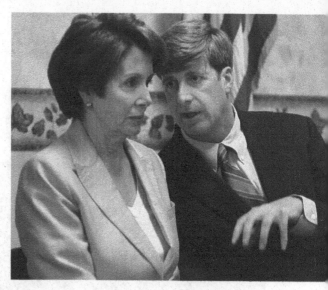

With Representative
Nancy Pelosi, before
giving a healthcare
address in Rhode Island;
as Speaker of the House,
she ushered through
the parity bill.
(AP Photo/Steven Senne)

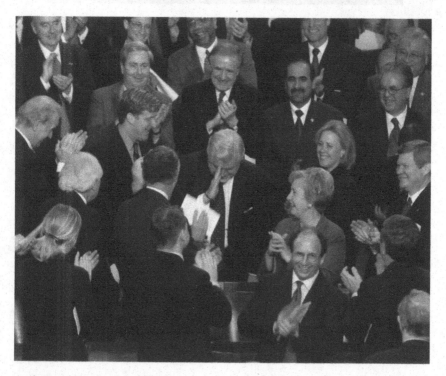

At the January 2002 State of the Union, when President George W. Bush acknowledged my father's contribution to the passage of the No Child Left Behind legislation; he is surrounded by, among others, his friends Joe Biden, at left, and Paul Wellstone, in front.

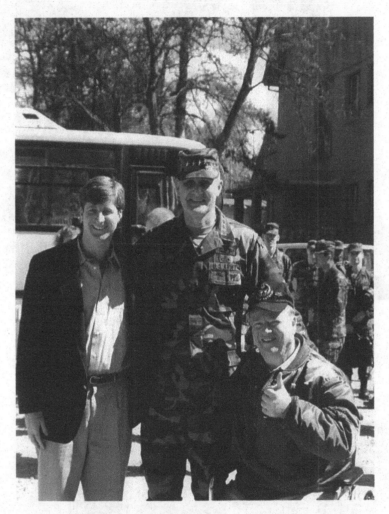

At Eagle Base, Bosnia and Herzegovina, with General Hugh Shelton, Chairman of the Joint Chiefs of Staff (center)—who taught me that in the military, mental healthcare is not a safety net but a "force multiplier"—and Senator Max Cleland, who was with me and my family during many battles, both legislative and personal.

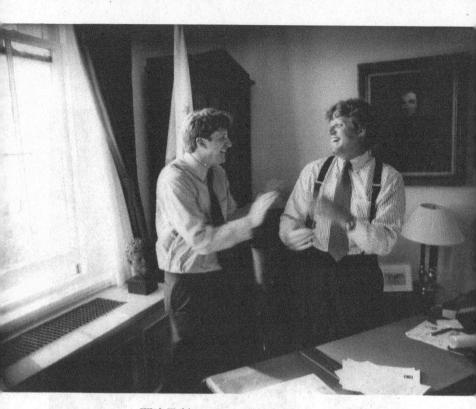

With Teddy, in my congressional office.

(Photograph by Callie Shell)

THE NEW YORK TIMES **NATIONAL** MONDAY, MAY 15, 2006

For a Kennedy, Fighting the Stigma of Mental Illness Becomes Personal

By SHERYL GAY STOLBERG

WASHINGTON, May 14 — Patrick J. Kennedy was keeping an uncomfortable secret.

Representative Kennedy, scion of America's most loved and hated Democratic clan, has been a passionate advocate for ending the stigma of mental illness; he told voters years ago of his treatment for depression and cocaine abuse. But when he slipped off to the Mayo Clinic last December to get help for addiction to prescription painkillers, he had trouble over coming that stigma himself.

When he crashed his Mustang convertible into a Capitol barricade in the middle of the night earlier this month, Mr. Kennedy, of Rhode Island, was thrust into a clash between personal privacy and political beliefs. Hours before he told the world

woman who said the two had argued while drinking on his yacht.

Mr. Kennedy's advisers say he now views these incidents, as well as his addiction and bout of binge drinking, through the prism of his bipolar disorder, a type of depression marked by extreme highs and lows. But some wonder whether this latest incident must be his last.

"I don't think anybody realized until now how serious his problems were," said M. Charles Bakst, a longtime political columnist for The Providence Journal. "Now it all makes sense, and you realize that this kid is on the brink. And I think if it happens again, you are going lower people say, not necessarily sourly or bitterly, but sadly, maybe, that public life isn't for him."

From the moment Patrick Joseph

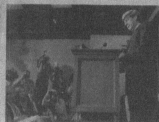

to become chairman of the Democratic Congressional Campaign Committee in 2000. It was a grueling year of fund-raising and travel, marked by both the Los Angeles airport and Coast Guard episodes.

It was also the year he disclosed, in an appearance with Tipper Gore, his bipolar disorder. The announcement was unplanned, but House members were not shocked.

After the 2000 elections, Mr. Kennedy was rewarded with a coveted seat on the House Appropriations Committee. He considered running for the Senate, but decided against it. And he has made mental health his signature issue.

"He found an attitude he was comfortable flying at," said Erik Smith, who was Mr. Kennedy's spokesman at the campaign committee.

The *New York Times* piece that came out while I was at the Mayo Clinic for treatment after the car crash, one of several that announced the new direction of my political career to focus on mental illness and addiction and use my own story more openly.

since we've lost President Kennedy, I've knelt down on my knees and prayed that this nation would live up to the promise of John Kennedy. I believe that Patrick Kennedy will and that's why I support him."

That's a lot for a guy just turning twenty-one to live up to.

While I was honored to have the support of Senator Pell and some other national figures from Rhode Island, such as retired Senator John Pastore, I found myself gravitating to more local politics, retail politics. I wasn't going into this to be a big outspoken public figure—I wanted to ring doorbells, hear people out, learn how day-to-day politics really worked. I was lucky enough to quickly make friends with Frank Di Paolo, the elder statesman of Providence politics and a lifelong Kennedy supporter. Frank owned and ran the Castle Spa, a diner in the district I was running in. I started eating breakfast there almost every day while campaigning, and he became my first character witness in the neighborhood when I was accused of being nothing but a carpetbagging student. He always said, "I have two boys and two beautiful girls, and my buddy Patrick, he's my third son."

Election Day was September 13—it was a primary, but since there were no Republican candidates, the Democratic winner would get the seat. It seemed like the entire Kennedy family descended on Providence to help out. We won, but I can't say the media was very impressed. The last line of the *Boston Globe* story about the election quoted a local bartender describing me as "a college kid who won't be around long." For a business owner in a town of college and university transients, that wasn't a completely unfair assumption.

When it came time for my swearing in, I was torn about what role, if any, my father should have in the events. He flew back from vacation in Hawaii to be there, and we arranged to borrow the Fitzgerald Bible—the same family Bible JFK had used at his inaugural—for my swearing in. But when Dad got there, I realized I didn't want him to be on the floor of the State House standing over me in every photo.

This was my maiden voyage as a very local politician in Rhode Island, and I wanted to be seen as a neighborhood guy, my own guy, and not just a Kennedy. I was constantly conflicted about my identity—I guess almost everyone is at that age—and I didn't want it to seem like my being elected was all part of this big plan masterminded at the Kennedy compound for us to take over. I wanted to make sure people were getting to know me.

So at the last minute, before we walked out to do the ceremony, I said to him, "You can't come on the floor with me." He was pretty shocked, especially since he had just flown fourteen hours to be there. But he understood. Afterward, we went to the secretary of state's private office and did another ceremonial swearing, with no press, just for my dad and me. We took a great picture of me with my hand on the family Bible and Dad behind me.

My family has always been very big on sending each other handwritten notes and signed photos to mark special occasions, and it was time for me to start doing the same. I wrote, "To Dad, my father & hero! Love, Patrick," and had it delivered to him.

IN THE FOLLOW-UP to my hospital stay for the surgery, my father's staff sent him a memo about an ongoing discussion about family medical bills. Apparently, since the beginning of my mother's illness, my father had been paying for all her care himself, by check, rather than putting in for any reimbursement from medical insurance and running the risk there would be a paper trail about her care. Ironically, he started doing this in the 1960s when federal employees actually had the only coverage available in America with full mental health parity—which was finally taken away only in the early eighties by the Reagan administration. But by 1987, with my mom's struggles with alcohol dependence well documented and their divorce long over, the staff decided to start submitting claims for my mom to medical insurance. (While my parents were divorced, they were still very much in each other's lives; my mom still always joined us for big family events at the Cape and was a fixture at the Thanksgiving table even after my father remarried.)

I'm guessing that during my lengthy hospital stay, somebody on his staff noticed that there had never been a medical insurance claim put in on me and decided that was ridiculous. So they tallied up all my unclaimed charges for 1987 and the ones ongoing for 1988 and finally submitted them for insurance.

What is particularly interesting about the correspondence—on which I was copied (and which I never looked at until recently)—is the way my dad's staffers explained to him the new managed care rules for mental healthcare coverage.

"Reimbursement of mental illness care is limited under the insurance policy," they wrote. "A MAXIMUM of 50 visits per calendar year are reimbursed at 70% of the usual and customary charges allowed; subject to a $75,000 MAXIMUM LIFETIME BENEFIT."

Between my rehab costs and my visits to Dr. Kramer, I can tell you that by the end of 1987 I would, at the age of twenty, already have gone through a shockingly significant percentage of my lifetime maximum benefit.

Chapter 8

My health was relatively stable as I finished my first two-year term in office. I started my second term in January of 1991, and as spring approached, I prepared to finally graduate from Providence at the age of twenty-three. I was still seeing Dr. Kramer, and whatever went wrong, we were able to deal with it. For a college student who did some weekend binge drinking—like almost everyone else—I was doing okay.

And then my dad and I met in Palm Beach for the Easter holiday.

This was the most investigated and publicized week of my life, after sexual assault charges were brought against my cousin William. I don't have much to add to the story of that night—except to say that when my father woke up my cousin and me and asked if we wanted to get a nightcap with him, I went along basically as the designated driver. I spent most of the evening nursing ginger ales.

It wasn't that I was so sober at the time. I was still defining sobriety as not using any illegal drugs. But I just didn't feel like drinking that night. The truth was, I did much of my drinking—and most of my dangerous drinking—alone, at night, at home.

For the first few weeks after the charges were filed, I did my best to hold it together, to be supportive of my family and responsible as a young politician. I gave interviews to major media and watched as the coverage focused first on my cousin and then on my father's lifestyle. That subject had been lingering in the press for over a year, since a devastating (although basically accurate) piece about his aggressively single lifestyle and its possible ramifications for his political authority had appeared in *GQ*.

Within two weeks, I could no longer handle the pressure. On April 15, the editor of the *Providence Journal* published an op-ed ripping my dad, entitled "Downhill All the Way." I was so livid that I drove over to the office of the *Journal*—which was, of course, the main publication I relied upon to cover my own political career. This was long before cell phones, so I went to the pay phone outside the *ProJo* building, called the editor, and started screaming and swearing at him. I dared him to come down and meet me on the street.

He very calmly said that if I had a problem with anything he had written, I was welcome to submit a letter to the editor.

I kept on screaming at him, yelling that he was scared I would beat him up. It started out as just totally mad blind rage, but soon I realized I was trembling, I was crying, *weeping* into the pay phone. I felt every cell of my body was in turmoil. This was about so much more than anger over an op-ed—it was the first time I really got in touch with what, in recovery, we say is that shame we carry within us. And I had never felt so *exposed* before. I didn't really have my own identity yet and I felt terrorized by not being able to separate from my parents' identities, as they were being so harshly criticized. My core of shame was being uncovered for the first time and I was melting down. And I was doing it on the phone with the editor of the *Journal*, the most important journalist in the world to me.

And that day, the editor of the *Journal* did the kindest thing:

nothing. He pretended none of this had ever happened. He never re-ported on the incident.

Sometimes it is what we *don't* do that changes people's lives.

I WAS, UNTIL PALM BEACH, a pretty low-profile politician—a member of the part-time General Assembly in the country's smallest state. After Palm Beach happened, there was press everywhere cover-ing almost anything that could have the word "Kennedy" in it.

Just days before I was scheduled to graduate from Providence in May, I was approached while entering the State House by reporters wanting comment on my mother—who had been arrested outside of Boston on a DUI. I had been planning a cookout for my constituents on my actual graduation day but then decided to cancel that because of the media attention. My parents attended the graduation, and that day went pretty well (until the Associated Press incorrectly reported I graduated with honors, and then issued a correction with the headline "Patrick Graduates, but NOT with Honors").

Over the next weeks, there was a national debate over whether or not my father was "an alcoholic" or if he "had a drinking problem." The debate included comments from many of his prominent Senate colleagues, most notably his best Republican friend, Senator Orrin Hatch, who admitted on the record that he had told my father he needed to stop drinking. My dad responded by repeatedly denying he had a problem.

On May 30, my mother pleaded guilty in Quincy to drunk driv-ing, after turning in her license for the third time. She immediately went to court-ordered rehab.

While this was all very public, my brother made a private decision. Just weeks after getting his master's at Yale, Teddy decided he would sign himself into the Institute of Living in Hartford for a three-week rehab. He and I were together with my dad at the Cape the weekend he told us. It was a huge blow to my dad. With me, Dad was kind of accepting—he seemed to associate my vulnerabilities with my mother. But with my brother, Teddy—well, Teddy was his namesake. He thought that would reflect on him. He was *not* happy.

I remember my father pulling me aside to discuss this. "Can you believe your brother?" he asked. "Does he really need to do that? Does he really think he's an alcoholic?" I remember that conversation like it was yesterday. I remember it mostly because I felt, for the first time, that, thank God, I was no longer alone with this stuff among my siblings.

So Teddy went to rehab. And when he came back, he was a pretty gung ho twelve-step guy. He even told the press he had received inpatient treatment. So my dad was forced to publicly confront this and comment.

"I'm very proud of the decision he has made," he told the *Globe*. "I hope everyone will respect it."

But Dad refused to budge on the issue of his own drinking. As the Senate reconvened in the fall, this was no longer just a Kennedy sobriety issue—some believed it was actually affecting public policy. That fall just happened to be when the Supreme Court nomination of Clarence Thomas was being debated—a nomination that my father and other Democrats completely opposed. It was, in fact, one of my father's staffers on the Senate Labor Committee, which he chaired, who had tracked down Thomas's former employee Anita Hill. But my father kept a low profile during most of the Judiciary Committee hearings, and when he did speak up in the Senate some of his longtime colleagues—including Arlen Specter and Orrin Hatch—called him out, suggesting he was hardly one to be accusing another of bad behavior. In what many then—and even more today—consider to have been one of the most unfortunate Supreme Court appointments in

American history, Thomas was approved in the Senate on October 15, 1991, by a vote of fifty-two to forty-eight. When the televised Thomas hearings were finished, my father's poll ratings had plummeted to the point where his reelection the next year was suddenly in question.

ALMOST TWO WEEKS AFTER the Thomas approval vote, the Institute of Politics at the Kennedy School at Harvard was celebrating its twenty-fifth anniversary in a two-day event. Dad was giving the opening address on Friday afternoon, and I was coming up the next morning to sit on a panel about young politicians. The evening before Dad's talk, word circulated that he would be delivering what the *Globe* called a "mystery speech." His office would not release an advance text.

I couldn't be there, but I was hopeful. After all, in the past six months both my older brother and my mother had very publicly faced their struggles with alcoholism, gone to rehab, and made a commitment to sobriety. For my father to follow them would have been not only the right thing to do personally but, honestly, the right thing to do politically as well.

But Dad just couldn't do it.

The best he could do was to acknowledge "the disappointment of my friends and many others who rely on me to fight the good fight" and to then admit, "I recognize my own shortcomings—the faults in the conduct of my private life. I realize that I alone am responsible for them, and I am the one who must confront them."

Many people thought this was his great mea culpa. To me, the speech reinforced the denial I had lived with most of my life.

I do understand that, for my father, it was earth-shattering that he would even remotely acknowledge any of this. And as I get older and further on in my own recovery, I feel a little more sympathetic because mostly this was a demonstration of how powerless we all are against addiction. In recovery we talk about a "moment of clarity" when we have reached a point of pitiful and incomprehensible demoralization. But other people can't force you into a moment of clarity, and they don't get to vote on when you should have one. You have to find it yourself.

My dad was the most resilient persevering human being that I have ever known. He had problems, and sure, some people would characterize him as an alcoholic. But, ultimately, it only mattered if he came to that realization himself. He managed his life in a way that was full of turmoil, but he always managed to survive, which reinforced his sense that this was manageable. His gifts of resiliency and strength were something I envied and for a long time wished I had. But, frankly, as I think about it these days, I am very glad I don't have those traits. I am glad to have a fuller realization of my powerlessness. What I once would have looked upon as weakness I now see as the key to empowerment.

But, at the time, my siblings and I were stuck. We had to decide: would we be true to ourselves or true to the family code of silence?

This is the struggle for all children growing up with the family disease of alcoholism. That is why many in recovery also attend some meetings of Al-Anon, the group for spouses, siblings, and friends of problem drinkers, which was founded by the wife of an AA member in 1951 and added a group for younger people, Alateen, in 1957. Some prefer meetings of ACOA, the Adult Children of Alcoholics organization, founded in 1978 by a group of twentysomething New Yorkers who had aged out of their Alateen group. ACOA focuses more on the challenges of our adult lives—providing twelve-step support with our struggles over the foundational emotional causes of our own insecurities—where Al-Anon is more about helping to cope with someone in your life engaged in active alcohol dependence. I am fortunate to have been helped by both groups.

IN EARLY DECEMBER OF 1991, my cousin went on trial for sexual assault in Palm Beach, in one of the first court proceedings ever covered live on national TV. My father and I both testified on Friday, December 6, and after my forty minutes on the stand—for which I had been excessively and expensively prepared—it would have been great if my involvement was almost at an end when he was acquitted.

Unfortunately, by then, the *National Enquirer* was covering me too. A guy I had briefly been in rehab with, back in 1986, sold his story of my treatment for cocaine addiction to the paper. The issue came out just as the trial was winding down. I prepared a statement and a letter to my constituents that we planned to release before the issue—in fact, the day after I testified in Florida. But my dad's large staff of political advisers convinced my extremely small staff this was a bad idea. The letter and statement instead came out just after the magazine. In both, I admitted to going to Spofford Hall and noted that "as a teenager I had started down the wrong path in dealing with the pressures of growing up. I mistakenly believed that experimenting with drugs and alcohol would alleviate them. I finally decided not to escape from those pressures but to confront them." I explained, "I have taken no drugs whatsoever since then" (true), and said, "I use alcohol only in moderation" (not exactly true, but since most of my binge drinking was alone, at night, to get to sleep, probably defensible).

While I was hopeful this letter and statement would find some sympathy with the voters in my college town, I was mostly concerned about the reaction of just one man. And it wasn't my father.

Frank Di Paolo, the godfather of Providence politics, was by then in his eighties and had become a complete surrogate political father to me. He had retired from running the Castle Spa, but he still cooked for me whenever he could. When I was in Providence, I always came to his house for Sunday dinner—usually homemade *pasta e fagioli*.

When I found out he had seen the *National Enquirer*, I was horrified. He was really old-school, just a gentleman of every sort. So I went to his house in the morning, and he was in the kitchen, at the stove, stirring the *pasta e fagioli* for dinner, stirring and stirring; he didn't turn around. I was thinking, *This is so awful*, and I knew that if he divorced me I could be through in local politics.

Finally he turned around.

"Son," he said, "I saw that story." And then he paused for a second. "That rat," he said, "that *rat*!"

At first I wasn't sure what he was talking about—was I the rat who had betrayed his trust, or was he talking about the guy who sold out to the *Enquirer*?

"That RAT!" he yelled. And then he turned his head and whispered, "You want me to do something about this?"

No, no, buddy, I said, that's all right. I love you and I'm just sorry for having let you down.

"You don't need to listen to those *gagoots* [idiots]!" he said. And then that was it. "What do you want to eat?"

He made me breakfast. Big thick slices of ham off the bone, an omelet big enough to feed a family of five. He smothered Italian toast with butter and put a big jar of grape jelly in front of me. I was in heaven. I couldn't get up for hours. By the time I did, I knew he and I could make this all right with the voters.

BUT THERE WAS still my dad to deal with—not about my scandal, but his. My siblings and I felt very strongly that Dad needed to do a lot better than the "shortcomings" speech. He needed to actually stop drinking for the first time since we had known him. This no longer felt like a private family issue—there were pundits writing about it in the paper every day, some of them his greatest admirers. It was like some kind of national intervention that he refused to attend.

This was also the time when my father started seriously dating Victoria Reggie, the Washington lawyer he would later marry. I acknowledge that the prospect of my dad's getting involved with someone did affect me—divorce and the potential for remarriage never stop being weird for the kids. But my main concern was that he take better care of his health.

Several weeks after the end of the Palm Beach trial, my dad was told that my siblings and I wanted to speak to him privately, in his study at the house in McLean. He had no way of knowing that we were planning a surprise intervention. I had been scribbling down notes wherever I was to get myself prepared for this—some of them on envelopes from my personal stationery, others on lined notebook pages or index cards—because, honestly, I was scared to death to actually confront my father.

At the last minute I wrote myself a little pep talk. Because my voice tended to rise and shake when I got nervous, I had been through thousands of dollars in presentation prep and vocal training for the Palm Beach trial. So I still had that high-priced advice in my head.

"Be firm," I wrote to myself. "No anger. No shrill voice. Not demanding. Keep to same point."

When the time came, we went back to Dad's private den, which had big comfortable couches; books everywhere; windows overlooking the Potomac; a high ceiling with an original harpoon from whaling days hanging from it; a scrimshaw coffee table made from planks from the USS *Massachusetts*; and a fireplace with a picture of my grandfather above it. It also had these big pocket doors, and I can still remember him sliding them shut behind us, so nobody else in the house would hear our conversation. He sat down in his favorite big, blue suede chair, and he was exactly in his comfort zone. And then we started talking.

Looking back, what we were saying was a pretty modest, watered-down intervention, nothing compared to what you could see today on A&E's *Intervention* any week. It was so anemic I'm not sure it even qualified as an intervention. We had our heads between our knees, almost, saying, "Dad, we're concerned, we're worried about you, and we think you're drinking too much."

And then we all cried.

He took it the exact opposite way we had hoped. What he heard was that we were abandoning him when he felt most vulnerable to the world and the judgments being made about him and his fitness as a father, as a senator, and as a man. He thought we were taking sides against him, siding with all "those people," the ones who didn't understand how difficult his life was and all that he had to shoulder and bear. We suddenly became part of the chorus of criticism that isolated him and made his life harder.

He was silent for a long time. He just looked at us and didn't say anything. Then he started talking briefly. "I've been seeing a priest," he said, "but you wouldn't know that. If you had bothered to *ask* me rather than just *accusing* me, you would have known I'm trying to get help."

So we were sitting there waiting for Dad to say something else to us. And suddenly he got up, slid open the pocket doors, and walked out of the room. That was it.

That was Monday, December 30. When I didn't hear back from him, I immediately sent him a follow-up note, reiterating the need for him to stop drinking. Then on New Year's Day, he sent me a six-page handwritten letter.

He began by explaining that it had been a difficult letter to write but that he wanted me to know that "I get the message, the point has been made." Then he pretty much proceeded to demonstrate that he hadn't received the message at all. He complained that we'd ambushed him, leaving him "no time to think what I might be able or willing to do—No just the hard fast pitch." He complained that we hadn't bothered to talk to the priest he was consulting or the doctor he claimed to have seen twice.

We had mentioned in the meeting that we thought his drinking was driving our family apart. He thought "the talk about the family was particularly disingenuous," saying, "What in heaven's sake does anyone think has been on my mind day and night, in restless dreams and sleepless nights—My God, Our family—my sisters and the cousins and the brutality of treatment to John and Bobby and I wonder how much I am to blame for all of this and I have to listen to 'What is happening to our family' from someone who rarely returned a phone call last fall and demonstrated little outreach during the most painful time."

He went on to say that he assumed from what we all said that we would not be staying with him for a while. So, he suggested that if I was in DC, I would stay with Kara, and at the Cape I would stay with my mother.

"That probably is a good idea for a while," he wrote. "Hopefully we can keep this in the family."

He explained that he would continue to "do anything for you politically just as before."

He ended this way: "This letter sounds like it's written in bitterness. It isn't. It's written with great disappointment and enormous sadness and I thought 1991 was over. Love, Dad."

Over the next weeks there was a lot of correspondence with my father. For every letter I sent there were dozens of handwritten drafts and false starts. But I was trying to be firm on one issue—he had to stop drinking and get help.

This was especially dramatic because Dad's sixtieth birthday was coming up at the end of February and his birthday parties were always particularly well lubricated. In early February, he sent me a note on Senate Armed Services Committee stationery, asking if I would come to his weekend of birthday celebrations and letting me know that Kara had agreed to attend and help. The letter ended, "I hope you are doing well, I miss you. Love, Dad."

I told him I wouldn't attend the parties unless he agreed to stop drinking. When he wouldn't agree to get treatment, I didn't go to any of his sixtieth-birthday parties.

No, 1991 wasn't going to be over for a long time.

Chapter 9

The Decade of the Brain started without me. This was hardly surprising at the time—I wasn't at all public about my own mental healthcare, and it wasn't a major issue yet for me politically. But when I later got deeply involved in mental health parity, it was clear that a lot of people I was working with had been doing this for a long time. And the Decade of the Brain—proclaimed by President George H. W. Bush but largely unfolding during the Clinton White House—was their shared reference point. It was when the worlds of mental health politics, economics, science, advocacy, and patienthood that we still live in today came of age; it was when the anger and outrage of medical discrimination against mental illness and addiction was first crystallized.

The Decade of the Brain had been declared in mid-1989, and in theory, the timing couldn't have been better. The idea was to do what we are still trying to do today—force the federal agencies and powerful institutions and clinicians and companies that focus on neurological illness and psychiatric illness to work together more and admit they are all dealing with the same brain. Unfortunately, the effort got off to a rocky start, because President Bush and Congress didn't attach any real increase in funding to it. When President Nixon declared his "War on Cancer" in 1971, it came with a $1.5 billion increase in funding over three years. (In 1990 dollars, a similar investment would have been around $5 billion; in today's dollars it would have been around $7 billion—which puts the recent $100 million–per–year funding of President Obama's new BRAIN Initiative into perspective.) So the Decade of the Brain wasn't even an underfunded mandate—there was really no mandate at all.

In fact, when the Decade of the Brain was proclaimed, the *New York Times* compared it not to the War on Cancer but to "National Prune Day, Tap Dance Day . . . [and] Dairy Goat Awareness Week" and asked whether it was time for Congress to stop commemorating and proclaiming so many things. So it was no surprise that when the National Institute of Mental Health (NIMH) and the National Institute of Neurological Disorders and Stroke (NINDS) met to create a strategic plan for the decade, they couldn't even agree on a way of working together.

One of the first big political moves of the Decade of the Brain involved bringing the medicine and science of mental health and addiction back under the umbrella of the National Institutes of Health (NIH), so it would hopefully be taken more seriously and funded more aggressively. This decision had been debated for many years—not only in terms of bringing the NIMH back to NIH, but whether or not the National Institute on Drug Abuse (NIDA) and the National Institute on Alcohol Abuse and Alcoholism (NIAAA) should become part of the NIH separately, or together as one addiction institute, or not at all. While these were political decisions, they had huge implications for how these diseases were viewed by the government and the public.

Finally, in 1992, the government broke up the nearly twenty-year-old Alcohol, Drug Abuse, and Mental Health Administration (ADAMHA)—which had, under one roof, all the "hard science" research into causes, treatments, cures, and preventions, as well as "softer" behavioral and social science research, training, and public education. NIMH, NIDA, and NIAAA went to NIH. (By the way, I share your utter disbelief that the world needs this many acronyms, but this is how we talk in government.) But since NIH only funded hard science, all the behavioral and social science, training, and education had to be moved to a new agency with a new acronym: the Substance Abuse and Mental Health Services Administration (SAMHSA, which we call "Sam-sa"—the H is silent). Yet with all this political and acronymic maneuvering there was, initially, no significant increase in government funding for brain disease research and treatment.

Still, there was enormous hope that all the people who would benefit from a real Decade of the Brain might be able to *will* it into being, even without additional government support. And, in many ways, they did. Luckily, the Decade of the Brain came at a moment of real hope in the treatment of mental illness: two of the breakthrough medications of the twentieth century had recently been approved.

Most Americans recall this as the time when everyone they knew started talking about the new drug Prozac, and the possibilities of an intriguing and controversial new class of widely used antidepressants. But people with family members suffering from intractable mental illness—especially schizophrenia and schizoaffective disorders—remember this as the moment when clozapine arrived. Marketed under the brand name Clozaril, it was the first "atypical antipsychotic" medication, able to cause an almost *Awakenings*-type response in many patients, making their visual, aural, olfactory, and other hallucinations either disappear or recede to the point where the patient could more easily understand they weren't real. (In mental healthcare, completely getting rid of symptoms is often not possible—the best we can hope for is medication and supportive therapy that allow those with the illnesses to have "insight" into their illness processes and see symptoms as nothing more than symptoms. So, as for the late mathematician John Nash in *A Beautiful Mind*, the hallucinations are still there but no longer controlling our actions; similarly, patients with "suicidal ideation" can understand that this is a medical symptom and not what it sometimes feels like, an existential call to self-destruction.)

On July 6, 1992, *Time* magazine ran a cover story about the clozapine revolution, with a picture of Brandon Fitch—a teenager with schizophrenia whose life had been turned around by the medication—attending his senior prom, rather than being in a psychiatric facility. Unfortunately, clozapine was extremely expensive and required regular blood testing because of an extremely rare but potentially dangerous side effect—so it was not being used by those who needed it the most, those already in state care or living at home and disabled.

The politics of both clozapine and Prozac soon came onto my radar. In the Rhode Island legislature, most bills having to do with mental illness were sponsored by Democratic Senator Rhoda Perry, who had family experience with these issues. In the 1993 session, she was trying to organize support for a bill concerning a relatively new concept, which was referred to as "insurance parity"—a very early version of what we now call "mental health parity." The bill was meant to address the disparate coverage limitations for mental illness and the absurdly low lifetime caps on care—which had existed for years but were made worse by the high cost of new brand-name psychiatric meds.

At that time, nobody even considered the possibility that all mental illnesses could be covered equally with other medical conditions. The best they could hope for was that the very sickest patients, who were hospitalized or disabled, might get better or closer-to-equal coverage—and, in this case, that this new drug clozapine, which was the equivalent of the first "chemotherapy" for schizophrenia, would be covered. While it was a national issue, healthcare is generally delivered at the state level, so each state had to pass its own form of "insurance parity," overseen by its own state insurance commissioner and attorney general.

Rhoda was sponsoring this legislation at the insistence of the local affiliate of an advocacy group that was starting to get traction nationwide: NAMI, which was then the National Alliance for the Mentally Ill and is now the National Alliance on Mental Illness. It was an organization mostly made up of family members of people with schizophrenia, many of whom were disabled, in and out of hospitals, homeless shelters, and jails. It had grown in ambition under the leadership of dynamo executive director Laurie Flynn and with the scientific encouragement of in-your-face schizophrenia researcher Dr. E. Fuller Torrey (who also donated the hardcover profits from his important early book *Surviving Schizophrenia* to NAMI). But much of NAMI's muscle in Washington came from its powerful ally in the US Senate: conservative New Mexico Republican Pete Domenici, who, along with his wife, Nancy, had struggled with the psychotic illness of their daughter Clare and treasured the support of fellow families in the same situation.

The local director of Rhode Island's AMI was a former schoolteacher named Bill Emmet, whose brother had schizophrenia and who, over the years, especially after their parents died, had gone from volunteering in this grassroots group to working for it full-time. Once Bill had Rhoda on board, he was looking for someone in the State House to sponsor the bill and was recommended to a newly elected young House member named Gordon Fox. It just so happened that Gordon Fox sat next to me in the State House. And that's why Bill Emmet decided that, while he was there lobbying Gordon, he would introduce himself to me and give me his pitch on "insurance parity."

It never occurred to me that one day I would be devoting my life to this cause. (Or that, twenty years later, I would hire Bill as the executive director of my parity initiative.)

Not long after, in June of 1993, my psychiatrist, Peter Kramer, published *Listening to Prozac*. I don't remember thinking at the time that this was going to be any huge deal. He had published an earlier book about psychotherapy, in 1989, which made no apparent impact on his life or our work together.

Peter had still never tried Prozac with me. Although he had previously tried me on imipramine, our therapy, then in its fourth year, was more focused on helping me with impulse control—to recognize and understand the consequences of trying to act on every feeling I had.

He was also focused on helping me develop a stronger and stronger sense of myself separate from my parents, and a sense of trust in other people. He saw me the way I would only much later see myself, as someone who never had a real sense of a safe, normal home. He always remembered the day I came into therapy and sang the song from *My Fair Lady* that I was going to perform for my singing and public speaking class at Providence—the one that begins, "All I want is a room somewhere . . ."

Dr. Kramer had helped me through college, and helped me through 1991 and the challenging period that followed. Just after my father turned sixty, he and Vicki announced their engagement and were soon married in a civil ceremony. Vicki moved into the McLean house with her two children from her first marriage: Curran and his younger sister, Caroline.

Over the next couple years, my mother grew increasingly ill—her longest period of sobriety now behind her—and by 1993 we were discussing some more drastic changes in her care, thinking that perhaps it was time for Don Juhl to move in with her for a while. For the first time, however, these conversations about her care were mostly between my mother, my siblings, and me. My dad was more of an outsider—except for his waning financial responsibility, he had moved on. He re-engaged in the discussion in part because it got mixed together with a more private conversation between my parents: my father hoped my mother would agree to an annulment so he and Vicki could get married in the Catholic Church.

As part of the discussions about my mother's health and the possible annulment, Mom came to understand that her divorce settlement might not be sufficient to cover her living and healthcare expenses. So she asked to revisit her ten-year-old divorce settlement, to make sure her care would never be a financial burder to my brother, sister, and me.

She had a pretty good idea of the possible expense of the care she was going to need for her alcoholism and depression, and the challenges she might have financially now that my dad was remarried. Ironically, she was facing some of the same issues of insurance discrimination and lifetime caps on care as a middle-class patient with schizophrenia. And as she became older, my siblings and I were just starting to realize we could be faced with the same kinds of issues concerning possible court-ordered care if she could not take care of herself. This was all, of course, a lot to sort out, especially since my relationship with my dad remained pretty frosty.

IN MARCH OF 1993, I moved to a new house—not far from where I had been living in Providence, but far enough that I became a resident of the First Congressional District, where some felt there was a vulnerable seat in the US Congress. I was making plans to test the waters for a move to DC after the 1994 midterm election.

On top of all this, in the summer of 1993, my laid-back therapist on a quiet street in Providence, Rhode Island, became an overnight bestselling author at the center of an incredibly harsh debate about the past and future of mental healthcare. While the press coverage of his book would suggest that it was a sales pitch for everyone to try Prozac and the new class of antidepressants, SSRIs, in fact the questions it

raised were much more complicated. In many ways, we're still struggling with them today. The book was written very much from the perspective of a lifelong psychodynamic psychotherapist who was actually
shocked at how well Prozac worked and who was wrestling with its
implications for his colleagues. The book was the first place where
many Americans heard the term Kramer had coined, "cosmetic psychopharmacology," and heard him ponder whether Prozac made some
people "better than well"—suggesting the drugs would be used not
just to treat illness but to enhance the performance of well people.

I'm sure these were interesting ideas for him to consider among his
fellow mental health professionals. And he had already been writing
about these ideas for a couple years in his *Psychiatric Times* columns,
using the same phrases, including "listening to Prozac." But by the
time the book came out there was already a small backlash against the
new antidepressant, which Kramer unwittingly helped fuel, as his
musings helped confirm the worst fears of a growing group of "antipsychiatry" advocates. Some of them came to their anger with mental
healthcare fairly, after experiences of their own or by family members
in overcrowded, underfunded state hospitals in the sixties, seventies,
and eighties. Others were followers of a small group of intellectuals
from the sixties, led by repentant psychiatrist Thomas Szasz, who
wrote a provocative book called *The Myth of Mental Illness.* Szasz's
work was then hijacked by the virulently antipsychiatry Church of
Scientology, which believed that mental illness didn't exist and all
treatments for it were a moneymaking scam. When Prozac turned out
to have side effects—like every other medication—they considered this
part of the "conspiracy."

Prozac helped an enormous number of people, not because it turned
out to be so much more effective than earlier antidepressants, but because it was much easier to take, and many more people who needed it
were willing to take it and remain on it. In every generation, this is still

the primary challenge of mental illness and addiction care. We desperately want new treatments and greater understanding of the processes of the brain. But we also know that the biggest struggle is convincing those who are ill to try any treatment at all, then get them on the right treatment (which can be a frustrating process of elimination), and then *keep* them on the right treatment—especially after they get some relief and start to think maybe they don't need treatment anymore. (This is also the same cycle we go through in recovery with sobriety.) The Prozac boom—which ultimately Peter's book did not create so much as it rode the crest of an already-formed wave—was a turning point in increasing the number of sick people willing to get treatment.

Did some take the pill who didn't need it? Of course. That's true for every popular new medication—especially since the 1990s, when the FDA began loosening restrictions on direct-to-consumer advertising of pharmaceuticals. And, in mental health, there was an additional change: after Prozac, primary care doctors started writing more and more prescriptions for psychoactive medications without having their patients consult mental health professionals. (From 1987 to 1997, the percentage of patients who got psychiatric meds from primary care docs doubled to nearly 75 percent; today nearly 80 percent of all antidepressants are prescribed by general practitioners, in most cases without making a psychiatric diagnosis.)

All these changes led to many patients being treated without much monitoring and with no psychotherapy—until something went terribly wrong—and it created a great deal of friction between the American Medical Association and the American Psychiatric Association, which they are still trying to work through today. Then the American Psychological Association added to the friction by lobbying—so far unsuccessfully—for their non-MD members to be able to write prescriptions for psychiatric drugs. (The hope for the future is a more collaborative care model that is patient centered and not controlled by one caregiver; since there aren't anywhere near enough mental health professionals, with or without MDs, to go around.)

Peter's book hit the *New York Times* bestseller list on July 18, 1993, and his life and practice were suddenly under a lot of media scrutiny. This spooked me, because I was already under a lot of local scrutiny myself, due to my likely candidacy for the US House of Representatives. During all the years I had gone to Peter for psychotherapy, I never actually parked in the small lot behind his office—I always left my car about ten blocks away and walked the rest of the way, so there was less chance someone would notice I was seeing a psychiatrist. But, that summer, people started asking me why they saw my car parked on the east side of Providence—that is, really, how small a state Rhode Island is. So I decided this would be a good time for us to stop our psychotherapy, and he agreed.

I was, as far as I could tell at the time, doing pretty well. In retrospect, however, I was trying to re-create my insides by re-creating my outside—getting my life validated on the surface while minimizing the confusion of my inner life. I was trying to create the image that I didn't have any problems and decided that if I didn't drink in public or use illegal drugs, that meant I was okay. But the whole time I was seeing Peter, I would binge-drink every couple of weeks—I would basically set aside a couple days for myself where it was safe to let it all go. And I certainly fought depression and had my hypomanic moments. But it was a way of life that I was able to maintain for a long while.

BY THIS TIME, the battle over the Clinton Health Security Act was in full swing. While this was all happening primarily at the federal level, I do remember visiting with Ira Magaziner—the Rhode Island–based national business consultant leading the healthcare charge with Hillary Clinton—as well as speaking on the floor of the Rhode Island

General Assembly to memorialize our support for the US Congress to pass healthcare reform.

My dad had been proposing bills for national health insurance since the early 1970s—it was his legislative holy grail. The Clinton Health Security Act began as a process to legislate full national health insurance during the temporary alignment of a Democratic White House with Democratic majorities in the Senate and House. But the initiative quickly got caught up in a lot of political issues, some policy, some process, some naïveté, some nothing more than attacks on Hillary and her leading role. The Clinton plan was incredibly ambitious and had a lot of moving parts—which later became a lot of moving targets.

When it came to mental illness and addiction, the Clinton Health Security Act had two basic steps that would unfold over eight years. It would begin with an immediate shift to very basic mental health and addiction coverage for all Americans (because more ambitious, comprehensive reform right away, according to their white paper, "could lead to chaos"). And then by 2001—when the Clintons expected to be leaving office—there would be full mental health and substance use disorder parity, no separate facilities for their treatment (because, by then, they would have been fully integrated into the rest of the healthcare system), and no prejudice against preexisting conditions or lifetime treatment limits.

It was a Decade of the Brain dream come true—as long as they could complete and pass the bill before the midterm election in 1994.

IN THE FALL OF 1993, my brother was getting married. His fiancée, Kiki Gershman, was a smart young psychiatrist at Yale and an assistant professor in the medical school. Teddy was in law school at UConn at the time, and was also working as director of a project to make homes safe from lead paint, a partnership between New Haven and

Yale medical school. Just before their mid-October wedding, he was interviewed about his relationship with Kiki by the *Boston Globe*. When they asked him about his past treatment for alcoholism, he was even more open about it than before.

"In my family and among my friends, I've seen what can happen when people don't address the problem," he told the paper. "I realized that nothing else could be right when that part was wrong. I'm glad I did it. It's been two and a half years since I've had a drink, and it was a great break. It agrees with me."

The wedding was on Block Island, Rhode Island. I was best man, Kara was one of the two bridesmaids, and Vicki's two children, Caroline and Curran, were the ring bearers. Among Teddy's ushers was his college roommate from Wesleyan, Akiva Goldsman, who was just starting to break through as a Hollywood screenplay writer; his adaptation of John Grisham's *The Client* was currently filming. The son of two mental health professionals in New York, he was also starting to look for a project that might allow him to dramatize the challenges of mental illness. Several years later, he would be hired by producer Brian Grazer to write the Oscar-winning screenplay for *A Beautiful Mind*.

NOT LONG AFTER THE WEDDING, my dad held a fund-raiser for my campaign for the US Congress at his house in McLean. Things weren't great between us, but this was work.

The truth was, he had done me a favor by pushing me away. The distance between us gave me some of the independence I needed to begin to construct my own life, my own narrative. I had made the decision to run for Congress myself: I didn't need his permission and I had never really sat down and talked to him about running, or even acknowledged I might need his blessing or support. Nobody else knew this, of course. But then, nobody knew my father and I were barely speaking at this point either. I would imagine that a number of the folks who signed on to support my candidacy just assumed I was coordinating with my dad and his office. Neither of us did anything to dissuade anyone's assumption that my father must have been enthusiastically behind me. Again, this was work.

Dick Gephardt, the Missouri Democrat who was then House Majority Leader, had held the first major fund-raiser for me in Washington several months before, and of course Dad was there—he had to show up; his son was running for Congress. Clearly, at some level, he had to have been proud of me. We just didn't give the press, or our supporters, any inkling of what was really going on between us.

But at this fall fund-raiser at the McLean house, there was one tiny inkling, a moment that, in retrospect, captures something of the friction. It was mentioned in pretty much every story about the event as a funny, benign, father-son interlude. Although, that's not exactly the way I remember it.

When I had first run for the Rhode Island General Assembly back in 1988, I had done a disastrous call-in radio appearance, in which I mistakenly described a VA hospital as being in the district I was running to represent—when it was just across the street that delineated the border for the next district. This geographical gaffe ignited a string of callers accusing me of being a carpetbagger who didn't even know the streets of the district and questioning how I could possibly represent its citizens.

At this party at my dad's, Rhode Island political leader Jack Reed—then a Congressman, now a US Senator—spoke nostalgically about the district I was running to represent in the House, saying it was dear to his heart and even noting that his grandmother had lived there. Her house, he said, was on Wisdom Avenue.

My dad couldn't resist a dig.

"D'ya know where that is, Patrick?"

Perhaps a little too anxiously, I started describing where Wisdom Avenue and every other nearby avenue and street were located. This got a laugh. But it wasn't that funny. It meant that some of the first national political stories about me would reprise an embarrassing anecdote that most people, otherwise, never would have known.

That said, at $500 a person, we raised $100,000 to start the campaign. That's what some people spent for their entire congressional races.

My young campaign staff was being run by longtime aide Tony Marcella, who was just a few years older than me. He had started in politics in Massachusetts as a staffer for the speaker of the State House and then as my dad's driver for his 1988 Senate campaign. Tony had come to Rhode Island as a volunteer on my first state rep run and now had worked his way up to being my most trusted employee.

I hired David Axelrod, a former Chicago political writer, as my media adviser. And I needed him, because while we led in the beginning, as 1994 progressed the races tightened. I also relied heavily on help from political supporters in Rhode Island, especially the new Majority Leader of the Rhode Island house, my longtime colleague George Caruolo. This was a midterm election after the Clintons had been in office for two years. The Democrat-controlled House and Senate had sputtered—the healthcare reform bill was stalled and would have to be tried again the next term—and the Republicans were gaining momentum. This was particularly bad for my father, who was in his first race since Palm Beach, facing Republican entrepreneur Mitt Romney. So it was, really, the first race of his career that it seemed possible he could lose.

WHILE I WAS POLLING AHEAD of my opponent, I was also starting to see for myself what it might be like to be a Kennedy in national office. During that campaign, I got my first really serious death threats.

I had experienced threats before. When I first ran for office, while still in college, the state police had heard about a threat and put a full protective detail on me. It only lasted ten days, because they caught the guy. Then, in 1989, when I was the primary sponsor of the state version of the Brady Bill, mandating a seven-day waiting period before purchasing firearms, there were more threats.

In the first week of my campaign for Congress, I received a call from Bill Barry, the ex–FBI agent who had been my Uncle Bobby's bodyguard and often helped with family security matters. He said that during recent FBI surveillance of a top Rhode Island official, someone had overheard discussion of a plan to undermine my candidacy by purposely crashing into my car when I was driving, and then to have cocaine planted in my car to be found at the accident scene. Bill told me it was time to stop driving myself anywhere and to hire a retired state trooper to drive me to campaign events.

All was quiet for much of the campaign, and then the last week, Bill Barry called me again. This time, he said there was a credible threat from a guy who said he was coming to Rhode Island to "get" me. He arranged for an extra security detail, and finally, the man who had made the threat was arrested—with a trunk full of guns. But, luckily, nothing else happened.

In the end, I was polling way ahead and went on to win by an eight-point margin. My father's race, on the other hand, remained tighter than he would have liked through the early fall. I remember him joking once on the phone about his poll numbers, saying, "If you get elected, make sure you don't forget me, I may need a job." Finally, in late October, he turned the corner with a smackdown performance against Mitt Romney at their debate at Faneuil Hall. After that, he was expected to win handily.

My family then had to decide where to be when the results came in—in Boston with my father or in Providence with me. Since they knew they couldn't be there for the results, Dad and Vicki drove down in the afternoon, after voting, to pre-congratulate me. But that night, Teddy and Kara and all the cousins were in Boston.

Only my mother came down to Providence to be onstage with me for my actual acceptance speech, and there was something kind of wonderful about that. I had grown up looking at pictures of Kennedy elections—for JFK, Bobby, and my father—where my mom was always a presence. She had been a go-to person for all those campaigns and all those election nights: strong and beautiful and committed. But that was a side of her I had never really seen in person, since for most of my life she had been defined by her illness. So to see her there, onstage with me as the historical figure she truly was but had never been to me, was a genuinely big deal. It was like having a flashback of a memory that wasn't actually real, like I was seeing myself in one of those family photos at my grandfather's house of the starts of all those political careers. It was a terrific way to begin my career as a national politician.

Besides my mother, I was flanked onstage by Senator Claiborne Pell, and we were surrounded by the people from Providence who had supported me since I was a twenty-year-old college-sophomore state rep, learning small-town, retail politics from people like Frank Di Paolo over *pasta e fagioli*. Now, at twenty-seven, I was going to be the youngest member of the United States Congress, representing the smallest state in the union.

But while my father and I were apart, we were both watching the same nightmare national TV coverage of the election. Republicans were capturing control of the House and Senate for the first time in over forty years. And I was about to join a Congress in which Newt Gingrich, who I considered at the time to be a right-wing bomb thrower, was going to be Speaker of the House. (Ironically, Newt and I became friends years later as he got more involved in brain research advocacy, but back then he was the ultimate political enemy.)

The only good news was that because the Democrats had lost a stunning fifty-four seats in the House—only two seats had gone from Republican to Democrat, and I was one of them—we had probably the smallest Democratic freshman class in the modern history of Congress. So we got a lot more attention than normal freshmen.

Newt announced his "Contract with America" and all the conservative legislation the Republicans were going to pass in the first hundred days—including a complete trashing of all the healthcare initiatives the Democrats had been working on for two years. The Health Security Act, which had stalled in Congress in the months before the election, was dead.

Clinton knew he had to double down on our base. So he quickly called a White House press conference to discuss raising the minimum wage. And he invited all the freshman Democrats to be there, along with the usual top leaders. I went down to the Cabinet Room as early as possible to get a good seat, right next to the President.

My dad, who was the chair of the Senate Labor Committee, arrived just before the meeting was about to start. Even after the election, I still hadn't really spoken to him very much. He walked in, saw me sitting there next to President Clinton, and said, "I can't believe this. How did *you* get in here?"

"Well, Dad," I said, grinning, "I actually got elected. I'm here as a Congressman."

And there wasn't even a beat. It was suddenly all behind us. Boom, we were simpatico. We were now . . . *colleagues*, not father and son— or, well, not *just* father and son. He was all right now. He had moved on. My dad was great about not holding a grudge. He had a strong temper but also a sense of life that was profound because he had seen so much of it—his big picture was really big.

But, also, he had won his election, and he had a sense of relief that he had closed that chapter of his life. Winning an election is like redemption.

Chapter 10

As the youngest member of Congress in 1995, I was doing my best to get acclimated and calm my nervousness. But it was a challenging time to grow up quickly in Washington, because the new Republican majority had given itself one hundred days to change everything—or at least to dismantle much of what Democrats like President Clinton and my father had been trying to build in the previous two years.

And eighteen days into those one hundred days, my grandmother Rose Kennedy died at the age of one hundred four. Gramma left forty-one great-grandchildren, myself and twenty-seven other grandchildren, and five of her own nine children—my father the youngest but, now more than ever, the patriarch.

So it did not feel like a good time for a brand-new Congressman to try to make a name for himself on big national issues, and I'm not sure I would have done that even if the Democrats were still in the majority. I felt very much like a local politician who had been sent to Washington to represent the needs of my district in Rhode Island, and that was the job I needed to learn how to do well first.

As the son of Ted Kennedy and the cousin of then-Congressman Joe Kennedy, I was immediately invited to appear at all the events—on evenings and weekends—where I could join them in networking on national issues. As the newest single Kennedy in Washington, there were also many more social pressures—and opportunities—than I was accustomed to. Nobody seemed to care that I had a serious girlfriend.

So, I decided that, as much as possible, I would keep my head down, focus on local issues, and spend my weekends back in Rhode Island, at home and with constituents. It was a political strategy but also a personal one. I felt safer and more in control in Providence than in Washington, and brought my Rhode Island campaign manager, Tony Marcella, with me as chief of staff. I also hired Terri Alford, the smart and maternal wife of a career naval officer, as my Washington receptionist; she went on to run my office and became an incredibly stabilizing figure in my life, working with me for my entire time in Congress.

When I lobbied for committee positions—which I did pretty hard, largely through my growing friendship with Dick Gephardt, who had just gone from House Majority Leader to House Minority Leader—I pushed not for traditional liberal Kennedy placements but a seat on the House Armed Services Committee. As I learned the ropes, I wanted to make sure I was in a position to protect jobs in Navy-related institutions and projects in my district: the Naval Undersea Warfare Center, the Naval War College, the Naval Surface Warfare Officers School Command, and the Naval Education/Training Center were all in the First Congressional District.

This was the beginning of my being seen as something of a hawk on defense issues. This notion was reinforced just a few months into my

first term, by a crystallizing trip I took to Fort Bragg in North Carolina for the thirty-year rededication of the John F. Kennedy Special
Warfare Center. That's where the US Army does training for Special
Forces (Green Beret/Special Ops), Civil Affairs and Psychological Operations, and where I first met my friend General Hugh Shelton, several years before he became Chairman of the Joint Chiefs of Staff.

What he told me that day, about Special Ops and mental health,
always stayed with me. He explained that Special Ops had the best
mental healthcare of any other branch of the service.

When I asked why, he said, "We don't look at mental healthcare as
a safety net. We look at it as a force multiplier."

ALL THE NEW STRESSES of being in a new job in a new place made
my bipolar disorder that much more challenging to manage and keep
secret. I had, by this time, also started overusing prescription painkillers. I had been introduced to them during and after my back surgery, and they seemed like the quickest and easiest way to stop feeling
pain and anxiety without technically breaking any laws or having alcohol on my breath. But mostly I drank, late at night, to get to sleep. I'd
do it at home, or at this bar, the Red River Grill, that was near my
apartment at Justice Court, walking distance to the Capitol.

Part of the challenge of these illnesses is that they can make you
feel anxious and unstable where there is no real external reason to feel
that way. But I had lots of reasons to feel stressed, if not completely
terrified.

The first time I rose to speak in the House, for example, I forgot
to request unanimous consent to extend my remarks—a violation of
parliamentary procedure—and then a veteran colleague had to tell
me to try looking into the camera when I spoke. Behind my back, but
not always out of earshot, my elders and detractors referred to me as

"Congressboy" rather than Congressman. The press called me "the un-Kennedy" and said that the "charisma gene had eluded" me.

My staff, some of whom had come with me from Providence, were still learning how to function in the nation's capital; when they weren't sure what to do, they would quietly call someone on my dad's veteran staff for advice. But while his staff was helpful, there were lessons my father wanted me to learn myself. I had run up a substantial debt campaigning, which I knew he could help me pay off by sponsoring a couple of big fund-raising events. While I now realize he was probably right to force me to figure out how to solve this problem, I recall being very angry with him about this at the time.

I was, in some ways, a very old twenty-seven, and in other ways a very young twenty-seven. This was, after all, my first true full-time job.

Still, even with my steep learning curve, it was a good time to be one of thirteen freshman Democrats in the House, when the conservative "Contract with America" made every vote for our party really count.

ONE OF THE MOST RESONANT experiences of that first year was the trip to Israel in November for the funeral of assassinated Israeli Prime Minister Yitzhak Rabin. I was part of the large US delegation, which included twenty-one other House members and my father and sixteen of his Senate colleagues.

Before we left, my dad and I made a visit to Arlington National Cemetery, to the graves of his brothers. Rabin's death felt, in so many ways, like the deaths of my uncles—not just the murder of an incredible human being but the attempted murder of a cause, uniquely led by this inspiring individual through the power of his own personal narrative. When he was taken, the dream was taken. My father decided it would be appropriate to carry dirt from Arlington to sprinkle on Rabin's grave. Because of his back problems, he couldn't really even bend over. So I knelt down and scooped up some earth from around JFK's gravesite and put it in a Ziploc sandwich bag we had brought. And then I walked down the path to Uncle Bobby's grave and did the same thing.

We sat together on the plane to Israel, on Air Force Two. It was the first time we had traveled together in a long time and since nobody else had family members with them, the trip also became a bit of a father-son bonding experience. It was actually a good thing I was there, because he had a hard time with the funeral. It was very crowded, and I think he just struggled with the painful symbolism of Rabin's assassination. All the other heads of state tossed dirt from the grave site onto the coffin, and we were waiting until the end, with our little Ziploc bag. And then at a certain point he was pushing me, saying, "Now, now, now, go put the dirt in."

I can still hear his voice saying it, "Now, now, now!" I think that dirt actually helped him emotionally navigate the situation; it gave him something else to focus on.

I was surprised by how difficult that funeral was for him. Growing up, I remember going with him to so many funerals, so many visits to the homes of families of the fallen. When someone dies, the Kennedys are seen as experts in how to deal with it. My dad gave so many eulogies, sat in so many living rooms, and walked through so many houses like he was a family member. I think the most powerful thing I witnessed as his son was the consolation he gave those who were suffering the unbearable loss of a young person—usually a son—who died serving our country. He had incredible empathy, because he always brought with him the experience of losing so many family members tragically, suddenly, and in their prime.

So I was not surprised when, after the funeral, many of Rabin's family members and friends wanted to talk to my father about how a family and country deal with assassination, how the legacy of a public figure can be maintained after his murder. It was unusual to be an expert on such trauma. Especially back then, when the impact of trauma was so little understood and appreciated.

It is amazing, actually, how the world of PTSD and trauma-based mental illness has changed over the last two decades. Today, because of the overwhelming evidence of how PTSD has hurt a generation of American veterans, the controversies concern mostly how to lower the PTSD-driven suicide rate and how best to treat this unique set of illnesses. When Rabin died, there was very little understanding of the role of trauma-based illnesses. And except for Vietnam veterans, many patients who suffered from post-traumatic illnesses had their traumas questioned, downplayed, or even denied; they were sometimes told it didn't matter if their traumas were real or imaginary, for the purposes of treatment, something we would never consider saying to someone traumatized in combat. I think, honestly, most Americans didn't really take PTSD very seriously until after 9/11, when the traumas and their impact were undeniable, and shared by so many.

THIS WAS A VERY DRAMATIC and fascinating time in the politics of mental health, and I wish I had felt more comfortable being as directly involved as I would have liked. While I quietly supported funding for various mental health causes and joined groups of cosponsors of some bills, I was afraid to try to lead—because someone might ask me what personal reason I had for making this a priority. I was mortified by the prospect that someone would find out I was getting any kind of psychiatric or psychological care, because I had successfully convinced the press that my time in rehab as a teen was a brief youthful indiscretion that was only made public by someone seeking money during the Palm Beach coverage.

My party line was that I had never used illegal drugs or abused alcohol since my high school visit to Spofford Hall. I just assumed nobody would notice if, every once in a while, I drank more than my share of shots at the Red River Grill and then called in to my office the next morning to postpone my first appointments.

I deferred to others, more established than me and more comfortable being "out" about their mental illnesses and addictions, who were creating a whole new national dialogue about mental illness. Bob Boorstin, the thirtysomething former *New York Times* political reporter turned consultant and speechwriter who was working with the Clintons on healthcare, was probably the youngest, most prominent person willing to come *way* out about his hospitalization for bipolar disorder and the challenge of managing a mental illness and a career. From his earliest days in the Clinton White House, he openly discussed his first manic-psychotic episode, in 1987, which took place while he was working on the Dukakis campaign. And he was a unique spokesman for the emotional politics of having a mental illness and the Washington politics of getting his care covered.

Boorstin was close friends with Dr. Kay Redfield Jamison, the prominent psychiatry professor at Johns Hopkins who had recently co-authored the authoritative textbook on my disease—which she still liked to refer to, old-school, as "manic-depressive illness." But only a handful of colleagues in mental health knew that she had struggled with the disease herself for years. In April of 1995, just months after I started in Congress, she stunned the medical and political worlds of Washington—where she and her husband, schizophrenia researcher Dr. Richard J. Wyatt, were well-known—by "coming out" to the *Washington Post Magazine* and announcing an upcoming "memoir of madness" called *An Unquiet Mind*. It became an overnight bestseller, showing just how many people were desperate to know more about mental illness and talk about the real world of its care.

Kay was involved with a mood disorders conference held annually at Hopkins—founded by her colleague Dr. Ray DePaulo and known in the District but not nationally—where several older, prominent people recently had come out, including *60 Minutes* correspondent Mike Wallace, Dick Cavett, and author William Styron. (The first public person to come out in a big way with bipolar disorder was actress Patty Duke, in her 1987 autobiography and in a bold 1992 book just about her experience with the illness.)

These brave people began coming out to help fight stigma, increase appropriations for the NIMH, and support the mental health provisions of the Clinton healthcare plan. But after the Republican revolution they were also trying to save the largely bipartisan gains of the previous years. I admired them and never imagined I would join them—I really didn't yet see what was wrong with me through the same medical prism they did. They were fighting—and possibly endangering their own privacy and careers—so that the public, and the business and political establishments, might one day see their symptoms as just one more medical problem that deserved to be covered and respected like cancer and diabetes.

I wasn't yet ready to take responsibility for my own illness, for my own health. When I look back at my journals during this time, I didn't really understand much about myself or what was wrong with me. So it was probably a good thing I wasn't anywhere near ready to be "out."

DURING MY FIRST YEAR in office, I kept a pretty low profile in Congress and, politically, tried to stay closer to the middle of the road than was my nature. I turned down pretty much all national media requests. When CNN asked me to be on a panel of legislators—including my father and Chris Dodd—talking about how liberals would deal with the new conservative majority, I turned it down; correspondent Candy

Crowley announced on the air that the reason I said no was because I wasn't a liberal.

Then one day in late March of 1996, I decided I had to stop being so cautious. We were in the middle of a debate about one of the more infamous bills during the Gingrich era, the Gun Crime Enforcement and Second Amendment Restoration Act of 1996, which, based on heavy lobbying by the NRA, proposed lifting the ban on many semi-automatic assault weapons and large-capacity ammunition-feeding devices that President Clinton had signed just two years earlier (and I had passed in the Rhode Island legislature). One of the active Republican cosponsors of the bill was Rules Committee chairman Gerald Solomon from the district around Lake Placid, New York. He was thirty-seven years my elder and none too happy when I asked for two minutes to address the bill and just *went off* on him.

I started a little shakily—describing the conservative logic of the bill as "just bogus."

Then I started building up a head of steam, yelling, "I cannot *believe* . . . you have the nerve to bring this bill up," especially since only a week earlier there had been a horrific school shooting incident, in which sixteen five-year-old students and their teacher had been murdered at the Dunblane Primary School in Scotland.

"Families like mine all across this country know all too well what damage weapons can do," I said. "And you want to *arm our people even more*? You want to add *more magazines* to the assault weapons so they can spray and kill even *more people*?

"Shame on you. What in the world are you *thinking* when you are opening up the debate on this issue? Mr. Speaker, this is nothing but a sham, to come on this floor and say you are going to have an open and fair debate about assault weapons. My God, all I have to say to you is, play with the devil, die with the devil.

"There are families out there, Mr. Speaker, and the gentleman will *never* know what it is like, because they do not have someone in their family killed. It is not the person who is killed, it is the whole family that is affected."

After I finished by loudly announcing that the assault weapons ban should stay in place, Solomon asked to speak. He said he had great respect for me and my family but added, "I am going to tell him [me] something: when he stands up and questions the integrity of those of us that have this bill on the floor, the gentleman ought to be a little more careful. And *let me tell you why!*"

As I began walking away from the microphone at the front of the chamber, I yelled, "Yeah, go ahead, tell me why."

And then he just started screaming, "My wife lives alone five days a week in a rural area in upstate New York! She has a right to defend herself when I am not there, son, and don't you ever forget it. *Don't . . . you . . . ever . . . forget . . . it!*"

As I walked away, a number of reporters heard Solomon dare me to "step outside" with him. It was the lead story on all three networks that night. And it was, in retrospect, the day I first found my voice as a Congressman, the day some of my colleagues started thinking, *Maybe there's a* there *there.*

While the media noted that I appeared to be invoking my own family's experience on the House floor, the truth was I was angered almost as much for my girlfriend, Kate Lowenstein, who had lost her father—well-known New York civil rights and antiwar activist Allard Lowenstein—to gun violence almost exactly sixteen years before, in March of 1980, when she was just nine years old. Al Lowenstein had been a close friend of my father and my uncles, and Dad had given one of his eulogies. He was buried near JFK and Bobby in Arlington (I put a stone on his gravestone the day we came to get the dirt for Rabin's funeral). Al was murdered in his New York office by Dennis Sweeney, a former protégé of his who was known to have been suffering from schizophrenia. Kate and her older brother had been active in making sure Sweeney was treated as mentally ill by the courts. They became early experts and advocates against the death penalty and for a more progressive version of the insanity plea.

More recently, Kate had found herself in a different situation, actively opposing unsupervised furloughs for her father's killer, fearing for her family's safety and the public's. But, regardless of the challenges of death penalty issues (which became her life's work at Murder Victims' Families for Human Rights) and the complex mental health issues, there was no room for ambiguity in her family's feelings about gun control. Or mine.

Chapter 11

Just a few weeks after my yelling match on the floor of the House, mental health parity got its first serious airing on the floor of the US Senate. It's not that the idea of such equality of coverage for mental illness had never come up before in Congress, but this was a political turning point for the idea—and for the phrase "mental health parity" itself. It came in the form of a last-minute amendment to a health insurance bill my father was trying to get passed, which eventually became the Health Insurance Portability and Accountability Act (and created the infamous HIPAA regulations that so aggressively restrict access to patient information).

As soon as the Clinton healthcare act had died in 1994—and with it, the chances for equality for mental illness and addiction treatment to be part of a larger healthcare reform package that also prevented any preexisting conditions from affecting coverage—a handful of stand-alone strategies had been suggested and debated. Parity seemed like a pretty basic concept, but it actually wasn't: there were a lot of possible moving parts, each of which came with its own economic and political price tag.

One of the biggest issues was what exactly would be covered by a parity law, and how this parity could be created and enforced. Would it cover only what the government called "serious mental illnesses" (a definition that was more limited in 1996 than it is today, including only schizophrenia, bipolar disorder, and the most disabling clinical depression)? Would parity cover what the government called "all mental illnesses"—which, in theory, included any condition listed in the *DSM* (a list that was different and somewhat more limited in 1996 than it is now)? Would parity include all addictions and substance use disorders (which, in 1996, some leading mental health advocates were still claiming were not actually diseases)? Would parity cover a menu of evidence-based treatments from different caregivers in different settings that worked for different patients—the equivalent of covering surgery, medication, outpatient physical therapy, inpatient rehab, and other treatments for a knee injury—or would it mostly be parity for generic psychopharmacology, a little short-term outpatient therapy, and maybe a few days in a hospital after a suicide attempt?

Would parity cover private insurance plans that already included mental health coverage? Would it mandate that all private insurance plans cover mental health, since some of them did not? Would it cover all federally funded health insurance—Medicare, Medicaid, Veterans Health Administration, federal employee coverage—and all publicly funded insurance at the state level?

And what would "parity" actually mean, once the law got beyond banning denial of coverage based on preexisting conditions, and disparate copays and lifetime caps for mental healthcare? How would the parity law remedy problems like the shortages in qualified caregivers in various parts of the country, and shortages of mental health beds and facilities for inpatient and outpatient care? If mental healthcare stopped being separate from all other medicine, how would a law force it to be better integrated into the practices of various specialists and generalists?

And would any of these changes actually lessen the stigma of mental health diagnoses and mental healthcare to the point where most of the people who needed help would get it—and once diagnosed and treated, would remain in treatment? Because, historically, no matter how effective treatments were and how much better they got, the majority of people refused to get, or stay in, care.

Given the deep political divides between the answers to these questions—made even deeper by a Republican-controlled Congress that had already shut down the federal government twice for a total of twenty-six days—it was especially significant that the mental health parity amendment was cosponsored by perhaps the two most diametrically opposed members of the Senate. On the Republican side there was card-carrying conservative Pete Domenici and on the Democratic side, card-carrying liberal Paul Wellstone from Minnesota—who I was getting to know because he was my neighbor in Justice Court, so we sometimes walked home together from work.

Domenici was already becoming well-known for his heroic public calls for increased research funding for the NIMH. Because his family's advocacy grew out of his daughter's struggle with schizoaffective disorder—which made anyone's short list of the most "serious" mental illnesses—he tended to want the strongest possible parity for the smallest possible group of the most seriously ill and disabled patients. And he was completely against including substance use disorders in parity.

Wellstone was a well-known liberal on healthcare issues but had only recently begun speaking about the reason for his interest in mental health parity. In the 1950s, his older brother Stephen had been hospitalized repeatedly for mental illness, and his care had nearly bankrupted the family. He vividly recalled being eleven years old and visiting Stephen—who was then nineteen—at Western State Hospital in Staunton, Virginia, and realizing that the way patients were being treated was terribly wrong. He considered that the crystallizing experience of his life, which made him want to go into politics, so he could stop people struggling with mental illness from being "put into parentheses." While Stephen had been originally diagnosed as suffering from schizophrenia—as almost all hospitalized patients were in the fifties—he was later rediagnosed with bipolar disorder and responded well to modern treatment with medication and supportive therapy. But he still had to struggle to function again and rejoin society, and he and his family were haunted by the blatant discrimination against him. Wellstone supported the broadest possible parity, including all mental illnesses and substance use disorders.

Between the two of them, they had built a bipartisan coalition of senators who had personal interests in mental illness and crafted an amendment. It was based on a bill they had proposed the year before, the Equitable Health Care for Severe Mental Illnesses Act, which had never made it out of conference. Their proposed amendment primarily impacted only larger employers with private insurance that already included mental healthcare, preventing them from putting annual or lifetime caps on care. The bill they proposed to amend just happened to be a health insurance reform act my father had cosponsored with Kansas Republican Nancy Kassebaum.

The amendment was notable in Washington because of the scene it caused on the floor of the Senate on the evening of April 18, 1996. In utter desperation to get their issue heard, several senators began pouring their hearts out concerning friends and family members devastated by mental illness.

Pete Domenici began:

Nobody is at fault because somebody has schizophrenia and acts differently and reasons differently. They are just as sick as your neighbor who has cancer. Yet only two percent of all individuals with mental illnesses are covered by insurance which provides benefits equal to the coverage for physical illnesses. . . . Through caps that are irresponsible but save money so insurance companies do it in their own self-interest, only two percent of Americans with mental illness are covered with the same degree of coverage as if they got tuberculosis or cancer instead of manic-depression or schizophrenia. You can walk down any street in urban America and you will find them. It is time to give these people access to care they need, and as you see them in urban America sleeping on grates and other things, you should realize that they probably started out as wonderful teenage children in some beautiful family. And when the costs got prohibitive and the behavior uncontrollable, they are abandoned.

Domenici yielded the floor to Wellstone, who spoke equally eloquently and, at the very end, personally. "I do not usually do this on the floor of the Senate," he said, "but I would like to dedicate my remarks to my brother who has struggled with mental illness almost his whole life. He is doing great now."

Alan Simpson, the Republican Senator from Wyoming, then got up and told about the suicide of his niece.

We did not get or understand the signals in time, and the signals were very clear as we all look back now out of sheer guilt and anguish. She was tough-minded, independent, loving, strong, and forceful. . . . She began to withdraw, and then she went into some religious and almost cultish activities, and she had a child. And that is a beautiful child. I know that child. . . . And after years of reaching out to us in her way and us not hearing and us not knowing, she one day decisively purchased a pistol and a few hours later purchased the ammunition and went to an isolated field, removed her shoes, sat in a crouched position . . . and blew her chest away.

She [had been] taking medication, and it was working. But then something, something unknown, entered her mind and her life and she decided not to take the medication—knowing what would happen if she did not—and then her tragic plan of ultimate rejection came to pass.

Simpson was followed by North Dakota Democrat Kent Conrad, who talked about a young woman who was the beloved receptionist at the state tax commissioner's office when both he and his fellow senator Byron Dorgan had worked there. "She was a beautiful and vibrant young woman. She was somebody who absolutely lit up an office. One day, she just went off the deep end with a mental illness that none of us knew that she had. Pictures were speaking to her. She had all kinds of aberrant thoughts. It led to her institutionalization. It led to her attempting to take her own life. That was a young woman, because of a suicide attempt, who did enormous damage to herself from which she will never fully recover. That young woman had a mental illness, and that illness deserved to be treated like any other illness."

It is not so unusual anymore to hear this kind of testimony in Congress. But to hear this from senators, late in the evening on the floor of the Senate in 1996, was a revelation.

Almost equally shocking was that after the senators spoke so movingly, my father got up and moved that their amendment be tabled.

He said he was completely in agreement with them in theory, but he thought the amendment would undermine the chances for his main piece of legislation to get through Congress and be signed into law. But Domenici and Wellstone refused to withdraw the amendment, so the motion to table mental health parity was put to a dramatic vote. My father and Senator Kassebaum, along with Chris Dodd, Tom Daschle, Bill Frist, Harry Reid, John McCain, and others, voted to have the parity amendment tabled.

They were soundly defeated, 65 to 33.

The motion was, at least temporarily, attached to the bill. But the amendment ended up being taken out of the HIPAA legislation at the very last minute, on August 1.

The very next day, Domenici and Wellstone reintroduced it as a stand-alone bill, the Mental Health Parity Act of 1996—which was the official beginning of using the phrase "mental health parity" for the movement to end medical discrimination against brain disorders. They proposed this new "parity" be accomplished through changes to the federal Employee Retirement Income Security Act (ERISA), which defined the rules of many retirement and healthcare plans and, because it was under the Department of Labor and not the Department of Health and Human Services, would more quickly and broadly be effective. (Since healthcare is largely dispensed at the state level, state health laws can be different than federal laws, yet many federal labor healthcare protections cross state boundaries.)

When President Clinton signed the HIPAA bill on August 21, he made it a point to express his "disappointment that the Congress dropped from this legislation the mental health parity provision that received such bipartisan support in the Senate," adding, "Individuals with mental illness have long suffered from discrimination in health plans that impose severe financial burdens on top of the illnesses they already face. I urge the Congress to act at the earliest opportunity to require parity in health insurance coverage for mental health services."

At that point, one of my colleagues in the House—longtime California Democratic Congressman Pete Stark—made a last-minute attempt to beef up the mental health parity protections, introducing a bill closer to what Paul Wellstone had originally wanted. It would have amended the Internal Revenue Code to force all group health plans to have full parity—covering all *DSM* diagnoses—and, more important, would have restructured the Medicare health benefit for full parity. (Because Medicare is the largest single health insurer in the nation, a change in the Medicare health benefit is followed by all insurers.) But the House instead followed the lead of Republican Marge Roukema from New Jersey—the longest-serving woman in the House and one of the first representatives openly interested in mental health issues (in part because her husband was a psychiatrist). Her bill was pretty close to the Senate bill, and that's where we ended up.

A month later, the parity bill was attached to a veterans appropriation bill and was quickly signed into law. The final version was pretty watered down. It only included "serious mental illnesses," it didn't include substance use disorders at all, and the final version even allowed employers to shift the new costs to employees by raising their overall copayments and deductibles.

"We didn't even get half a loaf, we just got crumbs," Paul Wellstone later told a colleague. "But," he said, "it's a start."

The era of mental health parity as a political struggle—a way of trying to end medical discrimination through legislation, just like the civil rights movement—had officially begun.

THIS ORIGINAL mental health parity act was limited, largely because of fear of skyrocketing costs and lack of political will. But the truth was, the mental health community itself was deeply divided, and the public's perception of mental healthcare as scientific and evidence based was under attack.

Prozac and the antidepressants that came after it became wonder drugs for some patients and for almost all pharmaceutical companies. The drugs also became a convenient target for those who didn't "believe" in mental healthcare or mental illness—or had been victims of substandard or outdated care when they needed help the most—and who focused their attacks on some of the understated side effects of the new medications (as if all drugs, new and old, weren't supposed to have side effects) and the huge profits the drug companies were making, especially with "me-too" drugs. Ironically, they focused much of their attention on one particular phenomenon—a slight uptick in suicidal ideation and suicide attempts in the first weeks after some patients began responding to antidepressants. There is always some risk of suicide at every stage of a mood disorder—even the moment when symptoms improve slightly with treatment. But the antipsychiatry forces, who believed that the illnesses were caused by the medications, used this small uptick to attack biologically based mental healthcare itself.

Some of these antipsychiatry attacks were encouraged by psychologists, social workers, counselors, and others who treated patients only with various "talk therapies" and distrusted the growing psychiatric drug culture. But the world of psychotherapy was also being rocked by a huge controversy about so-called false memories of abuse that parents claimed their teenage and grown children's therapists were "implanting" during treatment. This "false memory" controversy was an attack on certain techniques used in certain forms of intensive psychotherapy—mostly clinical hypnosis. But it was also an attack on what was coming to be called "trauma-based therapy," and the challenge of figuring out how to treat a newly appreciated range of post-traumatic stress disorders. Most people agreed that the trauma of war, or the trauma of sexual or other physical abuse, could trigger mental illness, and throughout the history of mental healthcare, practitioners and patients were taught that memories can be powerful and debilitating without being completely accurate. So it was shocking when parents began suing therapists claiming they were deliberately destroying families by blindly overbelieving patients.

This was also the period when electroconvulsive therapy (ECT) was beginning to make a comeback. Unlike in the harsh early days of the technique—which was used before there were any practical medications for mental illness, and before much was known about the seizures it triggered—ECT was now done at much, much lower doses, and with full anesthesia to minimize the negative effects of the treatment and maximize its unique antidepressant effect. But it still scared some people (mostly people who didn't need it).

These controversies, while overblown by the media, did serve to reinforce to some people the notion that mental healthcare wasn't yet ready for parity. But that was, of course, part of the discrimination. There were similarly bitter controversies in many areas of medical care, from cholesterol and cardiovascular disease to cancer, about treatments that were overused or overpriced. But only when it came to mental health was the public given the impression that it was okay to question the care itself, and even to wonder just how "medical" the diseases really were.

Chapter 12

A s all this was happening, my own mental health was getting worse. But I was getting really good at hiding it.

Because I did not have a strong opponent coming into the 1996 election, I decided to spend time on the road to help the Democratic Party win back the House, campaigning and raising money for thirty-five different candidates across the country. My thinking was that if I one day wanted to be involved in making policy on national issues— or even if I just wanted more political capital to protect my district and my state—the best thing I could do while this young and inexperienced was to use the fact that people wanted to hear a Kennedy speak about rebuilding the Democratic majority in the Congress. This would also help my House mentor, Dick Gephardt, who of course wanted to be Majority Leader again but also was thinking about the White House.

I worked incredibly hard for the party all over the country, hoping my local constituents would understand that this would ultimately help them as well. (Some in the local press understood better than others.) But the traveling drained me, isolated me, and made me more depressed and anxious than usual.

And constantly staying in hotels made for too many empty nights alone with too many temptations. I drank too much, and honestly, I was not a faithful boyfriend. Hypersexuality can be a symptom of bipolar disorder, seeking the release of sexual compulsions can be its own addictive behavior, and the role that sex plays in mental illness and addiction is something that we still don't talk enough about or research enough. Sexual dysfunction and overdrive can hinder the process of connecting to other people and increase shame, both of which can get in the way of treatment and recovery. And being unfaithful is also cruel. I'm not going to use my illness as my sole explanation for my behavior—I was also too immature and insecure to be in a committed relationship and didn't even know what one looked like. But I am solely responsible for the infidelities that blew up that relationship.

When I admitted to Kate what I had done and begged for her forgiveness, she decided we should spend some time apart. When that time apart extended from the start of summer into when she was about to start law school in the fall and I hadn't convinced her—or myself—that I was ready to marry and settle down, she said we should start seeing other people. I was devastated.

This had really been my first long-term, pretty serious relationship, and I hadn't realized just how important she was to me and to my basic daily stability in Washington—until she was gone.

I started falling apart. As part of my attempt to not fall apart—and to try to document and break certain patterns of behavior—I decided to start keeping a diary. So I have a pretty good record of how I unraveled.

My staff recognized a change in me. I was clearly more depressed, or more *something*, because I had never said out loud to any of them that I suffered from depression. They knew I had a therapist, because they had to block out times for me to see him. But they didn't really understand the depths of my illness and what exactly I was being treated for. At the time I honestly didn't realize how they saw me. I thought I was doing a pretty good job of appearing pretty normal. In fact, my swinging moods and occasional morning hangovers became predictable enough that my schedule was built around those cycles. And the smart lobbyists—especially those in mental health and addiction, some of whom were in recovery themselves and understood what was going on better than I did—just called ahead before any meeting to see if I was okay and offered the staff the option of rescheduling so there was minimal friction.

Since I've been fully committed to recovery over the past few years, I've recently had the chance to talk to my former staff about what they thought was going on back then. One said he assumed I was going to therapy to "be on the couch" discussing "stuff" about "your dad." This was based on the assumption that psychotherapy was something I decided to do for self-improvement, not something I needed in order to treat a medical condition.

What is amazing as I look back at this time is how functional I was able to remain. One thing people who don't suffer from mental illness often don't understand about these diseases is how long—how many days, weeks, months—people can suffer from symptoms that are extremely painful and debilitating but just bearable enough to stay ahead of.

When people have depressive or manic or psychotic breakdowns, or make suicide attempts, the people around them are often surprised they "didn't see it coming." But that's because it is rare for the person with mental illness to be open and honest in real time about what is happening, what is "coming." It is hard sometimes to admit to ourselves how often these illnesses are encroaching on our lives before we reach the point of emergency.

It is hard to admit how abnormal our normal can be.

Like many people who suffer from mood disorders, I was elevating the dramas of my life all out of proportion. I became fixated on my breakup with my girlfriend, mentally yanking myself back and forth about whether or not I was ready for marriage and whether I had destroyed my only chance at happiness.

I talked about this with my dad, but that only made it worse. He didn't seem to get upset enough about what I was upset by, and this infuriated me. But sometimes, I had to admit to myself that the real problem I had with him were the questions I wasn't brave enough to ask. I had just blown a relationship because I had cheated—and took that cheating to mean that this probably wasn't the right relationship for me, or the right time to be in it. So what I really wanted to know was how these issues had played out in his life.

Of course, who ever asks their dad about that? Even if their dad has been asked the same question dozens of times by the press.

As I had since I was a teenager, I started writing my father letters that I was never going to send, as therapy. One day I wrote, "Dear Dad, with all you've been through I wish you could talk to me, really talk to me, about what advice you have for me to have a fuller, more intimate and meaningful life. How to cope with life's challenges and really talk . . . I guess I need to live and love more women and can never get away from the challenge of dealing with my internal boogey man and quell the unsettling desires."

Only weeks after I wrote this, my cousin John Kennedy Jr. got married, in a very private ceremony. Almost immediately, the press decided that, although the country was in the middle of a presidential election, it was important to do some stories speculating on who would be the family's most eligible bachelor—or, as the *New York Post* asked, who would "inherit John-John's hunky mantle." Everyone from the *Post* to the Nashville *Tennessean* to, even, *Roll Call*, our Capitol Hill insiders' paper, nominated me. They did this even though the *Tennessean* said I was "the family geek" and *Roll Call* ran a cartoon about a "Kennedy Closeout Sale" and said I was the "only one left" and "ready to be your mystery date."

I joked about this to the press—it was funny, and what else was I going to do? But it couldn't have come at a more painful time.

Two weeks later, I wrote, "I have been on automatic pilot for the last ten days or so and I've wanted to lose track of myself but it hasn't been possible. I feel as though I am holding my breath emotionally and have yet to exhale after my breakup with Kate. . . . I feel like I'm losing it. . . . [I'm so] loosely wrapped . . . that anything, people or events, can pull my strings and I could unravel. I feel my self-esteem shrinking in the face of unhappy news or difficult times . . . I missed my plane and . . . the panic over it was enough to send me into tears."

Still, I managed to function. The President was reelected in November, and while we didn't get back control of the House or Senate, we made some progress in both. And it was pretty clear that Newt Gingrich would not remain as Speaker too much longer.

MY FIRST SERIOUS INVOLVEMENT in national healthcare issues in Congress grew out of a situation that was very local: an ailing nonprofit hospital system in Providence, the Roger Williams Medical Center, was being eyed for purchase by Nashville-based Columbia/ HCA—the new giant in the growing and feared field of for-profit hospitals. We worried that meant there would be no guarantees the hospital would continue to offer the kind of free care for the indigent that Providence required. We were against for-profit hospitals in theory, a struggle that now seems very out-of-date, since we now realize there can be good and bad nonprofit and for-profit hospitals. However, this particular chain had a number of specific allegations against it already, and in retrospect, it still seems like it was worth challenging them.

Because this proposed takeover wasn't a national issue, I didn't have to worry about the Republican majority in the House. Instead, we brought national Democratic attention to the issues, even bringing Congressman Pete Stark from California in to speak against it.

The only real downside for me, politically, was that the sale was supported by Rhode Island's senior US Senator, John Chafee, a moderate Republican. I had a good relationship with the Senator even though many thought I should run against him as soon as I reached the minimum age of thirty.

I may have been the only Democrat in New England who *didn't* think I should run for Chafee's Senate seat. I realized early on that the nature of my illness could prevent me from taking that next step, where there was more pressure, and more danger of getting sicker and being exposed.

Working with colleagues in Congress and former colleagues in the State House, we were able to help craft a bill that would make it so restrictive for a for-profit hospital company to come into Rhode Island and buy a non-profit hospital that it wouldn't be worth it. The governor vetoed the bill, but we had enough support to override the veto.

Not long after, federal authorities announced they had been investigating Columbia/HCA for defrauding state and federal healthcare programs, and a whistleblower who had reported the company had been sent back in to gather more evidence. Eventually there were resignations, plea agreements, and a large fine.

THIS WAS ONE of the first in what became a series of healthcare—related investigations by the regional offices of the US Attorney, and state Attorneys General—many of which were seen as taking the place of the federal regulations and oversight that had been undermined by the Republicans in Congress. These investigations looked at corrupt practices in hospital care, and individual physicians overcharging or phantom-billing for services.

Eventually, whistleblowers helped state and federal authorities to investigate illegal drug company promotion, especially in cases where expensive new mental health drugs were promoted for uses that had not been approved by the FDA. When a medication is approved by the FDA, it is usually approved to treat only one illness, which is listed on the label—at least initially. Once approved, however, it may be tried by physicians to see if it will work for other illnesses.

But drug companies are not allowed to actively promote this "off-label" use, or even to nudge the word-of-mouth. They are supposed to, instead, pay to have the drug tested for those other uses and apply for additional "indications" on the label. Some of these off-label experimentations lead doctors to discover a much more important use for a medication than the one it was originally approved for—some antiepilepsy drugs, for example, have turned out to have much broader applications in treating bipolar disorder. However, because these off-label uses have not yet been thoroughly tested, they can easily lead to problems.

For example, there is a class of medications called atypical antipsychotics—which began when Clozaril (clozapine) proved there was a more effective way to treat schizophrenia, schizoaffective disorder, and the psychotic symptoms of severe bipolar disorder. Clozaril was revolutionary and effective but since it carried a small risk of blood disease and required regular blood testing, drug companies set out to create other atypical antipsychotics that might not require blood testing—and they came up with Risperdal, Seroquel, and several others. While perhaps not quite as effective as Clozaril, they were much easier to take—which meant more patients who needed them might stay on them. And if these drugs had primarily been prescribed for patients with severe mental illnesses who needed them, they would likely have been pretty successful and probably largely uncontroversial.

However, after the runaway success of Prozac—which dovetailed with the relaxing of FDA rules that had all but prevented medications from being advertised on television—mental health drugs started to be prescribed and advertised more aggressively. Physicians—some trained in mental healthcare, many just primary care docs—began trying them on patients with different diagnoses, with varying success. And pharmaceutical company sales reps started spreading the news of physicians who claimed to have good results, even though those results were anecdotal and had not been verified in clinical trials.

This kind of off-label promotion is illegal, and it can be dangerous. Many adults were tried on the drugs who didn't need a medication that powerful, and then many children with behavioral problems were tried on them, under the mistaken assumption they had an adolescent form of bipolar disorder and needed a baby dose of these medications (which would be a little bit like giving baby doses of skin cancer chemotherapy to kids with acne). With more of the drugs being given to more people, more patients were exposed to potential side effects—which turned out to include early onset diabetes and, in some males, growth of breasts.

Now, if you had schizophrenia and these drugs were the only ones that dampened your severe symptoms, you might actually consider the possibility of diabetes and male breasts to be a risk worth taking. Treatment-resistant schizophrenia is one of the most debilitating diseases known to man. But, certainly, those risks were not worth taking for the much larger group of people without such severe illnesses.

However, that isn't why the companies were prosecuted. They were prosecuted for illegally promoting these off-label uses. And these whistleblower prosecutions would lead to some of the largest multibillion-dollar settlements in history.

While there have been illegal promotion guilty pleas involving other drugs for other diseases, these prosecutions have clearly had the greatest effect on mental health care. The headlines from the cases have fed a social prejudice that mental health drugs are haphazardly and overzealously prescribed. They have served to compound stigma. I am very concerned about the health and economic impact of overprescribing and illegal promotion of medications. But I am also concerned about the millions of Americans with mental illnesses who need medication and refuse to take it, or won't even go get evaluated or diagnosed because of stigma and discrimination.

These prosecutions are also part of the reason that many drug companies have cut back or eliminated their research and development programs for new mental health medications; the other reason is that drugs for central nervous system conditions have generally taken longer to get approved than drugs for other body systems, and a smaller percentage of them are approved at all. So, only a handful of companies are still trying to develop new drugs for brain diseases, and there is a shortage of new drug "targets" for their research. The situation is so dire that the Institute of Medicine held a symposium recently just to discuss how to get the pharmaceutical industry interested again in the broad unmet needs in central nervous system medications.

You may have issues with big business–like companies. A lot of people do. But you should have even bigger issues with those companies getting out of the business of trying to treat or cure your medical problems.

Chapter 13

In mid-November of 1998, I was summoned to the office of Steve Elmendorf, who was chief of staff for my House mentor, Dick Gephardt. I walked over to his office, which was in the back of the Minority Leader's suite, and he ushered me in and closed the door.

He told me how much Dick loved me and appreciated what I had done for the party. And he said Dick wanted me to become the chairman of the Democratic Congressional Campaign Committee, the party's political and fund-raising arm for the House. It was a proposition beyond my wildest dreams: a leadership position rarely offered to someone so young. I had just turned thirty-one, and this would make me the fifth-ranking Democrat in the House.

There was, however, one catch.

"If you do this," he said, "you can't drink."

Amazingly, I do not recall feeling freaked out by this in the least, which gives a pretty good indication of how little insight I had into my illness; the level of self-delusion and pretending that goes on with these diseases is really astonishing. I didn't feel exposed or scared, and

I didn't see this for what it was—my first-ever intervention, by some-one who held my professional future in his hands.

My reaction was to say to him, and to myself, "Okay, I got it."

It was as if he had told me I had to lose a few pounds or shave off a bad mustache. I never for one minute thought, *I must have a pretty serious problem if the House Minority Leader is this worried about it.* I just had no concept of how much my bipolar disorder and my drink-ing had impacted my life.

I also didn't know if Gephardt knew, or if his younger chief of staff had heard the gossip and was trying to run interference for him. I un-derstood that the word must have been out that "Patrick really ties one on." Of course, I already realized that in Washington everyone knows everything. I just, somehow, believed that was true for everyone else but *me*. I had grown up in a family culture where we continued to deny, even to ourselves, what everyone else seemed to already know.

But, in all honesty, this had little to do with being a Kennedy and much more to do with being an addict. This is how all addicts are. The denial is so huge, the self-perception so skewed. And the problem wors-ens so gradually that it's like being in water and you don't notice the temperature is rising a degree at a time until you realize, *Oh my God, it's boiling, and I'm cooked!*

So, at a moment when many people might have been scared straight, shocked into some kind of self-realization—and would have considered taking immediate action, getting serious help—I just matter-of-factly agreed to stop drinking. As if that meant I could, or that the underly-ing reasons I was self-medicating with alcohol would just go away.

THIS WAS ALL HAPPENING, in part, because the Democrats had done well enough in the midterm election that Newt Gingrich stepped down as Speaker of the House. Dick decided that he would not challenge Al Gore for the Democratic nomination for President, but instead dedicate all his efforts to winning back the House and becoming Speaker. Since we were now only eleven seats behind, we would only need six more seats in the next election to retake the majority—an ambitious but not impossible goal. Besides the amount of money I raised, I would be judged by whether or not we won back those six seats.

There was also another incentive to do well. I was being given a new committee assignment, the most coveted committee assignment: Appropriations. But in order to make sure nobody screamed about my being too low on the seniority ladder to get that assignment, I agreed to suspend my membership in the new committee until after I had finished my two years at the DCCC.

So, in January of 1999 I became the chairman of the DCCC, overseeing a staff of 126 and spending all my free time—and some of my not-free time—traveling all over the country raising money for Democratic congressional candidates to win back the House.

This was a job I was born to do. When the task was stoking Democratic pride and filling party coffers, that's when the power of this name I inherited, which elevated me in ways I have spent my life trying to fully understand, was perfectly clear. We dramatically increased the levels of donations we sought. Before I took over the DCCC, the highest donation we asked for was $15,000 in "hard money" to join our "Speaker's Club." I initiated "Team 2000," a "soft money" campaign for those who donated at least $100,000. They would be rewarded with special events, including the opportunity to attend a special clambake and tour at our family compound in Hyannis Port. Democrats were still trying to legislate against the growth of soft money in elections, but we just couldn't let the Republicans keep killing us in that area while awaiting campaign finance reform.

We raised a lot of money and helped a lot of candidates. And because of that, everyone was willing to ignore that I periodically didn't look so well. Mostly, I kept my illness to myself. But, looking back, it is amazing how much people were willing to ignore or explain away.

IN MY OWN MIND, of course, I hadn't agreed to stop drinking so much as to stop drinking in public. For the most part, I kept that promise for the two years I ran the DCCC. But that was also when I started abusing prescription narcotic painkillers.

I was not alone. While narcotic painkillers were not new, the FDA recently had approved OxyContin, a new, more powerful time-release pill version of oxycodone, the compound found in Percocet and other medications. The drug was approved in 1995 for serious pain management of cancer and the worst cases of arthritis—and labeled as a dangerous, highly addictive Schedule II drug. But as soon as it started being marketed in 1996, OxyContin began being used off-label for other types of pain management and being abused as a street drug.

The risk of dependence was especially high with the larger-dose pills. The drug was available in ten-, twenty-, forty-, and eighty-milligram pills—and, in 2000, they briefly added a one-hundred-sixty-milligram pill (which was quickly forced off the market because of absurd levels of abuse). What made Oxy so effective as a painkiller was exactly what made it so addictive: it was very powerful and remained that way for up to twelve hours. For those who couldn't wait for the time release, they would chew the pills before swallowing them to break up the coating, or smash the pills and snort them.

Like most people with chronic back pain, I was no stranger to pain medicine. And it's not like I didn't need pain relief. My back had never been quite right after the surgery to remove that tumor, and I shared chronic back pain with almost every male member of my family. I just didn't need quite as much pain relief as I was starting to give myself.

———

Four months after I was put in charge of the DCCC, I was on Air Force One with President Clinton, Dick Gephardt, and others, heading to a major fund-raiser in Massachusetts, where we would meet my father and John Kerry. The event was at the home of Alan Solomont, a longtime family friend and former healthcare company director who was very active in philanthropy and had recently served as the finance chair of the DCCC. (He was later the US Ambassador to Spain.) It was a very important fund-raiser, very close to home in a lot of ways.

I had taken OxyContin for my back pain that morning. Among its other effects, Oxy really diminishes your motor skills—and I am a little uncoordinated to begin with. But it doesn't make you appear intoxicated, so I had the false impression that I seemed okay.

During the flight, I went to the bathroom. And as I was washing up, I stuffed a paper towel too far into the disposal bin, which had a lid that popped up on a spring. So my left hand got stuck in there. And since I was feeling no pain, I tried to yank it out.

In the process, I ripped off the whole top of my middle finger.

That I felt. But mostly I shrieked because I looked down and saw there was blood all over the bathroom. I wrapped my finger with a paper towel and it was still bleeding like crazy. My heart was pounding; I couldn't believe this was happening. But since I wasn't in pain— I could barely feel anything—it was like I was a third-party witness to my own disaster.

So I quietly went up to some of the Secret Service and showed them my hand. They brought me to this room on the plane that got repurposed for major medical emergencies. When I walked in it didn't look like anything but a little room, but then they started pulling out shelves and operating tables and pulling down lights, and suddenly it was transformed into a surgical suite in a trauma center.

The physician who accompanied the President was there, and he didn't miss a beat. He turned on the lights, held my hand down, and all the injections were ready in a split second. Next thing I knew they were suturing me up. And, of course, I was pretending like this was really hurting me. Because I knew that in the closet they had lots of narcotics.

Soon President Clinton looked in on me. He couldn't believe what was going on; he'd never seen anything like this before on Air Force One. He teased me a little bit, and I said, "Mr. President, now I can say I was operated on at thirty thousand feet on Air Force One."

And he just said, "Oh my God, this is really something . . ."

They finished sewing me up, bandaged me, and handed me a jar of Percocets. The physician said, "Be sure not to take too many of these."

And as I did with every other doctor who said that to me—and, over the years, there were many—I responded, "Okay." I couldn't wait to get out of his line of sight so I could take even more.

In Boston we were met by a big motorcade. We got to the event, and my dad and John Kerry and others were already there; my escapade getting my hand sewn up was all the buzz.

And then I collapsed.

I was taken to a side room in the house and when I came to, the advance people told me that if I didn't feel up to speaking, the president said it was okay. This was probably their polite way of telling me to sit this one out. And I completely ignored them.

So, when everyone was supposed to go on, I got up and walked to the stage with them. My job was to introduce Dick Gephardt and do my stump speech.

Instead I got up there with my bandaged middle finger—I was really flying by then, I had taken a few more pills—and I said, "It's good to be here. Some of you may have learned I had a mishap on Air Force One and had to get stitches."

And then I showed my hand, with the bandaged middle finger.

"As you know," I continued, "one of our jobs is to come up with effective messaging to take back the House from the Republicans and their right-wing agenda. But sometimes you can't deliver the message in any other way but to give them, y'know, a hand signal."

The mere notion I would do this in front of the President, my father, the top donors for the party, is appalling, frightening. But I was feeling no pain at the time. I remember thinking it was all pretty funny.

And, regardless of my behavior, the dinner was a great success and raised $800,000. And the next morning we got back on the road to do more fund-raising.

DURING THE WINTER AND SPRING of 1999, the world of brain diseases was preparing for the first-ever White House Conference on Mental Health, to be held in June. It was, as much as anything, an acknowledgment that the Decade of the Brain was almost over, as was the Clinton presidency—and for all their ambitious goals for improving the care of mental illness and increasing research into its treatment and cure, they hadn't made enough progress.

The conference was also meant to introduce the important role mental health would play if Al Gore were elected president. And the timing of the conference—just before the official announcement that he was running—was no coincidence.

But there was no mistaking that this was primarily a labor of love for Tipper Gore, who wanted to make it clear that mental health would be her primary concern if she got to be First Lady but also wanted to make a difference right away just in case there wasn't a Gore presidency. The planning was elaborate, because Tipper held many regional meetings as a warm-up to the national conference and also insisted that the main event be simulcast by satellite—which, back in 1999, was a considerable undertaking—to six thousand locations across the country. The President was also arranging to announce a broad array of executive orders at the conference, which would attempt to make a significant impact on the main issues being addressed.

If it was not already clear that such a conference was long overdue, a major tragedy made the point horrifically and poignantly. On April 20, thirteen students and faculty were killed, and more than twenty were injured, at Columbine High School in Littleton, Colorado, by two heavily armed students who then took their own lives. The assault did not immediately instigate a discussion about mental illness, as more recent shootings have—it took a longer time to figure out what had happened and why.

As the conference approached, Tipper also made a bold revelation. She had, for years, been explaining that her deep interest in mental illness had grown out of her own academic studies—she had two degrees in psychology, although she never practiced—and the fact that her mother had suffered serious depressions. But then, several weeks before the White House conference, Tipper did a Q & A with *USA Today* in which she revealed an even more personal reason why mental health was her main concern. She said that she had been treated for depression with psychotherapy and medication ten years earlier, in the aftermath of her six-year-old son's severe injuries in an auto accident. In 1999, that kind of revelation from a public figure was still big news.

THE CONFERENCE ITSELF, held on June 7, lasted only one hour and thirty-nine minutes. But it was a fantastically concentrated burst of science, policy, and advocacy. I still recall sitting in the packed room at Howard University—with innumerable members of Congress, leaders of government agencies, and power players in the mental health care-giver and patient advocacy communities—being amazed at how much cutting-edge information and smart medical politics were crammed into such a short period of time.

The presentations were carefully orchestrated, with Tipper moving three high-powered conversations deftly onward. The first was moderated by her and included moving testimony from three successfully treated patients, including Mike Wallace from *60 Minutes*, who was now speaking openly about his three major bouts with depression (the first one had come during a high-profile lawsuit against CBS; the other two, he explained, happened mostly because he kept going off his medication). Then the Vice President walked stage right and moderated a conversation about how families and communities and businesses can respond to mental health issues, with a mother from his home state who had to navigate the system for her bipolar child, and the medical director of Bank One Corporation, who discussed how offering better mental health coverage to the company's employees saved them money. He also spoke via satellite link to Surgeon General Dr. David Satcher, who was joining the discussion—along with a large audience—from Atlanta.

Then Hillary Clinton walked to stage left and talked about science and treatment with Dr. Steven Hyman—the outspoken young biological psychiatry researcher who, at age forty-six, had been the director of the National Institute of Mental Health for three years and was being talked about as a possible candidate to run the entire National Institutes of Health in a Gore administration (which would have been the first time a brain scientist ever ran the entire organization). Hyman showed some of the slides that had been making such an impact at recent medical conferences—images that for the first time allowed even a layperson who didn't "believe" in mental illness to see the undeniable differences in the brains of people suffering from depression and schizophrenia. Hillary moved on to child psychiatry expert Dr. Harold Koplewicz from NYU and then to my House colleague from Michigan Lynn Rivers. She was the nation's highest-ranking elected official who was open about suffering from mental illness, having revealed her bipolar disorder in 1994 on a call-in radio show during her first campaign for Congress.

Then the President got up and gave a very moving address, which included announcements of several changes he could make immediately, with just his executive authority. He was mandating that federal civil service hiring could no longer have different disability standards for people with physical, developmental, and mental disabilities: previously, people with autism or Down syndrome had better disability protections than people with schizophrenia and mood disorders.

And he was righting a wrong that my uncle had originally addressed in the early sixties, only to have his effort reversed by President Reagan. He ordered the nation's largest private insurer, the Federal Employees Health Benefits Program, which covered over nine million Americans in three hundred health plans, to begin providing full parity for mental health conditions, "equal coverage for mental and physical illnesses," beginning in 2001.

The President also called for congressional hearings on mental health parity for the rest of insured Americans—knowing, of course, that this was going to take much longer to achieve and that it couldn't be accomplished with just a stroke of his pen.

OVER THE NEXT FEW WEEKS after the conference, the NIMH unveiled a new $7.3 million study that would, for the first time, explore in depth the prevalence of mental illness in the US and the treatments currently in use. This was information that nobody had and the only way to have a benchmark from which to improve, as well as a way of assessing what mental health parity might actually mean in practice. NIMH also announced $61 million in new funding for two large much-needed clinical trials: one to examine the relative effectiveness of antipsychotic medications, the other to study long-term effects of different sequences of drug therapy and psychotherapy for treatment-resistant depression.

Surgeon General David Satcher also began a major initiative on suicide in July. This was surprising only because his office was still working on the first-ever US Surgeon General's report on mental illness, which had been under way for nearly two years. But with growing public concern about the aftermath of Columbine, he decided to make a surgical strike on the issue of teen suicide, which had become the third-leading cause of death among young people (and, unfortunately, is now their second-leading cause of death).

Choosing suicide as a focal point was an interesting approach: I have personally left many large mental health conferences—where there are many well-meaning factions competing to get their illnesses or treatment approaches or facilities funded—thinking that the one thing all brain diseases ultimately have in common is that, for too many of their patients, their end point is a suicide attempt. Working backward from suicide is a way of being very inclusive to all mental health and addiction care, and it's also a way of working to prevent our biggest shared fear and medical emergency.

Everyone mourns when someone takes their own life—which we now describe as "completing suicide" because "committing" suggests a crime. But the truth is that up until that life is lost, people sometimes minimize the risk of self-harm or treat certain statements and actions too cavalierly. If a person is alive and in treatment for mental illness, even if the patient is vocal about having suicidal thoughts and plans, there is often too much discussion among family members, teachers, and even caregivers about how "real" or how "serious" the symptoms really are. How many times have we heard people parse whether or not a suicide attempt was "serious" or just "a cry for help," as if those were two different things.

I am extremely fortunate that suicidal ideation and behavior have not been components of my illnesses. So while I have been self-destructive, I am not plagued with the compulsion toward self-harm. This is one of the luckier aspects of my genetic loading for brain disease. Because given my poor impulse control over much of my young life, if I were often feeling suicidal, I might not still be here.

MOST OF MY RECOLLECTIONS of the summer of 1999, however, are overwhelmed by a deeply personal loss: the death of my cousin John Kennedy Jr. John was seven years older than me, so growing up, he was part of that older generation of cousins.

We had become closer during recent years after he founded the great new political magazine, *George,* in 1995. The magazine's offices were in New York, but John was frequently in DC. It was great having him in town more often, bringing a young, irreverent voice to Washington culture during a period of generational and political upheaval.

Besides the articles in the magazine, he also did a number of promotional events that were great fun. In fact, the last time I saw him was June 17 at the US Airways Center, because he asked me to be part of a politicians-versus-pundits road race to raise money for breast cancer research, co-sponsored by BMW and the Susan G. Komen foundation. It was me, Jesse Jackson Jr., and several other Democrats, along with Republicans Mary Bono, Jim DeMint, and Lindsay Graham, racing in BMW 3 sedans around the parking lot against Ann Coulter, Laura Ingraham, Juan Williams, and others. John couldn't drive in the race himself because his leg was in a cast—he had recently broken it while paragliding.

In mid-July, the week of my thirty-second birthday, I was scheduled to spend the weekend in California for Democratic fund-raising events. I wasn't happy about this, because it was going to prevent me from being at the Cape, where most of my family was assembling for the wedding of my cousin Rory. I landed in San Francisco and was whisked to a fund-raiser, after which I went to bed. Early Saturday morning, I received word that John's plane was missing and immediately arranged to fly home. I didn't get to Hyannis until late Saturday afternoon. By then Rory's wedding had been postponed, and the family gathering had been transformed into a vigil for John, his wife, Carolyn, and his sister-in-law, Lauren. But since a small bit of wreckage from their plane had already been found, prospects were grim.

Early Wednesday morning, we received word that the divers had found something. A helicopter came to pick up my father, my brother, and me, landing on the front lawn of the main house and taking us to the Coast Guard station on Martha's Vineyard. We were transported on a Coast Guard cutter to the site, and by around two o'clock in the afternoon we were on the Navy salvage ship, the USS *Grasp*, whose divers and robot cameras were working over one hundred feet below the surface.

Over the previous few days, we had been consumed—and perhaps even a little distracted—by the technical details of the search, which were provided to us in the depersonalized language the military adopts when looking for anyone or anything. But when we were out on that cutter, just my brother and me flanking my dad, it was starting to become more and more real. I thought about how many tragedies like this my father had been forced to confront and process: his older brother Joe and his older sister "Kick" dying in plane crashes in the 1940s; his older brothers Jack and Bobby being shot to death in the 1960s. I understood, intellectually, how those traumas had formed him and my family over the decades. But I had no real understanding of that moment of incomprehensible pain and isolation, what it probably felt like when my father flashed back—until we heard on the radio that they were going to start bringing up what they had found and the winch began cranking.

My father couldn't really react except to put his hand on my shoulder. He was so deep inside himself that he just shut down. He couldn't comprehend what we were witnessing; it was too much, so raw. The only comfort I could take from being with him at that moment is that we were *really with him*—in a way that only a grown child, or a brother, can be.

IN THE FALL OF 1999, the preliminary draft of the first-ever Surgeon General's report on mental health began quietly circulating for comment. This five-hundred-page report had involved an incredibly accomplished cast of characters from all corners of mental healthcare, the current and the upcoming best and brightest. They all devoted hundreds of hours to this landmark enterprise, an attempt to create one large document that, in plain language, explained the challenging history of treating brain diseases and the current state of treatment, research, facilities, caregivers, and patients, and offered for the first time a smart conceptual road map for change.

All Americans should read this report. It's smart and provocative and comprehensive, and in many cases can help patients, families, and caregivers better understand what is known and not known about these illnesses and the efficacy of various treatments, and also help them not to be surprised or shocked by controversies everyone working in the field already knows about.

So, with the White House Conference on Mental Health, the

Surgeon General's report, new executive orders to combat medical discrimination against mental illness, and a popular incumbent Vice President running for President on a platform of prioritizing care for brain diseases, things looked very promising for a second, even better Decade of the Brain. All we had to do was win the election.

Chapter 14

On Tuesday, February 29, 2000, at the Woonsocket Senior Center in northeastern Rhode Island, my life took a dramatic turn.

I was hosting a campaign appearance by Tipper Gore for some two hundred senior citizens. Woonsocket was an old industrial town on the northern end of my district, politically important because it was a powerful Democratic stronghold and housed the corporate headquarters of the CVS drugstore chain. It was also close enough to Boston that my mom decided to join us.

This event wasn't supposed to be anything special, just a chance for Tipper to give her stump speech on mental health and for me to speak generally about the problem of stigma.

I had no plans to share anything personal that day. In fact, I was not feeling or looking well: I get especially seasonally depressed in the darker days of winter, and I was taking too many Oxys.

During the Q & A session after Tipper's remarks, I got on a roll talking about the stigma of depression. Here I was in a room full of senior citizens concerned about this subject—many, I assume, because they were suffering—and sitting with my mom, who had been remarkably open about her alcoholism but still, even privately, had trouble admitting she was depressed.

I was already well-known to my staff and my House colleagues for going off script in public appearances and pushing the envelope. One of my top aides came to refer to me as "the Ratchet" because I was never satisfied with normal messaging and, in front of a microphone, always wanted to "ratchet" things up. But none of them knew—nor did I—what I was about to say.

"I myself have suffered from depression," I blurted out. "I have been treated by psychiatrists."

There was a hush in the room.

Finally, I said, "Oh, my God, it's out! That's another skeleton in the closet!"

When that produced a chuckle, I kept going: "Yes, I am on a lot of different medications for, among other things, depression. I have suffered with depression since I was young. But I'm here to tell you, thank God I got treatment, because I wouldn't be as strong as I am today if I didn't get that treatment."

"People with depression are suffering, but they're suffering in silence," Tipper said. "Tell yourself to get help. Don't suffer in silence." And then we got back to the messages we had come to deliver.

After the event, reporters had more questions that, honestly, I really wasn't up for answering. I didn't feel that great, I was sort of in shock over what I had just done, and I didn't want to give out any more information. I also didn't want it to appear as unplanned as it was, so I did my best to spin it as if this were all part of my plan, as my staff rolled their eyes. I told Charlie Bakst, the *Providence Journal* reporter who covered me the most, that I had decided to reveal this ahead of time, which is why I had invited my mom, who had suffered with alcoholism and depression. I told him that if I was going to tell senior citizens to get treatment and push past the stigma of mental illness, "I ought to walk the walk."

My mom told him she thought it was "wonderful" that I had spoken out. And then she had a great Mom line with so many meanings.

"People like honesty," she told the reporter.

So they immediately asked her whether she was seeing a psychiatrist. She said she hadn't seen one in five years but "would call one tomorrow if I needed one. But I'm so lucky—I can afford one. A lot of people can't."

The reporters pressed me for the name of my psychiatrist, the names of the drugs I was taking. I didn't want to go there. I just tried to keep on message.

"I hope that my admission that I get help and that it makes me a stronger person—along with Tipper's admission and others who are coming out—will help make more people realize there is nothing to be ashamed of. It should be treated as a private issue, but for the purpose of breaking the stigma, I have no problem saying that."

When I got back to Washington that night, I dashed off a handwritten note to Bill Emmet, who had been the first person who ever talked to me about mental health parity, back in Rhode Island. He was now in Washington too, as deputy executive director of NAMI. I wrote, "Dear Bill, I've always admired your work, and now you know why."

He was called for comment after a local radio show made fun of me the next day for my public admission—basically saying that since I was a Kennedy, what did I have "to be depressed about?"

"Mental illness is a biological brain disorder!" Bill shot back. "Saying Patrick has nothing to be depressed about is like saying Patrick has no reason to have heart disease, no reason to have cancer. Stigma is very real, and it's going to take a lot more public officials to burn away the stigma!"

Other media, however, did get it. The *Boston Globe*, which was not always so friendly to me, did a really nice op-ed that said, "Representative Patrick Kennedy performed an important service when he told a Rhode Island political gathering that he has been treating depression with medications. In doing so, he demonstrated that it is possible to lead a successful career while coping with a mental condition requiring medical treatment—an example to counter the stigma still applied to those who suffer with mental illnesses."

WHILE THIS WAS ALL VERY KIND, I *wasn't* coping with my mental condition. Not really. The fact that I had just blurted out private information about my treatment was, arguably, a *symptom* of my mental condition (as was, probably, running for public office at the age of twenty when I was still a college student).

Also, when you have what is called a "dual diagnosis"—one that involves a mood disorder and a substance use disorder—it is easy to use one to cover for the other. At that time, my mood shifts were probably secondary to, and being fueled by, my overuse of narcotic painkillers (in public) and my drinking (in private). And because of the broad cycles in my moods, while it was true I had suffered "depressions," they really had been part of the swings of bipolar disorder.

But from a political standpoint, it was easier to admit to depression. People were less upset by it.

I didn't understand any of this at the time. I was not aware back then what I was doing—mental illnesses, of course, can affect perception, cognition, the things the brain does easily and efficiently when it is working properly.

In public life, once you say something out loud, you can't take it back. But you can use it to your political advantage—and as a way of deflecting what you didn't say. So, for the next couple years, I never went beyond the handful of facts I revealed that day in Woonsocket to anyone. That was true even among my closest staff members, who were shocked by what I did that day, and probably further shocked when I didn't say anything more about it to any of them.

They knew that, from then on, in any conversation about mental illness, I would repeat only the two facts I had publicly shared: that I had been treated for depression with medication and therapy, and I had always parked far from my doctor's office to avoid my car being noticed in the lot of a psychiatrist. But they also suspected there was a lot more going on that I wouldn't talk about.

LESS THAN A MONTH AFTER I "came out," I was in Los Angeles for eleven hours for a quick fund-raiser, after which I broke my own rule about drinking in public and really regretted it.

It was the Sunday of the Oscars. I had begun the day early doing events in Delaware and Maryland and then boarded a plane in Philly with my staff to get to LA by one P.M., to do an event there, and then fly immediately back to Boston on the 11:59 red-eye. After the LA fund-raiser, my staff stayed in California and I went to Elton John's Oscar party to raise money for AIDS treatment and research. I wasn't planning to stay long, but I was seated next to one of my musical heroes from youth, Debbie Harry from Blondie. And, as I had a couple drinks, I just had to tell her and Elton John my dad's "The Tide Is High" story, one of his very favorites from his repertoire about my formative years.

When I was twelve or thirteen, my parents used to chaperone little parties for my friends in our basement, little dances—although we obviously didn't encourage them to come down and check on us. My dad always told the story of opening the door to the basement, looking downstairs, and seeing that all the lights were turned off and he couldn't seem to find any of the kids, but a record kept playing over and over and over on the turntable. And that record was "The Tide Is High" by Blondie.

Because I just *had* to tell Debbie the album version of this story, and have another drink, I ended up leaving late for the airport and was in a rush when I got to LAX.

I was also nervous because I had to give a big controversial speech the morning after I flew back, as Providence struggled with the aftermath of a racially explosive incident. An off-duty African-American police sergeant was shot to death while trying to break up a fight at a diner, by two white police officers who mistook him for one of the armed suspects (even though he had been in the same academy class with one of the officers).

As if that wasn't horrible and combustible enough, the victim, Sergeant Cornel Young Jr., was well-known in the department. He was the oldest child of Major Cornel Young Sr., who had been the first African-American elevated to detective in the Providence police department—over the objection of some in the Fraternal Order of Police who felt he was being promoted prematurely because of race—and was now the highest-ranking African-American on the force. The shooting had taken place over two months before, but it was still unclear what would happen to the police officers and who should handle the investigation. Just before heading to LA, I had met with Young's mother and members of the local clergy, and told them I would report back to the community after speaking to national leaders interested in the situation, including the Congressional Black Caucus and the Civil Rights Division of the Justice Department.

With all this on my mind, I found a cab outside the Oscar party, arrived at LAX jumpy and still pretty drunk. And when I tried to hurry with my bag through the X-ray, they insisted it was too big to go through the machine and I needed to check it. I tried to explain that if I did that I would miss my flight and I had to be back in Rhode Island for congressional business—and I'm sure, in retrospect, I was being pretty obnoxious about all this. But the guard, a fifty-eight-year-old woman, said, "I don't care"—and why should she? She worked at LAX and I'm sure a lot of people tried to pull that "don't you know who I am" thing with her. And I just lost it. I tried flashing my congressional ID; I tried to stuff my bag through the X-ray and keep walking through, hoping that if it went through I could just pick it up and not argue with her and proceed to the gate.

This was before 9/11, so security wasn't exactly what it is today. But when I tried to force my way through the screening, she went to body-block me, and we both bounced into each other and almost fell over. Then I tried to push her away. Even though I was drunk and not in my right mind, there is no excuse for any of this behavior.

Suddenly I had a moment of clarity that this was going to be a disaster, that it would be on all the security cameras. This panicky feeling sobered me up for a second and I pulled out the bag, resigned myself to missing the flight, ran over to the check-in counter to check the bag, came back, and tried to apologize profusely to her.

I even gave her my card, which was probably an intoxicated mistake. But, at the time, I was certain I had made the situation right. I ran to make the flight—which I did make with minutes to spare—and as I sat down on the plane, I was convinced that I had beaten it, that I had talked my way out of it.

I got home, showered, and changed clothes and then immediately went to the Congdon Street Baptist Church in Providence, where the community was awaiting word about whether the Department of Justice would get involved in the shooting investigation and what Congressman John Lewis and others in the Black Caucus had advised. Politically, this was a situation where I had no choice but to either really anger the police union or really anger my African-American constituents. There was no middle ground. I followed my heart and focused on the needs of the Young family, and the concerns in the black community that there was racism involved in this shooting and there might need to be a special prosecutor.

While I would make that same choice again today, I probably could have tempered my remarks at the church, where I did get a little carried away. What I said from that pulpit was extremely well received in the black community and by the press. But I deliberately called out the police and incensed them by referring to Sergeant Young as having been "gunned down," and generally just saying things that played well in the church.

That day, I lost the police union's endorsement in about ten seconds—not just locally but nationally.

As FOR THE LAX INCIDENT, I completely forgot about it until more than a week later, when I heard the *National Enquirer* was doing a story about it. The guard was reportedly paid by the *Enquirer* to tell her story, after which she filed a report with the LAPD.

The whole incident did not slow me down—although perhaps it should have. And we returned to trying to win back the House—and doing everything we could to help with the efforts to win the Senate and elect another Democratic President.

I wanted Al Gore to win for reasons beyond just holding the White House for the party. I was convinced that he and Tipper had a uniquely strong and deep commitment to mental healthcare reform and brain disease research. Perhaps more important, they saw mental health as a stand-alone mission and not just part of more global healthcare reform. In May of 2000, Al and Tipper Gore doubled down on mental health, announcing an even more ambitious plan to spend $2.5 billion over ten years to make sure Americans had complete mental health parity. Their proposal was especially focused on parity for children's care and making sure that those disabled by mental illness had the same protections as everyone else with a disability.

While I don't want to oversell what the Gores might have been able to accomplish, I still imagine what might have happened if a couple this committed to mental health, addiction, and neuroscience had made it to the Oval Office.

In June, there was a one-year anniversary celebration of the White House Conference on Mental Health, which Tipper used to announce the launch of the National Mental Health Awareness Campaign. She sent me a very kind note that day, thanking me for my "deep commitment to mental health issues." It reminded me that unlike the year before at the conference, when I was mostly seen as just another interested Congressman, I was now being invited into the small group of Washington insiders who were openly and passionately interested in the politics of mental health.

I remember this as a time that seemed full of incredible promise for mental health. And, for me, this period was infused by the competing dramas of my two full-time jobs—as Congressman and DCCC chair—and my recent experience "coming out" with my depression, combined with my overwhelming obfuscation of what was really going on with me medically.

Most people come out with their mental illness or addiction when they are in recovery, when they are relatively well. It would have been reasonable for people close to me to assume that I wouldn't have come out if that weren't true. But, of course, it wasn't.

In a way, you could say that I came out part of the way to get everyone off my back—enough that if, say, I got into a scuffle with an airport security guard, that might be blamed on my depression without anyone's asking if I had been drunk. Gaming the system this way also could minimize the surprise the next time I got in trouble—which happened in July at Cape Cod.

One of the tricks I used to keep myself from drinking during my time with the DCCC was to fantasize about the few times when I wouldn't have to work, when it might be safe to let loose. The biggest of these opportunities was the week at the end of July when the Republicans had their national convention in Philadelphia—that's when I could take time off. I rented a forty-two-foot sailboat and planned to go sailing around Cape Cod.

I was really looking forward to getting away because I was, in the weeks prior to the break, under the microscope even more than usual. A political science professor at Brown, Darrell West, had given himself the thankless job of writing a completely unauthorized biography of me for an educational press. *Patrick Kennedy: The Rise to Power* featured a cover of me looking about twelve years old being interviewed in front of my first congressional campaign office. The experience of having a book written about me at such an absurdly young age—I was just about to turn thirty-three—was pretty strange. And, luckily, there was nothing about me in the book that was terribly controversial, although it did include a number of very funny quotes, some of the best from my mom. (When asked about the difference between campaigning for me and for my dad, she reportedly shot back, "Patrick says thank you.")

The day before I left, we held a big "Team 2000" clambake at our family house in Hyannis Port for about 450 big Democratic donors, featuring President Clinton. It was a nice send-off for my vacation.

The sailing trip didn't start well—the boat out of Mystic, Connecticut, was not ready when I arrived with my date, so we had to wait overnight before we could sail. That first day we got as far as Fisher's Island, where we anchored in a cove and then rowed a little dinghy in to have dinner at the Pequot Inn. I had way too much to drink—it was the first night I was actually free to drink in public in over eighteen months—and I met up with some friends there, which led to a big argument with my date. We were still arguing when we left a little after eleven P.M. and she decided to take the dinghy out to the boat herself. I stayed at the inn and continued to drink, figuring someone else would give me a ride out to the boat or I could just swim.

When I swam back to the boat several hours later, the dinghy was there and she wasn't. It was two in the morning and I was scared to death, imagining she had fallen off the boat. I didn't really know what to do; my head was spinning because every reason I could think of why she wasn't there was beyond comprehension.

After what seemed like an interminable amount of time, suddenly floodlights illuminated my boat and a big Coast Guard cutter was approaching, calling out to me on its PA system, "Congressman Kennedy, are you all right?"

When the Coast Guard boarded the boat, they proceeded to tell this wild story about how my date hadn't been able to turn on the lights when she got back to the boat, so she got worried and called an ex-boyfriend in Florida for help, and then he called the Coast Guard, suggesting she was in some kind of danger. They had actually sent the station's forty-one-foot rescue boat from the New London Coast Guard station, a half hour away, to come pick her up, and found her waiting on the deck with her bag packed. Later, back at New London, while waiting for a ride back to Boston, she suggested to the Coast Guard that there was some concern for my safety—I might be swimming drunk back to the boat. So at two thirty in the morning, the rescue boat was sent back. When they saw I was fine, they turned around and went back to New London.

And so ended the first day of my relaxing vacation.

Some friends joined me on the boat the next day, and I continued my vacation. There were some problems with the boat: it leaked, the engine had some issues, and it needed to be towed twice. Plus, I'm sure my friends and I partying probably didn't make the situation any bet-

ter. At the end of the week we left the boat—which we had not bothered to tidy up—anchored near Martha's Vineyard.

The boat rental company was mad at me. I was mad at them. I'm
sure they could have rented me a better boat, and I'm sure I could have
taken better care of the boat if I had been taking better care of myself.

I was just glad the whole incident was being kept quiet. My chief
of staff, Tony Marcella, was taking care of it. Tony had developed into
an extremely resourceful guy who was very adept at filling in the missing pieces of my life so that I could function. He often had to stand in
for me, speak for me, and in this case he could do so with firsthand
information about the situation—he had been one of the friends who
joined me on that boat for a week after my date left.

Tony had gotten me out of many jams worse than this one before. I
assumed he would figure out how to make it go away.

I HAD BEEN GOING to the Democratic National Convention for as
long as I could remember. But this was the first time I ever went as
a Democratic leader myself and not just Ted Kennedy's kid. The convention was being held in Los Angeles for the first time since my Uncle
Jack was nominated there in 1960, so it was an especially good year to
double down on the party connection with my family. We were all trying to do whatever it took to get Al Gore elected and hold the White
House; I had been dragging President Clinton to so many events over
the summer that he said, only half-jokingly, that he was campaigning
harder that year than he ever had for his own presidency (of course, he
was also campaigning for Hillary for Senate).

This year, my cousin Caroline was going to introduce my dad, as
her brother had previously, during his prime-time address. And, for
the first time, I was invited to give a speech—on opening day before
the live network coverage began, but still a great opportunity. I had

it all prepared—everything has to be on the teleprompter at the convention—but I decided while driving there in the van to rewrite it, so I could try to get some kind of call-and-response going at the end.

As we were pulling into the convention center, I still had the typescript balanced on my thigh, scribbling and crossing things out. The security team radioed ahead that I was in the building, referring to me by my party call sign, which was "Blue Jay"—because Leader Gephardt was "Cardinal," since he was from St. Louis.

I got onto the stage, and as I had hoped, the call-and-response got the attention of enough people that you could hear "With the Democrats, we *can* and we *will*" above the constant murmur of the crowd. When the day was over, security took the leadership back to the hotel, and you could hear them on the radio saying, "Taking Cardinal back to the nest but Blue Jay wants to go out and fly some more." They were right about that.

ONLY WEEKS AFTER THE CONVENTION, my mom suffered a major relapse. She had up-and-down periods over the previous eight years. Like many of us struggling with addictions, just when things begin to look promising, we sometimes sabotage ourselves. (Although I do sometimes wonder about this blaming language we use for "relapses" and "sabotage." If these are chronic illnesses, why not blame the illness for recurring and act less surprised when it does?) One of her upswings had been highlighted recently—perhaps a little too optimistically—in a big *Boston Globe Magazine* story about her. So it was particularly heartbreaking when, on a Sunday night in September, police got a call from a motorist following her blue Buick, which was reportedly swerving on the highway in Marstons Mills, not far from Hyannis. When police arrived, she would only give her first name, refused to show them her driver's license, and admitted having had wine.

While the reasons for any relapse are very complicated and very personal—I wouldn't pretend to understand my mom's any more than she would mine—I'm sure it didn't help that NBC was making a four-part miniseries called *Jackie, Ethel, Joan: The Women of Camelot*, which was based on a particularly salacious book and was known to feature a dramatization of my parents' marriage and divorce.

We got her back into treatment immediately and tried to push her court date back as far as we could—so it actually got scheduled for the morning of Election Day.

To add to the pressure, several days before the election, the charter boat company I was still arguing with about damages decided to "publicly threaten" to sue me.

After two years of raising a record $100 million to try to win the House, this was not how I had envisioned spending November 7, 2000—walking with my mom to the polls as reporters asked her to comment on her drunk-driving sentence and me to comment on my boating skills.

I guess I should have known with these harbingers that the election wasn't going to go as planned. Though the House remained under GOP control, we did manage to retain all the seats where incumbent Democrats hadn't run again, and picked up two other seats from the Republicans. Both my dad and I were reelected. As for the White House, that drama was going to drag on for weeks to come.

EVEN THOUGH I HAD DONE what the DCCC asked and broke every Democratic congressional fund-raising record, I was devastated that we failed to win back the House. And I decided right then that I needed a new mission. I needed to commit myself to an issue that was bigger than politics for me, an issue that would carry me into the new millennium, an issue where I could make a difference—not just as a Kennedy, but as me.

I talked to Dick Gephardt and told him I hoped to become the leading Democratic voice on mental health issues—and wanted to use the seat I was about to take on the Appropriations Committee to make a difference on mental illness and addiction. I also told this to the top political columnist at the *Providence Journal*, so all my constituents would know what I planned.

Of course, what I didn't tell them was how much I needed help with my own illness. With Election Day behind me, and the fear of being caught drinking lessened, I started letting loose. And as the press kept digging further into its coverage of my embarrassing boating excursion, things just got worse.

Several weeks later, I found myself on Air Force One again, accompanying President Clinton on his last trip in office, to Ireland, along with a large delegation that included Hillary, who had been elected Senator; my Aunt Jean Kennedy Smith, the former ambassador to Ireland; and my friend Senator Chris Dodd.

The trip took place at an important and infamous moment in the history of American politics. The day we left, the Supreme Court heard arguments in *Bush v. Gore*, the case that would determine the next President, and a lot about the presidency, by interpreting the dimpled chads of the Florida election. That morning, I had appeared in Palm Beach at a Democratic news conference at the Rose Garden—named after my grandmother—at the County Government Center, along with former Ohio Senator Howard Metzenbaum and two local Democrats who had been active in the recount controversy. I flew back to DC in time to be on Air Force One for the early evening departure, and we had a pretty good idea that by the time we reached Ireland, the Supreme Court would be about to rule.

So the atmosphere on the plane that evening was pretty charged. There was a lot of emotion and frivolity on that plane, and a lot of drinks being served. I was pounding rum and Cokes, and Jack and Cokes, while Martin O'Malley, then mayor of Baltimore, serenaded us with his guitar.

And I remember, somewhere just before landing in Shannon, I was in the Air Force One bathroom again. This time, I was throwing up.

Of course, I spent the next day with a splitting headache and feeling miserable, not at all enjoying what was an extraordinarily historic trip—the biggest official American trip to Ireland since my Uncle Jack went there in '63. And I was just nursing my wounds for the rest of the trip. I felt humiliated once I sobered up and realized that I probably had made an ass out of myself. People were probably talking privately about how out of control I was. But no one said a word to me.

That is, ultimately, one of the biggest and most constantly surprising and challenging problems concerning these illnesses, how so many people know what's going on but never say a word—because we don't know how, and we don't know if we should. That said, it was nobody's fault but my own that I wasn't taking care of myself.

Looking back, I can see this as the time where I was becoming just one more Washington politician with a mental health or substance use problem that needed to be navigated. There have always been senators and congressmen who people knew not to schedule meetings with early in the morning or late in the day, depending on the cycles of their illness. This doesn't happen just on Capitol Hill, of course, it happens at companies large and small and in families close and separated. It is one more way that these illnesses, already isolating because the brain isn't working quite properly and people aren't connecting quite normally, become even more isolating.

It also allows people like thirty-three-year-old me to tell ourselves the lie that we are doing fine and brilliantly hiding what is really going on.

Most people think they are hiding things much more brilliantly than they actually are. It is the things that everyone knows but can't acknowledge, the things hidden in plain sight, that can really hurt us. And that's especially sad because these are often the things that could really be treated if we spoke about them.

People often talk about "denial" like it's a passive thing, a path of least resistance. Denial is actually really aggressive. It's hard work. And I was doing quite a lot of it.

Chapter 15

A s 2001 began, I stepped down from the DCCC and stepped up to my position on the House Appropriations Committee, where I was placed on two important subcommittees: "Labor-H," which included everything under health, education, and labor; and CJS, which covered science, criminal justice, and commerce. This meant I'd be voting on the budgets for the Centers for Medicare & Medicaid Services (CMS), the Substance Abuse and Mental Health Services Administration (SAMHSA), and the entire Department of Health and Human Services (HHS), as well as the scientific budgets for NIH, NIMH, NIDA, and NIAAA, and the budget for the Department of Justice (DOJ), which included the Drug Enforcement Administration (DEA).

Combined, these budgets controlled pretty much every constituency and stakeholder affecting the wide world of brain disease. While I had been interacting with parts of these communities for years, this was the first time they would be actively lobbying me on budget matters. So we were all about to get to know each other much better.

Mostly, we were adjusting to the roller-coaster ride of the DCCC finally being over, the election being decided by the Supreme Court in December for George W. Bush.

Just weeks after he took office, President Bush made a point of inviting my family—including my father and Vicki; my cousin Kathleen Kennedy Townsend, the Lieutenant Governor of Maryland; and me—over to the White House for dinner and a screening of a new movie, *Thirteen Days*, about the Cuban Missile Crisis.

We ate ribs, cheeseburgers, and baked beans with the new First Family and did everything we could not to bring up the recent disputed election or what had happened earlier that very day—the controversial confirmation of John Ashcroft as Attorney General. President Bush was trying to mend fences, and it was time for me to step up and be a new member of the House Appropriations Committee. So I was respectful and, at the appropriate time, told him that I hoped I could count on him to support programs for mental health.

NOW THAT I WASN'T on the road for the DCCC, I was able to get back into a more normal life in Washington—which included weekly lunches with my father. We tried to make sure our staffs arranged for a time, usually on Wednesdays, when we could have lunch in his Senate "hideaway." Hideaways were private office spaces in the Capitol building that were given to senior senators, separate from the large public offices where they and their staff usually worked. My father had one of the most coveted hideaways, on the third floor of the Capitol, with gorgeous vaulted ceilings and amazing windows that overlooked the Mall, the Washington Monument, and the Lincoln Memorial. The carpets and walls were sea green, and the sitting area in front of the big white fireplace was organized around a long table made from a big piece of the rudder that had to be replaced on his wooden sailboat. While the room had comfy upholstered white wingback chairs, we usually ate in the sunny alcove at a round wooden table with smaller wooden armchairs, facing each other.

The hideaways had room service; we ordered from the kitchen, which was on the basement level, and food was brought up in an elevator. We always had soup, and then a sandwich or an entrée. My father was trying to take better care of himself—and his staff was under strict orders from Vicki to make sure he did. (This was one of the many ways Vicki helped him live a much healthier life.) So he would order a piece of chicken with no sauce, steamed vegetables, a protein shake, and some cottage cheese or slices of fruit. It killed him not to be able to have mayonnaise—he loved the mayonnaise. Of course, I would get a sandwich with mayo and french fries with ketchup. He would do his best to resist. And then I'd get a big tasty dessert, three scoops of ice cream and chocolate sauce, and when it arrived he would always laugh, and then break down and steal a scoop of it.

We would mostly talk about what was going on in the House and Senate, and sometimes a little gossip about the family. Those were such intimate times, the soft banter back and forth. On one level it seemed superficial, but I now see the connection we had while talking about superficial things, the little inflections and the body language that I just soaked up.

Honestly, I appreciate it more now that he's gone than I did then. Because back then, I read way too much into every little thing said and not said. But what I really wanted was for my father to come out and ask me how I *really* was: how are you really feeling, are you drinking at all, how's your love life, are you making enough time for yourself, all the things I couldn't tell anybody I was really worried about, obsessed with. I would go to therapy and talk about what my father and I never talked about—not that I was in any way working it through in therapy or getting any real insight into my problems or adjusting my perspectives. I was just complaining.

I've spent my whole life trying to unwind all of that, so I could understand why I felt so emotionally bounced around between my manic devotion to him and the way I could feel so absolutely dejected around him.

I had a lot invested in each glance, each stolen french fry or scoop of ice cream.

Since my dad was equally unable to express these feelings, Vicki tried to help. I started getting notes from her. When I did something good in public or on the House floor, invariably she would send a handwritten, hand-delivered note saying how proud my father and she were of me. But since the notes came from her, I was never sure how to interpret them—because I had never been married and just didn't understand the role spouses can play between family members who aren't great at communicating. Now that I'm happily married and understand the things Amy handles for us emotionally, as a couple, those notes make more sense. But at the time, they often felt like just one more layer of miscommunication between me and my father. One more thing about our relationship to obsess over.

So it was best to just eat our lunch and gossip about politics, which was—as I realized way too late—our form of intimacy.

THE 1996 MENTAL HEALTH PARITY ACT—which had not really created much in the way of parity itself but had inspired many states to create much better laws—was due to expire at the end of September of 2001. Over the past few years, there had been Senate and House attempts to improve and extend it—efforts to broaden its care for children, to extend its parity coverage to include addiction—but none of them had gotten any traction. So on March 15, 2001, Senators Wellstone and Domenici introduced a new version of it, Senate Bill 543, which required full parity for all *DSM* diagnoses, and we waited in the House for the Senate to hold hearings.

In the meantime, I held a four-hour public hearing in Providence at the State House with Surgeon General Dr. David Satcher, to try to raise awareness about the specific issues of children's mental health— the lack of proper funding for their care, and the inability of parents and schools to properly monitor early symptoms and commit to prevention and early treatment.

It was a challenge to get public and political attention to these issues. The press was mostly paying attention to my poll numbers, which had started to sag, and the ongoing legal struggle over my boat fiasco—even after I tried to take some wind out of their sails by poking fun at it, and myself, at the *Providence Journal* Follies, the annual get-together of Rhode Island press and politicians. (I arrived, late in the evening, as a surprise guest, dressed in a sailor's outfit and singing "Patrick the Sailor Man" to the tune of the old Popeye TV show theme.)

In April, I decided to make major changes in my team, relieving Tony Marcella as chief of staff in Washington and also replacing the manager of my congressional office in Rhode Island. This move was primarily about politics and poll numbers, confronting the inevitable backlash after I'd spent most of the previous two years away from home and in full attack mode against the Republicans. But those who knew Tony and me well understood there was a personal aspect to this that involved our mental health.

Tony and I had grown up together in politics, and he was my friend as well as my chief of staff. We had shared an apartment together; we had been in the political bunker together and had developed an unhealthy codependence.

His job was to be my protector. But while he liked crisis management and was good at it, sometimes we found ourselves in the center of storms we helped create. He had the ability to power through his hangovers better than me, while I would be in the back of the car trying to get it together to go to the next event. But, eventually, we spiraled out of control.

Some close to us might have described Tony as my enabler, but that sounds like I'm not taking responsibility for what I did, what I drank, what I took. And, honestly, neither of us really understood what we were doing and why. It took me years to see our behavior for what it was: addiction and self-medicating. At the time, I viewed Tony as something of a hypochondriac. He said he suffered from bad pain and some kind of nerve problems, which I wasn't sure I believed—even though, of course, I was saying the same thing. It was true I had my back issues, but also true I was exaggerating to get more medication than I needed. And when I decided to replace Tony as my chief of staff, it was very difficult but, I felt, necessary.

Several years later, I was stunned to find out that he had been diagnosed with amyotrophic lateral sclerosis (ALS), or "Lou Gehrig's disease." Many of the symptoms he had been complaining about—and presumably relieving through self-medication—were consistent with the early stages of that illness.

So he wasn't exaggerating. And I tell this story to remind myself and others of how easy it is to be judgmental of the medical complaints of others—especially those describing pain caused by something that isn't as easy to see as a wound or a broken leg.

BESIDES REPLACING my chief of staff in DC and my office manager in Rhode Island, I also brought back political consultant David Axelrod, who had helped me years before during my first run for Congress, and I enlisted a new polling team. We did a lot of focus groups and polling over the next months, and while I was not surprised that some voters considered some of my behavior immature and not particularly Congress-worthy, many of them described their feelings with an intriguing form of cautious optimism: they seemed to agree with me politically, and they hoped I would grow up. Even when they completely disagreed with me on something, they didn't hate me, they just thought I needed to grow up.

This is, in retrospect, the way I saw myself during this time. And I feel extremely fortunate that, somehow, people generally were willing to give me the benefit of the doubt. They assumed I wasn't such a bad guy; I was well-intentioned, just a little out of control sometimes.

Since I was publicly committing myself to be a leading voice in the politics of mental health, it was welcome news to see that this position polled really well. Voters were pleased that I was taking on mental illness and addiction—healthcare issues generally scored well, but mental health especially so. And even the voters who saw me as temperamental and immature were supportive of my being open about my treatment for depression.

In Washington my higher profile and new role at Appropriations meant diving into the very complex world of brain disease lobbying. This meant figuring out who was who, and who wanted what from budgets, and also who would support what for proposed laws.

With my new staff and expanded agenda, we were also writing and proposing more legislation. Our first major mental health bill, introduced in the summer of 2001, was the Foundations for Learning Act, which had thirty-seven other House cosponsors. It was a bill to establish a grant program to improve the mental and emotional health of schoolchildren by having money available for screening and treatment of at-risk kids and their parents. While it didn't initially get much traction beyond the House Education Committee, my father, who was managing the conference committee for President Bush's controversial No Child Left Behind law, got it added to that bill. So my first-ever piece of passed legislation can be found buried in subpart 14, section 5542, "Promotion of School Readiness Through Early Childhood Emotional and Social Development."

In the summer, the Senate Health, Education, Labor and Pensions (HELP) Committee held a hearing on mental health parity and ended up approving another watered-down version of parity, no stronger than the one before.

As we waited to see what would happen on both proposals, 9/11 brought life in America to a standstill.

In mental health politics, two things happened after 9/11. Our ideas about post-traumatic stress disorders were completely challenged, and clinical belief in this once-controversial diagnosis was much expanded, because now there were thousands of New Yorkers and Washingtonians who had, simultaneously, been through an incredibly traumatic experience, the existence of which could not be challenged.

Also, mental healthcare suddenly became a much bigger defense issue. It was the first time most Americans really understood how terrorism could be a psychological weapon of war and why mental health preparedness could be essential to national security. As the new department was added to the government, it became a "homeland security" issue, and when we later went to war in Iraq and Afghanistan, it grew even larger as a combat and veteran health issue.

At the time, however, we were really all just trying to recover our senses. Several weeks after 9/11, a letter containing anthrax was delivered to Senator Tom Daschle's office in Washington, setting off fear throughout every political office in the country. That same day, a secretary in my Pawtucket, Rhode Island, office discovered she had a rash and worried it might have been linked to a letter she had opened from

India that was supportive of US policy but did mention Osama bin Laden. Although it turned out later not to be anthrax, nine members of my Rhode Island staff went to hospitals to be examined and tested.

SADLY, THIS UNPRECEDENTED CHALLENGE to the nation's mental health did not result in any bipartisan support for better care. The original Mental Health Parity Act expired on the last day of the month 9/11 had taken place. The Congress didn't start to seriously discuss how it would be replaced until early December. This was the first of the parity debates in which I was prominently involved.

The major issues hadn't changed. Business lobbyists were still insisting they could never support a mental health parity law that could increase the cost of the nation's healthcare by their magic "1 percent" threshold.

I personally felt this was a false issue. The way that experts calculated this theoretical 1 percent increase was open to massive interpretation, used by those groups that could most afford lobbyists to argue that ending discrimination against diseases of the brain was too expensive.

I also felt that if it raised the costs over 1 percent, that was a small price to pay for the exponential improvement in Americans' quality of life and, for businesses, a dramatic decrease in the number of days lost to illness. It was a healthcare expenditure that would ultimately save lives and money.

The other issue was whether substance use disorder treatment would be included in parity. I believed in full parity for mental illness and addiction, and stood firmly on this point with my Senate friend Paul Wellstone. And, just as he had in 1996, Wellstone's Senate cosponsor, Pete Domenici—as well as a lot of other senators interested in healthcare, including my father—refused to include substance use disorders in parity and wanted only the most "serious" mental illnesses fully covered. It was mental health parity déjà vu all over again.

Domenici's position was supported—politically at least, because it seemed to have the best chance to win in a Republican-controlled government—by a powerful lobbying organization called the Coalition for Fairness in Mental Illness Coverage. It was a group whose members actually disagreed about a number of things and often lobbied against each other. Among the caregivers, the Coalition for Fairness spoke for the American Medical Association, the American Psychiatric Association, and the American Psychological Association; among the treatment facility and insurance community it spoke for the American Hospital Association, the Federation of American Hospitals, the National Association of Psychiatric Health Systems, and the American Managed Behavioral Healthcare Association; among the patient advocacy groups, it spoke for the National Alliance on Mental Illness and the National Mental Health Association—which is now called Mental Health America.

That was an awful lot of lobbying money and muscle to bring together to *oppose* full mental health parity. Especially since most of these people personally favored full parity. But they were all hedging their bets. They were so worried about what might not be politically possible that they were willing to side with an effort that could actually limit parity and *increase* stigma.

The Senate had attached a version of mental health parity, with no exemption based on its cost, to the bill that would fund the upcoming year of the Department of Health and Human Services. The House had not attached parity to its version of that funding bill, so we went into my first conference committee on mental health parity.

My colleague Nancy Johnson, Republican from Connecticut and chair of the House Ways and Means Health Subcommittee, proposed capping parity at a 1 percent rise in expenditures—although she said her experience with companies that had voluntarily adopted parity was that it never cost anything near that. Paul Wellstone and Pete Domenici wanted a threshold over 1 percent—and I was pushing for a threshold of 2 percent. Most of my Republican House colleagues were against the entire idea because they considered it anti-business, and those who modestly favored it were afraid of the costs. Republican Speaker Dennis Hastert proposed a novel way to block the legislation, claiming it shouldn't be attached to the funding bill at hand but instead needed the approval of three separate House committees—and, what a coincidence, the Republican chairs of each of these committees had written letters opposing it.

I worked as hard as I could in the House to get some parity traction. I failed.

Two weeks later, mental health parity died. It happened because my House colleagues on the conference committee voted along their exact strict party lines (a reminder of why I had spent the past two years fighting for a Democratic majority).

It was the beginning of my career as what the *Providence Journal* called "a legislative journeyman specializing in mental health issues . . . reconciled . . . to modest goals: a chunk of money for a local treatment program, an uncredited paragraph in someone else's bill, and a standby role promoting the mental-health lobby's long-shot priority of better health-insurance coverage. Plus, the less tangible attainment of giving voice to a needy constituency and gradually earning a name for that effort."

The life of a true Washington insider. Slow and steady, and a tiny glimmer of hope of actually winning the race.

Chapter 16

My dad turned seventy in February of 2002. Besides the usual big parties, he sent me, Teddy, and Kara a letter explaining, in detail, his estate planning. While it was useful to know what he had arranged for us, more important was that it explained more about how he had done his best to do right by my mother, who was really struggling with her alcoholism and depression again.

The letter ended, "Each of you has given me great pride, joy and love. If good fortune should be ours, I will live many more years to share that love with you."

I WAS DOING MY BEST to be a day-to-day Congressman and keep my mental health in check with a minimum of self-medicating beyond what I was prescribed. I also had new staff, and with an election coming—one thing about the House, every other year there's an election coming—we were focusing on constituent services and local issues ahead of what was predicted to be a tighter race for my seat than I'd ever had before.

In late April, President Bush came out and said he favored mental health parity—although he was very sketchy on how he planned to solve the Republican roadblock of cost. He impaneled what he called the New Freedom Commission on Mental Health, which was part of the New Freedom Initiative he had announced just after taking office, with the goal of improving the lives of all Americans with disabilities. He announced this new effort at the University of New Mexico, where he was appearing with Pete Domenici, and focused on the themes of ending stigma and fixing the fragmented system of mental healthcare delivery and unfair disparities in mental health insurance coverage. So it was clear that the New Freedom Commission was likely to address parity in the more limited, Republican fashion— or, to be fair, in a fashion that had any chance of being passed by a Republican majority.

Still, it was great to see another president speak publicly about mental health. And several weeks later, to punctuate the point, we held a "Parity Now!" rally on the West Lawn of the Capitol, where Senators Wellstone and Domenici appeared with me and my Republican House colleague Marge Roukema. It was one of Marge's last appearances on behalf of the issue she had spent so much time supporting, because she had decided not to run again for her seat.

In the fall, we were all involved in yet another round of parity law discussions likely to go nowhere. My local election was looking more promising after I had taken on a new chief of staff, Sean Richardson, a former member of Tom Daschle's leadership staff. But the big national news involved congressional hand-wringing over whether or not to authorize President Bush to go to war with Iraq.

My father broke ranks with the majority of Senate Democrats and voted against the authorization. I was perceived as breaking ranks with my father when I voted for it.

AND THEN, JUST A WEEK or two after that vote, after lunchtime on a Friday afternoon, came the horrible news: Paul Wellstone had been killed in a plane crash, along with his wife and daughter. They were on a short campaign ride from Minneapolis to Eveleth, Minnesota, and the twin-engine Beechcraft King Air A100 crashed in a swamp a quarter mile from the runway. The three of them had died on impact, along with all five others in the plane.

This was a stunning tragedy for so many reasons, but it was especially poignant to lose the most liberal member of the Senate at the age of fifty-eight at a time when every Democratic vote was so desperately needed. In the worlds of mental health and addiction—which were still very much divided politically—Wellstone had been the most powerful figure in government who insisted there could be no true mental health parity, no true end to the discrimination, unless addiction care was included.

For a decade in the Senate, he had been saving up chits for the day when he could call them all in and get the parity bill he wanted.

Suddenly, in an instant, he was gone.

We were all heartbroken. Paul was my neighbor and my friend; I loved him and we shared a passion for this cause. I wanted to do everything I could to continue his work on parity.

Besides mourning his loss, we had an immediate political problem: he couldn't remain on the ballot, and his seat was crucial to maintaining the very close party balance in the Senate. He had already been in a very close race, made closer by voting against the Iraq War. Former VP Walter Mondale was quickly put into Wellstone's spot on the ballot, but he ended up losing to a Republican challenger, which gave the GOP a clear majority in the Senate.

The Democrats actually lost four seats in the House in that 2002 election. I kept my seat, but we were worse off than before. Dick Gephardt decided not to run again for Minority Leader (and later not to run again for his seat), so we elevated Minority Whip Nancy Pelosi, making her the first woman to ever lead a major party in Congress.

Nancy was a strong, smart San Francisco liberal with a unique emotional presence not usually found at the highest levels of Washington—I hesitate to use the term "maternal" because she was that but so much more. She was a leader in the old-school tradition of really taking care of her members. She had kids my age and, like any prominent progressive of her era, had watched me grow up—actually, she was still watching me try to grow up—in politics.

I had first met her when I was only nine or ten. I was sent on a summer trip to California with a bunch of my classmates, and we arranged to stay in people's homes. Since I was allergic to almost everything, and my dad knew that the Pelosi house was smoke-free and pet-free, he asked if she would be willing to put me up, along with a few other kids. We pretty much went wild there, and I started a water fight in their elegant home, just barely missing all their wonderful art and other memorabilia. (Nancy always claimed she forgave me.) I had gotten to know her better during my time at the DCCC and while serving with her on Appropriations. Now she was the new boss.

OVER THAT CHRISTMAS, we found out that my sister, Kara, then forty-two, had lung cancer. It was a particularly challenging form of the cancer, so she; her husband, Michael; and their two young children, my niece and nephew Grace and Max, were facing quite a trial in the new year: ambitious surgery and then a course of chemotherapy. Just as my brother had, Kara went from Washington to Boston for all this care, making regular trips up to get her chemo at Dana Farber. Both treatments, thank God, were successful.

My mom's health, however, was getting worse and worse. She was now in her midsixties, a time that for some with addictions or mental illnesses can be associated with a lessening of symptoms as the body starts slowing down. But her drinking, depression, and anxiety were so advanced that while Kara was still recovering from cancer treatments, she, Teddy, and I were discussing the stunning possibility that we might have to take over our mother's medical care ourselves and become her legal guardians.

Over the next year, Mom was hospitalized for alcohol-related issues five different times in the inpatient unit at Mass General. During the last hospitalization, the caregivers at the hospital suggested we try something that was becoming popular in mental health and addiction care—a family contract, in which Mom acknowledged in writing her alcoholism and depression and the need for proper treatment to prevent a relapse. In this case, the contract was created as a precursor to what we felt needed to happen if inpatient treatment failed again: my brother, Teddy, would become her temporary guardian, and we would develop both a medical plan and an estate plan, so nobody could take financial advantage of my mom.

These legal matters are a part of the care of mental illness and substance use disorders that most people know little about. I know I didn't. The guardianships themselves were part of the family court system in each state. But before families reached this extreme point, there were a growing number of mental health courts in each state—and a variety of cities—that oversaw everything from involuntary inpatient commitments to court-ordered outpatient treatment with medicine (called "assisted outpatient treatment" or "outpatient commitment"). The mental health court system had been growing since 2000, when

Congress expanded funding for it with the America's Law Enforcement and Mental Health Project act. Sponsored by Republican Senator Mike DeWine from Ohio, the law helped deal with the exploding problem of mental illness in prison and the 25 to 40 percent of all Americans with mental illness who had some interaction with the criminal justice system. (I was involved in the funding of these mental health courts—as well as drug courts and veterans' courts—as part of my duties serving on the Justice Appropriations.) As my mother's case was being heard, a second mental health judicial bill, the Mentally Ill Offender Treatment and Crime Reduction Act, was on its way to approval.

Mom agreed that after being discharged from the hospital, she would go to the Hanley-Hazelden treatment center in West Palm Beach and complete the twenty-eight-day program there. Then we would speak again. But when she returned, nothing had improved. So the next step was getting a statement from her doctor that her illness was so incapacitating that she was incapable of caring for her personal and financial affairs.

I would say this was heartbreaking, but I'm not sure any of us could actually afford to make contact with how we really felt. Even in our lives, this was off any scale.

The doctor wrote that even during her times of sobriety she didn't seem to have enough insight into her illness to appreciate the repercussions of her drinking. He worried about her decision-making processes and her understanding of the consequences of her actions.

I can't imagine what it must have been like for my mom to read this assessment and go through this harsh legal process. And through the history of court-ordered treatment, every family has had to balance the medical need with the real possibility that their loved one will never truly forgive them for the measures required to help save their lives. In the future, perhaps people with mental illnesses and addictions will rely more on advance directives—signed when they are well—so that when court-ordered care is truly needed, they can be reminded it was they who once thought it was a good idea. That would certainly help in some situations. But court-ordered care and medical guardianship are always going to be emotionally scarring. All we can do is acknowledge the scars and try to help heal them.

WHILE BROAD MENTAL HEALTH REFORM was still pretty much on the shelf, there was suddenly a dramatic push in the Senate for new legislation to prevent the epidemic of teen suicides. There had been interest in this area for some time, but it took the personal tragedy of a prominent member of the Senate to actually get action: the suicide of Garrett Lee Smith, the son of Oregon Republican Gordon Smith, on September 8, 2003, the eve of his twenty-second birthday. Garrett had been struggling with bipolar disorder. His parents and sister were aware of the struggle, and he was receiving treatment, which is why his death had been especially devastating.

Six months after Garrett's death, Gordon Smith gave some of the most heart-wrenching testimony ever heard in a Senate committee hearing about his son and his loss. It was so moving and persuasive, on a subject so difficult for the public and politicians, that several of his colleagues decided to take decisive action. They combined two separate bills they were hoping to get through that session—one to increase mental health services for college students, the other to expand youth suicide early intervention and prevention—and named the resulting legislation the Garrett Lee Smith Memorial Act. When the bill came up for a vote on the Senate floor on July 8, 2004, Smith's fellow legislators were so moved by his courage and his open heart that they too shared personal experiences during the debate.

Democratic Senator Harry Reid of Nevada, then Minority Whip, rose and spoke about his father's suicide. While some senators knew he had lost his father this way, some thirty years before, they had never heard him speak so openly about it. He described how, in 1972 when he was Lieutenant Governor, he had been visiting at Muhammad Ali's Nevada training camp, and when he returned to his office his receptionist said his mother was on the phone.

"I picked up the phone," he recalled, and he heard his mother say, "Your pop shot himself." Later he realized that his father had been planning it for a while, and the last time he saw him—a week before—he had given his son one of his prized possessions, an ore specimen from his days as a miner. Reid had first revealed his father's suicide at a hearing for the Senate Special Committee on Aging in the 1990s, moved to reveal his own story after hearing Mike Wallace talk about his experience with depression.

After Reid's moving testimony, his predecessor as Minority Whip, Oklahoma Republican Don Nickles, rose to admit that he had experienced a similar loss, a fact that few of his colleagues knew.

"My father also committed suicide," Nickles said. "I am not going to go into the details, but it is a lot of pain."

The bill, which would appropriate $82 million over three years for prevention and treatment, passed the Senate unanimously and without amendment—no one would dare. And then it was sent on to the House, where equally swift passage was expected.

Several years before, the House had been through a similar tragedy: the seventeen-year-old namesake son of Michigan Democrat Bart Stupak had died of a self-inflicted gunshot wound. House members had chartered a plane to his funeral. In the aftermath, however, Bart had focused his legislative attention less on suicide itself than on a psychiatric adverse drug reaction to an acne medicine, which he believed was the trigger of his son's depression. (There are many common medications—including the top-selling class of antibiotics, the quinolones—that can, in some patients, trigger depression, psychosis, and suicidal ideation; the FDA was already making label changes on the drug, Accutane, that Bart Stupak Jr. had used.)

And, if that wasn't enough to garner support for the Garrett Lee Smith law, less than three weeks after the Senate passed the bill, the sixteen-year-old son of another of our House colleagues, Kansas Republican Todd Tiahrt, took his own life.

That's why I was so amazed when Senator Gordon Smith called me one day in early September, worried about passage of the Garrett Lee Smith Memorial Act in the House and hopeful I could help him. A group of right-wing representatives whom we referred to as the CATs (because they had been called the Conservative Action Team before rebranding as the Republican Study Group) were trying to block the bill by adding all sorts of ideological amendments to it. According to the book he later wrote about his son, *Remembering Garrett*, when Gordon—a conservative-leaning Republican himself—tried to talk to the CATs, he was told, "We don't pass bills over here that Democrats want," and "Preventing suicide is the business of parents and not the federal government." When he tried to explain that the government spent hundreds of millions on "physical health" and it was time to be equally concerned about mental health—something he had personally come to understand "only too painfully and too late"—they just stared at him blankly. And when he told them President Bush had already said he was anxious to sign the bill, they said, "Don't take this personally, it's just politics."

He said, "It's hard not to take it personally when the bill is named after your dead son!"

The CATs' last resort was to add a provision they knew would be a poison pill. They had been attempting for some time to change many school-related programs that had "opt out" clauses for religious objections so that, instead, the law would require every student to "opt in" with parental permission, which would dramatically reduce participation. They believed that if they could get this opt-in clause into *any* education-related law, the precedent could be more broadly used.

Until this could get worked out, Senator Smith wanted my help in keeping the Democrats together on supporting the bill—since, even though the Republicans were in the majority, their split on CATs issues meant our votes would make the difference. If the Democrats helped pass it, he was sure he could get the opt-in amendment removed in conference committee. As it turned out, he couldn't deliver on that, but the conservative Republican chair of the House Energy and Commerce Committee, Joe Barton of Texas, did the next best thing: he changed the opt-in language so it could never apply to any other bill but this one, and created emergency provisions so suicidial students could be treated without being expected to ask their parents to opt-in. We were able to keep the Democratic supporters on board, and the bill was finally passed.

It was one of the most satisfying moments that those of us on the Hill who were interested in mental healthcare had experienced in quite some time.

I WAS NOW in an interesting position in Congress. I was one of the go-to guys on mental health and addiction, but nobody really knew how much I was struggling with my illnesses. Because I had become way too good at it.

I saw a psychiatrist who gave me a cocktail of meds—lithium, Wellbutrin, Lamictal—and listened to me talk about my insecurities, my issues with my parents, and my inability to create lasting relationships; I would tell him when I went on a weekend drinking spree, which happened maybe a dozen times a year, but I didn't admit to all the narcotic painkillers I was getting from other doctors, even the doctors who took care of us in Congress.

Since the 2002 election, my chief of staff, Sean Richardson, had been wondering—more out loud than others who had worked for me—why my behavior was so erratic. Initially he thought I was more young and impulsive than unhealthy, and he suspected that maybe I created situations that got a little out of control because I liked them and thought I could be more effective that way. He knew I liked to "ratchet it up."

In the summer of 2004, my back started hurting more than usual, and I increased my use of any opioid painkiller I could get. They helped with pain, they helped with sleep, and I moved around so much in the summer between DC, Rhode Island, and the Cape that I could always find a doctor who would sympathize with my stories of my prescriptions running out.

By the fall, something had changed. This was noticed first, I suspect, by some of the mental health and addiction lobbyists—many of whom were in treatment or recovery themselves, so they had good brain disease radar—but my staff was also becoming more worried. Finally, one day in the late fall I was home at my apartment for lunch and a package arrived at the office from the Attending Physician at the Capitol. My office manager opened it and Sean, just in passing, asked to see what it was. He looked into the package, assuming it was asthma inhalers or something, and saw it was a bottle of OxyContin. And, for some reason, it was suddenly crystal clear to him what had been going on. He called me at home and said he needed to come speak to me in person, right away.

He arrived, very upset, and started telling a story about an uncle of his who was a heroin addict. The family had convinced his Uncle Joe to go for treatment but there wasn't a bed immediately available and during the wait he ended up killing himself. This experience had really helped shape who Sean had grown up to be, and he still wondered if he could have helped his uncle. So, even though he had no idea if I was going to fire him for saying this, he had to tell me that he thought I was addicted to narcotic painkillers and I needed help. Immediately. And he was going to take care of the details and get me through it.

Honestly, I felt an incredible sense of relief. I just said, "Okay, let's go." He told me to stay in the apartment while he jogged back to the office to talk to my staff, to my personal financial manager, to my dad and Vicki, and to Dr. Larry Horowitz. It was decided that we would not go public with this hospitalization, even though we realized the risk if it later leaked out.

Within twelve hours, I was on a plane to Sierra Tucson in Arizona for a thirty-day "medical evaluation." When I checked in, I gave my name as "Patrick Bennett," using my mother's maiden name, just as she always had in rehab. I even signed my name that way, "Patrick J. Bennett."

After all those years of being afraid of ending up as ill as my mother, here I was.

WHILE I LOOKED PERFECTLY NORMAL when I arrived at Sierra Tucson, within a few hours I began to show signs of opiate withdrawal and soon I was severely depressed.

I began a full testing and treatment regime, and then started group therapy. I was, naturally, concerned about confidentiality in group discussions, since my mother and I had both already been betrayed in the tabloids by people with whom we'd been in treatment. After about five days, I was just too nervous that something was going to leak out about my being there and told them I wanted to continue with an individual psychiatrist, preferably back home in an outpatient setting.

After eight days there, and my growing nervousness about my privacy, they agreed that I could leave, even though I wasn't done detoxing yet. On top of my regular meds, they gave me a prescription for Suboxone, which had only recently been approved in the US after years of use in Europe. Suboxone is a combination of a synthetic opiate, buprenorphine, and a fascinating drug called naloxone, which can immediately reverse the narcotic effects of opiates in the brain (which is why it is, increasingly, used by police and other first responders to save people who have overdosed). Suboxone helps people detox from addiction to opiates and for some patients is a better choice than the traditional methadone. (Methadone is stronger and itself more addictive, and is still preferred for patients with the heaviest addictions to heroin and prescription opiates). When I was done with the Suboxone I could take naltrexone, an older medication used to prevent opiate dependence (or relapse into dependence) by blocking the euphoric effects of the drugs. This was the first time I had ever taken meds like these. They were part of an expanding addiction pharmacology that was coming to be referred to as "medication-assisted treatment" (MAT). This included drugs for alcoholism as well, starting with the older medication Antabuse (disulfiram), which made patients ill if they consumed alcohol.

All I knew about addiction treatment was what I had gone through once as a teenager and had seen my mom go through many times: you detoxed by just stopping and suffering. In the world of traditional twelve-step recovery, taking any medication in place of drugs or alcohol was considered strictly taboo. But it was a taboo that addiction medicine was trying to change, because for some people, it worked better.

My home detox took a little longer than planned because the minute I got back to my apartment, I took all the prescription opiates I still had left there. I decided to change psychiatrists, and I tried going to

AA meetings but they weren't for me at the time—I was too scared of word getting out that I was in recovery. So I did my best to stay on my meds and in therapy. It was challenging, since the anti-addiction meds are very sedating, and I went from being borderline manic during the day to occasionally nodding off. I was fighting depression and anxiety.

THE MONTH AFTER I returned from treatment at Sierra Tucson, my Aunt Rosemary died in a Wisconsin hospital at the age of eighty-six, with my father and my aunts by her side. By this time the family and media were more open about her developmental disability and the tragedy of her lobotomy, but people still didn't seem to understand the last lesson Aunt Rosemary had to teach us. She wasn't given a lobotomy because of her developmental disability, which had been relatively stable since her birth; her case actually illustrated perfectly how a certain percentage of the entire population, regardless of their other conditions, will develop mental illness in their late teens and early twenties.

This medical challenge is still a huge, underappreciated problem. There are many psychiatrists and psychologists who simply will not see a patient with an intellectual disability. And there are many parents and family members of people with intellectual disabilities who still refuse to believe that postadolescent changes in their behavior could be from psychiatric illness. While it is still unclear just how treatable or reversible the kind of brain damage Aunt Rosemary experienced at birth might one day turn out to be, we already know that, today, her mental illness would likely have been very treatable.

This is, I think, another lesson we can learn from Aunt Rosemary, whose story has already helped destigmatize the world of intellectual disabilities by inspiring Special Olympics and turning shame into something positive worldwide. I hope, one day, that improved diagno-

sis and treatment of mental illnesses for those with developmental disabilities will also be part of her legacy.

ONLY WEEKS AFTER ROSEMARY DIED, word leaked to the press
about Mom's medical guardianship, which still had not been finalized.
She was terribly embarrassed and angry, and while we thought the
situation was getting under control, it then got much worse. I didn't
think, after all these years, it could get any more painful—for her or
for us. I was wrong.

Late at night on a Tuesday evening at the end of March, she was
found lying in the street with a concussion and a broken shoulder,
and at three A.M. she was taken to Tufts New England Medical Center
and later transferred to Mass General, where I met her and spent the
rest of the night sleeping in her room.

I had to speak to the press about this, trying to explain both what
was happening to my mother and that our extreme course of action
was not as uncommon as the press believed—the world of addiction and mental illness is filled with people who are so symptomatic
and unable to care for themselves that family needs to intervene. I also
told the truth, which was that while the press had heard about only
this incident, there had been many other nights like this when my
mom ended up in the ER, which had been kept private.

We weren't trying to spin any story. We were trying to save our
mother's life. We had spent a long time in denial about the true seri-
ousness of her condition. We were in denial not because we had no
idea there was a problem—of course we did—but because sometimes
you learn to tolerate as "normal" what a normal person never would.
What most people see as a crisis, you come to see as just another bump
in the road. When we had started the guardianship proceedings the

year before, the only thing her doctors said to us was, "What took you so long?"

DURING THIS DIFFICULT TIME with my mother's health, one thing happened that I did not then appreciate would matter so much.

Just a week after the initial report about my mom's concussion and hospitalization, I was sent a handwritten note by a House colleague who I did not know very well. His name was Jim Ramstad, and he was a moderate Republican representing Minnesota's Third Congressional District, just outside of Minneapolis.

Tall and mild-mannered, Jim was twenty years older than me— when I was a kid, he was already a lawyer who was serving in the National Guard during Vietnam. I primarily knew him as one of the small group of legislators who usually cosponsored bills concerning alcohol and drug dependence policy. The year before, he and I had founded the Addiction, Treatment and Recovery Caucus in the House, which was attempting to get addiction treatment either its own insurance parity or connect it to mental health parity. But we were not close friends or anything. As far as he knew, I was interested in addiction politics mostly because of my mother and because of the connection between substance use and mental illness.

Jim was not a big public talker, but he was consistently on record about why he cared so much about addiction: he had been a recovering alcoholic since 1981. And just as my staff had already heard me talk a thousand times about parking far away from my therapist's office so nobody would know I was in treatment, Jim's staff had been hearing for much longer about the night of July 31, 1981, when he woke up, hung over, in a jail cell in Sioux Falls, South Dakota, and realized he suffered from alcoholism and needed treatment. He was, at the time, in his first year as an elected official in the Minnesota State Senate, and was told by his staff that the only way to save his career was to say he and the Sioux Falls police had "an unfortunate misunderstanding." Instead, he publicly announced he was going for inpatient treatment at St. Mary's Hospital in Minneapolis and afterward that he was in twelve-step recovery. And he was then amazed by just how many people pulled him aside and said, "Now that you're in the club, welcome aboard, brother"—and how his public admission didn't hurt his reelection in the least.

In the world of politics, we write a lot of notes: once you're elected, you live like a perpetual newlywed, creating an almost endless stream of thank-you notes. On April 5, Jim Ramstad sat down and handwrote this note to me:

> *Dear Patrick,*
>
> *Your mother and you are in my thoughts and prayers, as I know how difficult it is. I'm here for you if I can be helpful in any way, so don't hesitate to call. As you know, I've been there!*
>
> > *Your friend,*
> > *Jim*

I had no idea that this note, which arrived among piles of others from colleagues, friends, and constituents, would predict the course of my personal and professional life.

Chapter 17

During all this turmoil with my mother's illness, the press was focusing a lot on whether or not I would run for the Senate. I had
never actually wanted to run for the Senate—or, rather, whenever I
considered it, I quickly realized that the additional media scrutiny
could present an insurmountable challenge, and with my illnesses I was
safer in the House. I remembered what it was like when my dad ran for
President, and how the pressure on a candidate was so much more than
what he was accustomed to in the Senate. I always remembered that
Roger Mudd interview; it was a symbol of what could happen when
you tried to move to the next rung on the political ladder (and also an
early indicator of how the media would expand its focus on the private
lives of public officials). But my dad really wanted me to run for Senate, so he would occasionally float the idea independently. And when
you're in public office, if people start speculating about whether you
would run for higher office, it's sometimes best to let the speculation
keep bubbling because people take you a little bit more seriously.

While we were handling my mom's hospitalization, I decided to
finally burst the press bubble and announce I wouldn't run for Senate

and was very happy to run again for my House seat. Without any other information, the press assumed I was doing this because I was choosing my mother's care over my political ambitions.

In fact, the life I needed to save at that moment was my own.

My family and staff did a very good job of keeping it quiet that, two weeks after my mom was hospitalized, I checked into the Mayo Clinic in Minnesota, one of the only places in the country that specialized in treatment of "dual diagnosis" patients.

I was admitted to the medical side of Mayo complaining of back pain. But, just as the first doctor I saw described me in his notes as a "pleasant, medically complicated gentleman," my chronic back pain wasn't the real reason for my visit. Between the pressure of work and the emotional strain of my sister's cancer and my mother's advanced illness, I had stopped taking the Suboxone or the naltrexone to prevent narcotic dependence and had again started taking Percocets for my back pain and my brain pain. I was swallowing up to twenty of them a day, and then sometimes would wake up in the middle of the night withdrawing and needing more. I had crossed the line with opiates.

The only lucky thing about this was that I had no problem getting Percocets by prescription, or paying for them. What was happening with a lot of people like me, who were addicted to opioids, is that they slowly, invariably were making the transition to heroin—which was much cheaper and, from what I heard, more powerful and pleasurable. I was, honestly, afraid I would like heroin too much to try it.

Although I had not been admitted to the mental health wing of Mayo—for fear I'd be discovered there—I was really honest with the doctors I met with, in a way I hadn't been before in more regular care. In general, my overall moods were pretty bad and my anxiety levels were off the charts. (I really had chosen the most unlikely profession for someone with an anxiety disorder.) When I wasn't working I really couldn't deal with being around people—and was often faking it when

I was around them during the day. You get good at that with these ill-nesses. Too good.

I also managed my private life so I could remain isolated. So I hadn't dated anyone regularly in nearly two years.

The physician at Mayo had a really interesting observation about me that nobody had ever suggested before. He felt that besides my bipolar disorder and addictions, I had a chronic anxiety disorder—the symptoms of which were sometimes being misinterpreted as asthma attacks. This sounded accurate to me as a patient, and I was relieved it might offer a better chance of getting all my symptoms under control. But in the political world of mental health, I knew to keep a secondary anxiety diagnosis to myself. Bipolar disorder, my primary diagnose, was considered a "serious mental illness." Anxiety disorders still were not, so if I admitted to having one, I'd be more likely to hear critical, stigmatizing "snap out of it" feedback.

Interestingly, during this time, the American Psychiatric Associa-tion was starting the process that would eventually lead to a new *Diag-nostic and Statistical Manual* (*DSM*). At that point, they were setting up a massive international literature search and analysis, convening thirteen international research planning conferences, with over four hundred experts from thirty-nine countries, in cooperation with the World Health Organization (WHO) Division of Mental Health, the World Psychiatric Association, the National Institute of Mental Health (NIMH), the National Institute on Drug Abuse (NIDA), and the Na-tional Institute on Alcohol Abuse and Alcoholism (NIAAA).

One of the major global changes they were contemplating for the new *DSM* was simplifying diagnosis by viewing mental illnesses on a "spec-trum" and recognizing that, when symptoms were most pronounced and disabling, all mental illnesses could be "serious" by the definition of society (and government). And just as many could be treated before be-coming more serious and even possibly prevented.

But that new paradigm was years from being published (the new *DSM* came out in 2013) and even longer from being accepted. So, while I was quietly starting to be treated for anxiety as well, in public settings I would continue describing my diagnosis as addiction and a mood disorder. Nobody would question whether these were "serious."

I spent six days at Mayo, getting detoxed and getting my meds checked and changed. And then I went back to my life as a Congressman, trying to improve the care of the diseases from which I suffered.

BESIDES TRYING IN EVERY SESSION of Congress to pass a new mental health parity act, we had a number of other legislative efforts meant to improve the world of brain diseases. Not long after President Bush took office, the NIMH commissioned a consulting firm to look again at the cost of making mental health parity the law of the land. And then the Robert Wood Johnson Foundation convened a sort of health actuary Woodstock workshop to explore the same issue. These two efforts combined to create a whole new way of crunching the numbers for our side, which was then accepted by the Congressional Budget Office, which does statistical analysis at congressional request. So, from 2002 on, the official CBO figure for the increased cost of mental health parity was 0.9 percent—which was under the political magic number.

That still wasn't enough to get parity passed in a Republican-controlled Congress—especially since, now, we were calling our House bill the Senator Paul Wellstone Mental Health Equitable Treatment Act in Paul's memory and were including substance use disorders, which would increase the cost. But it was a big step in the right direction.

So was the creation, in 2003, of a new advocacy partnership called the Campaign for Mental Health Reform. Inspired by the success of the Campaign for Tobacco-Free Kids, the Campaign for Mental

Health Reform was the brainchild of my friend and colleague Andy Hyman. Andy was a healthcare lawyer who had worked in several high-ranking positions at the Department of Health and Human Services (HHS) during the Clinton administration, and was then director of government relations and legislative counsel for the National Association of State Mental Health Program Directors—a very influential group representing the mental health executives overseeing all publicly funded care in every state. The campaign was started by that organization, NAMI, the Bazelon Center for Mental Health Law, and Mental Health America but included the CEOs of almost every major player in the field. It was run by my advocate friend from Rhode Island and NAMI, Bill Emmet, along with Andy.

I also proposed several pieces of legislation with strong mental health and family themes. One was the Keeping Families Together Act, which would combat an utterly appalling problem we were hearing more about: states were forcing families to give up custody of their children with serious mental illnesses as a condition of providing them treatment. We also proposed the Child Health Care Crisis Relief Act to address the critical shortage of mental health professionals with experience treating children, creating incentives to recruit and retain psychiatrists, psychologists, social workers, psychiatric nurses, and others already able to provide care to younger patients; the legislation would also create programs to train a new, larger generation of caregivers for children. We proposed the Positive Aging Act to help with the crisis of seniors with undiagnosed and untreated mental illnesses. And we also proposed the first major PTSD treatment bill for veterans, the Comprehensive Assistance for Veterans Exposed to Traumatic Stressors Act.

I had also introduced the sweeping 21st Century Health Information Act, a bill that would dramatically transform how healthcare information was captured, stored, and analyzed—locally, regionally, and nationally. It was an expanded version of a previous bill I had championed, the Josie King Act, in memory of an eighteen-month-old girl who died on Martha's Vineyard because of medical errors and massive health information screwups. The 21st Century Health Information Act—which especially would have revolutionized how mental health and addiction records were kept—was cosponsored by a relatively new face on the brain disease political scene, Representative Tim Murphy, a Republican psychologist from Western Pennsylvania who was very interested in mental health legislation. (One of the biggest challenges of encouraging medical information technology is that, even today, we still have separate rules for records concerning mental illness care and addiction care, because of extra privacy restrictions, including those from an old section of the Code of Federal Regulations, 42 CFR, Part 2. These were all probably well-meaning when put into place but now prevent the easy flow of crucial information between caregivers and block true parity from being achieved. Today, my own personal physician still can't easily access my rehab records because of these restrictions.)

All I could do was try to keep the appropriations and legislation coming, and try to maintain my own health and sanity. And since my siblings and I were now my mother's medical guardians, we were also overseeing her health aggressively for the first time. In early October, just as Breast Cancer Awareness Month was getting under way, she discovered she had a lump in her breast and we helped make sure she got immediate care. Because it was found early, only a lumpectomy was required.

Unfortunately, my health was harder to get under control. When I wasn't feeling well, I had a tendency to take too many pills, and not always for the reasons they were prescribed. So I found myself haphazardly taking Suboxone, which was supposed to help me get off of opiates, because I thought its sedating side effects would help me with my anxiety. And then, to counteract that, I would take a lot of stimulants and drink a lot of coffee to stay awake and alert at work—which I, basically, was able to do. The irony is that this was happening during the intense Capitol Hill meetings in which major cuts were being made in the budgets of all the agencies that were charged with improving mental healthcare and drug and alcohol addiction treatment.

I remember being in an Appropriations meeting about increasing DEA funding to help attack the rise of OxyContin dependence, while I was sitting there with Oxy pills in my pocket. I made it a point to keep whatever pills I was taking in a Bayer aspirin bottle, so anyone who saw me take one would assume I was treating a garden-variety headache. (Since I also sat on the committees appropriating for DEA, I did wonder why Oxy dependence was being treated primarily as a law enforcement issue rather than a health issue.)

Amid this daily grind of self-medicating, I would intermittently go out for a planned "lost night" to blow off all the stress. I went out with friends, had five Glenlivets right away, almost blacked out, and then just kept drinking; it wasn't uncommon for me to have fifteen or twenty drinks in an evening. I had a car waiting for me to take me home. Then I would sleep a few hours before getting up and going to work. I remember after one of these nights I had to wake up and give a speech to a group of drug and alcohol counselors.

As the 2005 holidays approached, I got it into my head that I needed to go to Liberia in January on a "CODEL"—short for "congressional delegation," a government-paid trip to inform legislation. I did have a substantial Liberian population in my district, but this would have been a very challenging and probably dangerous time to go. Even the State Department was saying they couldn't guarantee my security, but I was hell-bent on making this trip across Africa. My staff was scared for my safety, and my chief of staff, Sean Richardson—the only one who knew anything concrete about my health challenges—was worried I would get sicker over there, and also possibly run out of whatever prescription drugs I was overusing.

Sean had just recently lost his father to cancer and was trying to be home for the holidays with his family but instead was on the phone with me about Africa. I finally called him Christmas Eve and he was sitting in the car in his in-laws' driveway begging me to cancel this trip—because he was sure that if I went, I was never coming back.

"I just lost my dad and I'm not losing you, too," he said. And I finally just caved in, broke down, apologized for being so unreasonable, and asked him to get me back into treatment somewhere.

TWO DAYS AFTER CHRISTMAS, I was admitted to the Mayo Clinic for the second time in eight months. Again I insisted on being treated on the medical side (which is the patient's choice) so, if I were discovered, nobody could easily prove I had come for mental healthcare; I could be detoxed without anyone finding out just how deeply depressed I was and how manic I could be. I was also taking an enormous number of medications. The list was staggering:

> Lithium carbonate, 300 mg three times a day for bipolar
>   disorder
> Lamictal, 200 mg three times a day for bipolar disorder
> Prozac, 20 mg daily for depression
> Wellbutrin, 75 mg tablets, three tabs in the morning, three
>   at noon, for depression
> Buprenorphine, 16 mg four times daily (my chart said
>   "for back pain" but this was to help me avoid narcotic
>   pain meds)
> Docusate, 240 mg, three tabs four times daily for constipation
>   from buprenorphine

Clonazepam, 0.5 mg once or twice daily for sleep or anxiety
    (my chart said "rarely uses but primarily for sleep")
Ambien, 20 mg about once a week, as necessary for sleep
Caffeine, 200 mg tablets, about three tabs daily for alertness in
    morning
Alka-Seltzer in the morning for dyspepsia
Ibuprofen, 600 mg three times a day for back pain
Proventil HFA, two pills four times a day or as needed for
    shortness of breath
Advair 500/50, one puff twice daily for asthma
Singulair, 10 mg at night for vasomotor rhinitis
Intal inhaler, two puffs before exercise for asthma

The doctors on the medical side did their best to try to convince me I needed to transfer over to the Intensive Addiction Program, which meant moving into another building, the Generose Building, and technically being in rehab. I just couldn't bring myself to do it. After eight days of being told I really needed to be in the addiction program, we agreed on a ridiculous compromise—I would stay in the medical wing but join the day program at Generose, which was primarily for people who lived nearby and were sleeping in their own homes.

I was still having issues being in group sessions; I just felt nervous sharing any real truth (especially after my name tag disappeared a couple times from my breakfast tray and I became convinced someone was saving up information to sell my story). As I detoxed and participated in the longest intensive treatment of my life, I was also thinking that I had quite a history of unresolved feelings of rage. We discussed whether anger management could be part of my treatment.

On my sixteenth day at Mayo, I had a revelation. During an individual therapy session, the psychiatrist started talking to me about cognitive-behavioral therapy (CBT). He explained that CBT was a type of short-term, practical, goal-directed therapy that focused not so much on bringing up and examining painful memories but instead on identifying certain present-day behaviors and the sometimes distorted thinking that fueled them, trying to modify beliefs and relate to others in different ways—and by doing so changing behaviors.

CBT had been pioneered in the early 1960s by a psychiatrist at Penn named Dr. Aaron "Tim" Beck. I had certainly heard of CBT because it was growing in popularity—especially among clinical psychologists, who now vastly outnumbered the psychiatrists who had almost exclusively done psychotherapy until the 1970s. In the growing area of mental health managed care, CBT was also the only psychotherapy that had been studied in depth for efficacy in clinical trials— just like medications were studied, because Tim Beck was very practical about not only his therapy itself but how it would be reimbursed.

I knew some of this already, at least from a mental health policy standpoint: this type of result-oriented psychotherapy was a large part of what we were arguing needed to be covered under mental health parity. Ironically, however, I had to admit that while some considered me the nation's leading advocate for cutting-edge mental healthcare, I had never in my life had one session of cognitive therapy. I had always had more supportive and psychoanalytic psychotherapy, during which, except for the part of the session in which my meds were checked, I was free to drone on about who in my family I was still most angry at. It was often my dad, for old wounds that wouldn't heal.

So, for the first time ever, I spent most of a therapy session talking about strategies for managing my moods, and ways of identifying anxiety-provoking thoughts and stopping myself from acting on them. We talked about how I could stop worrying about the possibility of appearing anxious in social situations, and by doing so maybe actually be less anxious. I'm not saying this solved all or any of my problems immediately, but it was, for me, a unique and healthy approach. I was sent back to the medical wing with homework for my next session—which is very common in CBT but nothing I had ever done before. I was told to start creating a list of positive activities I could engage in to help manage my anxiety.

I could exercise, but in my years in Washington I had never managed to do that consistently. I went through periods where I swam in the Capitol pool—which is below the Capitol basketball court and the weight room where members of Congress blow off steam. I also sometimes went running around the Mall. But I had found it hard to stay on a schedule, and when it came to running, I was also a little bit afraid to be seen in public doing it badly—since I come from a family of hard-core exercisers. I would often run in a floppy hat and sunglasses so nobody would notice me shuffling among the monuments.

When it was possible, I always wanted to be sailing—which was for me, just as it was for my dad, a way to relax and focus on the here and now. In spite of my sailing fiascos, there were many more uneventful sails across the Sakonnet River between my home in Portsmouth and Sachuest Point, on the other side of my congressional district in Little Compton, Rhode Island.

These were all things I could do more but didn't. Generally, I neither relaxed on weekends nor did things that might energize or reenergize me during the week. Instead, I would burn myself out with alcohol and worry about what was coming during the next week.

Working out or sailing more would not change the fact that I had a mental illness. But it seemed like there might be a better way to help me stay on my treatments and face daily life with more optimism, control, and self-awareness.

As my time at Mayo was coming to an end—I had to get back to Washington—there was discussion in sessions of other issues I hadn't spent much time considering in therapy, like the role of forgiveness and spirituality in my recovery. Even though I was still in the day program—which was, in retrospect, still a sign I wasn't completely committed to treatment and my own recovery—I attended the medallion-closure ceremony with my peers from the inpatient unit. When I left Mayo after what had turned into a full month there, I felt healthy and optimistic.

TWO WEEKS LATER, I was standing in front of a packed crowd at the National Press Club, talking about a new report called "The State of Depression in America" funded by the Depression and Bipolar Support Alliance (DBSA). Long based in Chicago, but now also working out of DC, DBSA (formerly the National Depressive and Manic-Depressive Association) had, for years, been the nation's major advocacy group for mood disorders. Even though it correctly called itself "the leading patient-directed national organization focusing on the most prevalent mental illnesses," DBSA was less politically powerful than NAMI, which did its best to speak in Washington for all serious mental illness but skewed toward families with members disabled by schizophrenia and the most debilitating mood disorders. DBSA was, primarily, a national web of support groups for mood disorder patients who could care for themselves; NAMI had started as a political force largely for patients who could not always take care of themselves, and was run more by parents, family members, and researchers than actual consumers.

We were releasing the report in the aftermath of President Bush's last State of the Union address, in which he mentioned mental illness a total of zero times, followed by a budget proposal that cut $88 million in funding for mental health programs in SAMHSA, NIMH, NIDA, and NIAAA. I appeared at the Press Club event along with Mike Wallace from *60 Minutes* and a number of top mood disorder experts.

It was the beginning of what was expected to be a jam-packed spring of events and legislative proposals to try to push the lack of mental health parity—and the solutions to this problem—onto the front pages of the nation's newspapers and the top of lawmakers' agendas. I was, during this time, doing everything I could to function at the highest level during the day and take the best care of myself during whatever free time I had.

After leaving Mayo, I had enrolled in the day program in Fairfax at CAPS, a well-regarded mental health facility. It was the first time I had ever tried a day program as an outpatient, the way they are supposed to be used. For an outpatient, a day program—also referred to as a "partial hospitalization program" (PHP)—is somewhere between a forty-five-minute outpatient psychotherapy session or twelve-step meeting and a full day of inpatient care. It's a more intensive way to spend part of a morning, afternoon, or evening in treatment while still maintaining your work and life, less fully one-on-one than psychotherapy but more multifaceted and medical than a recovery meeting. Someday, people with mental illness and addiction will use day programs much more often and effectively. In our current model of treatment—which offers mostly acute care for these chronic illnesses—most patients with coverage bounce between inpatient stays and then just being out in the world jousting with everything.

I also liked the day program because it felt a little safer than attending an AA meeting closer to where I lived and worked. However, because CAPS was further away, I started going less frequently.

I was committed, during this time, to not abusing prescription painkillers. And I didn't. But I was still occasionally drinking at night. And, because I was having trouble sleeping, I started taking Ambien again. That would have gotten me in trouble at CAPS if I had told them, so I didn't. And then I felt bad I was lying to my rehab counselors, who are the last people in the world from whom you need to keep secrets. So I finally just quit the program.

————

AT THE END OF MARCH, the *New England Journal of Medicine* published a landmark study we had been anticipating for some time; the unprovocative title, "Behavioral Health Insurance Parity for Federal Employees," belied just how politically provocative it was. Written by a team led by Dr. Howard Goldman, a psychiatry professor at the University of Maryland, and Harvard health economist Dr. Richard Frank, the article analyzed the recent experience of the federal government's insurance plan for its employees, which President Clinton had ordered to establish mental health and addiction parity in 1999. The study compared seven federal employee health plans that had added parity and paired the findings with results over the same period of seven other plans—not covering federal employees, but insuring a similar group of patients—that did not offer parity. The findings were a surprise even to us, because in many cases the plans with mental health parity hadn't seen any increases in costs at all; some even saw decreases.

Interestingly, the study also didn't find any evidence of the dreaded "moral hazard," an insurance economics concept that was often brought up by opponents of parity. "Moral hazard" refers to a phenomenon—real or imagined—where if people have increased coverage for any medical problem, they will use it, even if they don't need it, just because they can. It is a particularly troubling concept to use when discussing mental health and addiction care, where the real problems are the dramatic underutilization and underavailability of care, and the challenge of keeping patients who can get care in treatment.

The percentage of Americans who, each year, have a mental illness or substance use disorder yet refuse to treat it is actually measured by the government. In general, in any given year, about one-third of the people with the most serious, debilitating illnesses do not have any treatment at all; in the broader category of people diagnosed with any mental illness, that number is actually over one-half.

We hoped the study would show that parity didn't increase costs more than 1 percent—and it didn't, although of course experts representing the businesses that would have to add coverage criticized the methodology. But there were actually more mixed feelings about the fact that utilization didn't dramatically increase when there were fewer financial impediments. Because this meant that even with parity, a lot of people suffering from mental illness and addiction were still not getting the treatment they needed and deserved.

Politically, however, that battle was far down the road. We could worry about such morally hazardous concerns after we actually made parity law—or at least got some of the other bills passed that we had proposed so many times in so many Congresses.

For example, the day this study came out, I was on the floor of the House trying to raise interest—for the third straight session—for my proposed legislation to improve child and adolescent mental healthcare by increasing the number of caregivers hired in that area of behavioral health, and incentivizing a larger next generation of caregivers with college loan forgiveness. I brought with me to the House floor a young woman from South Dakota who had developed bipolar disorder as a teen—which is when it begins to manifest itself in many people—and ended up dropping out of school and attempting suicide. Why? Because when her family tried to get her psychiatric help, they were told that since there was a severe caregiver shortage she would need to wait four months for an appointment.

"Millions of American families need hope," I hollered. "Millions of them need help. The number of suicides is twice the rate of homicides in this country; thirty-six thousand people take their lives every year successfully. Every day in this country, one thousand three hundred eighty-five people attempt suicide. It is the third leading cause of death for young people. . . . This year alone, fourteen hundred college students will successfully take their lives. Mr. Speaker, we need to make sure that we have adequate personnel to *make sure* that the services are delivered, and the services will *never* be delivered unless there are *enough people to deliver them!*"

SEVERAL DAYS LATER, I had my first appointment with a new psychiatrist at George Washington University Medical Center. I did my intake meeting with him but then didn't show up the next week for my first actual session. At the last minute I had to be in Rhode Island for meetings.

In fact, at the time I would have been meeting the psychiatrist, I was in my district office in Providence being hit in the mouth with a hammer. I was doing a presentation with an out-of-state manufacturer who was thinking of opening a factory in my district, to manufacture a type of shock-absorbing gel, used in vests and saddles and shoe inserts. He put one of these pads on my glass-top desk and prepared to hit it with a hammer to demonstrate its shock-absorbing powers. But when he swung the hammer, the head flew off and hit me in the face. There was blood everywhere, and I ended up in the hospital getting six stitches in what was now my very stiff upper lip.

They offered me opiate painkillers, which I took, and a prescription for more, which I went out the next morning to fill. I unwisely drove myself—in the car I kept at my home in Portsmouth, a late-model silver Ford Crown Victoria—over to my local CVS. On the way over I was observed swerving a bit on the road, and when I tried to turn quickly into the CVS parking lot, I pulled right in front of another driver, whose car crashed into mine.

I was in a total panic because I realized I was under the influence. I got out of the car, and there was an older woman in the parking lot who had seen the whole thing—in fact, I apparently had almost hit her car a few minutes before, and she was angry. As I got out of my car, she asked if I realized I could have hit her. Then she saw I was swaying and my eyes were a little glazed. And instead of acting like a jerk, as she probably expected, I contritely said, "I'm sorry for the fuss."

Both she and the guy who I caused to hit my car recognized me—after all, I was their Congressman—and I guess they either felt sorry for me or didn't want to be bothered with all the aggravation of making what would have been a perfectly warranted accusation against me. From the moment the police arrived to take our statements, I was convinced I would be arrested. But the police officer wrote "appeared normal" under "condition of the driver" and left me with paperwork for my auto insurance. I went into the drugstore, filled my prescription, and drove home.

Honestly, I couldn't believe I didn't get arrested.

But nineteen days later, I wasn't so lucky.

Or, maybe, I was actually luckier.

Chapter 18

After my crash at the Capitol, everyone wanted to know if I had been drunk that night. I wasn't, but people who understand these illnesses realize that was the wrong question. Both addiction and depression come in cycles of waves, which you think you have adjusted to until a bigger one knocks you down. It isn't all that revealing to chart how that last wave hit; it's more important to understand what you were doing out there in the water in the first place.

So the real story of the week that forever changed my life starts not on the Wednesday before I crashed, but two days earlier, on the Amtrak Acela coming back from New York after a long day of meetings. During that three-hour ride, I drank—to the best of my recollection—eight straight vodkas from those little one-ounce travel bottles before arriving at Union Station.

I felt awful the next day, for all the obvious reasons, but there was also one developing medical issue: a lot of pain and discomfort in my whole lower abdomen. So in the early evening I went to the Attending Physician for the Congress and was given Phenergan liquid. It helped the pain and was a little sedating, so I took it again before bed.

The next day I had a lot of meetings, because a lot of mental health advocates were in town lobbying on the Hill. In between meetings, I was on the House floor voting on everything from increased accountability and transparency for lobbyists, to prohibitions on price gouging in the sale of gasoline and other fuels, to amending the Internal Revenue Code and ERISA to reform pension funding rules.

I then left to say a few words at a reception in the Rayburn Building for the "National Council"—the nickname of the National Council for Behavioral Health, one of the more powerful and ambitious forces in mental health. The National Council represented every state community mental health organization in the country. (Back then, in 2006, that was about 1,300 organizations with some 250,000 caregivers and staff; today they represent over 2,000 organizations and over 750,000 caregivers and staff.) In the two years since its new executive director, Linda Rosenberg, had taken over, the National Council had become a much more prominent political player, pushing to develop the kind of muscle that once only NAMI could exert. Linda had advocates in town from all over the country for their "Hill Day."

I was scheduled to meet with her again the next morning, along with the executive directors of several other major mental health groups representing the leadership of the formidable Campaign for Mental Health Reform, which was now in its third year of being the most organized effort ever to lobby for change in behavioral healthcare. So, basically, a lot of people who mattered to me politically in the world of brain healthcare and advocacy were in town.

Because it would be a bad idea to be seen drinking at a National Council reception, before I went I walked around the corner to the Hawk 'n' Dove. I went to the back room bar and, as I always did, ordered a drink that was dark—Jack and Coke—so it could be mistaken for a soft drink. It turned out the female bartender also worked as an IT specialist for one of my congressional colleagues, so we talked a little politics, I watched a few minutes of the baseball game they had on—it was about 6:30 P.M.—and then I had a second drink and left.

After the National Council reception, I returned to the House floor to vote on one last bill, concerning maritime and cargo security, and was done a little after nine P.M. I called a woman I had been dating to see if she wanted to come over. She arrived around ten, and before we went to sleep I took my meds.

As always, there were a lot of them, including Ambien, which I took to help me sleep. I generally took two ten-milligram pills, somewhat higher than the standard 12.5-milligram dose recommended at the time but still considered safe. Seven weeks earlier, the *Washington Post* had actually run a big story in its Tuesday health section about a dramatic rise in side effects of Ambien, including sleepwalking and sleep-driving and even sleep-shoplifting. (While doctors were already wondering if these effects were dose related, it wasn't until 2013 that the FDA officially announced that dosing for this drug was too high across the board and cut all the recommended doses in half.)

But the truth was, I had been taking twenty milligrams of Ambien to sleep on and off for many months and had never had a problem. I took it when I knew I needed to sleep soundly because I had an early morning meeting.

The only new med I was taking that night was the Phenergan, which I had been gulping for my stomach all day. The drug was not known to interact with Ambien, but it was itself capable of making people drowsy.

We were asleep before midnight. And when I woke up the next morning and went to work my life had completely changed.

THE IRONY OF MY THREE A.M. car crash into a Capitol barrier is that it was pretty much the only disaster of my professional life that *wasn't* caused by excessive use of alcohol or opioid painkillers. It really was a case of sleep-driving because of the Ambien and the Phenergan. So there were plenty of people close to me who were sure I could get out of this just by telling the pharmacological truth.

But as that Thursday unfolded, and I found myself locked in my office trying to avoid the dozens of cameras waiting outside, I realized this might be my only chance to tell the actual truth, the bigger truth.

I was an alcoholic; I was a drug addict; I had bipolar disorder and anxiety disorder, and I hadn't been properly treating any of them. And for the first time in my life, at the age of thirty-eight, I just wanted to stop lying about all of this. Because it is the lies and the secrets that eventually kill you.

When word broke of the unfolding controversy, I was on the floor of the House and was called to come to one of the private phone booths in the cloakroom. One of the first things I heard my chief of staff say to me on the phone was, "Is there something you want to tell me?"

Finally, the answer was yes.

I realized I had been living, for as long as I could remember, with this constant fear of being found out, of the other shoe finally dropping. Now, *every* other shoe was dropping; it was raining wingtips and boat shoes. On top of everything else, part of what was driving the story was my long-ago-damaged relationship with the police unions: when they found out the Capitol Police brass had handled my case the way they would have handled the case of any Congressman or Senator in that situation—with more dignity than I deserved, perhaps, but by just taking me home to sleep it off, without breath or blood tests—they raised the specter of "special treatment," which pushes every possible political button. While, in politics, we all know that what goes around comes around, it's rare for so much to come around at precisely the same moment.

And that's why, honestly, my feelings of dread started giving way to an overwhelming sense of relief. I had been waiting for this day my entire life. As long as I could remember, I had been trying to please people and manage their expectations so I could, just by a little, exceed them. I isolated myself when my feelings were overwhelming—which happened more often than anyone would have believed for someone so public—and I kept my emotional and spiritual distance from people so they couldn't destroy me. At the same time, I had been seeking out self-destructive, exhilarating, risky situations that would take me out of the anguish of being all alone. All this was built on the question I constantly asked myself: "Is anybody going to find out?"

I remember sitting in my office with a growing feeling of freedom. I felt so overwhelmed that I just *let go*, first with a nervous-giddy laugh and then with a much more profound release. I finally didn't have to white-knuckle my life anymore. I no longer had to worry about the small stuff I had spent my life obsessing over, because the fight was finished. I had, at the same time, lost and won.

FRIDAY MORNING, I arranged to read a brief prepared statement to the press before leaving for Minnesota to be treated at the Mayo Clinic. In the statement, I revealed much more than I needed to and much more than my advisers advised me to. I explained that I had been struggling with the challenges of addiction and depression my entire adult life—as did the millions of Americans to whom I had dedicated my public service. I admitted for the first time that I had been treated for addiction to prescription pain medication and that I had spent the recent holiday recess at Mayo trying to address that problem.

I expressed my genuine confusion about what had happened on Wednesday night. I admitted I had no memory of getting out of bed, driving to the Capitol, being pulled over by police, or being cited for driving infractions.

But I was not trying to use that as an excuse. "That's not how I want to live my life," I said, "and it's not how I want to represent the people of Rhode Island. . . . I am deeply concerned about my reaction to the medication, and my lack of knowledge of the accident that evening. But I do know enough that I know that I need help."

The statement ended, "I hope that my openness today and in the past, and my acknowledgment that I need help, will give others the courage to get help if they need it. I am blessed to have a loving family who is in my corner every step of the way. And I'm grateful to my friends, both here and in Rhode Island, for reaching out to me at this time."

But while it took every ounce of restraint I had to stick to the prepared statement—which my staff had never, ever seen me do before—I did finally deviate on the last line.

I was supposed to say, "Thank you for your prayers and your support."

Instead, I looked right into the cameras and said, "And I'd like to call, once again, for passage of mental health parity. Thank you."

On the way to National Airport, I had the driver bring me by my dad's house for a minute. We sat on the back porch—me, my father, Vicki, their dogs—and there wasn't a whole lot anyone could say. By then there was no more talk of "fendah bendahs" and damage containment. I had escalated everything myself, answered questions the press hadn't even thought to ask yet. There was no turning back.

I remember my father saying, "You did a good job today. You're doing the right thing." And then I had to get going so I could make my plane.

As I left town, the two people who meant the most to my political future stood up for me in strong public statements.

From my dad:

I love Patrick very much and am very proud of him. All of us in the family admire his courage in speaking publicly about very personal issues and fully support his decision to seek treatment. He has taken full responsibility for events that occurred Wednesday evening, and he will continue to cooperate fully in any investigation.

I have the rare and special honor of being able to serve with my son in the Congress, and I have enormous respect for the work Patrick has done. The people of the 1st District of Rhode Island have a tireless champion for the issues they care about, and today I hope they join me in feeling pride and respect for a courageous man who has admitted to a problem and taken bold action to correct it.

And from Nancy Pelosi:

Congressman Patrick Kennedy's statement today was one of honesty and courage. I hope it will serve as inspiration and encouragement to all the families in America who are facing the challenges of addiction and depression.

No one in the country has been a better advocate than Patrick Kennedy for the parity of mental health services—to end the discrimination by insurance companies against people struggling with mental illness.

I have told Patrick I am so proud of his brave statement today and for his leadership and service to his country every day. I pray

for him and his family during this difficult time, and look forward
to his return to Washington.

I ARRIVED at Mayo late Friday afternoon. This time, I wasn't going to
make the mistake of doing the "just visiting" version of rehab in fear of
being found out. I checked into the Intensive Addiction Program in the
Generose Building as an inpatient, making sure I had nowhere to hide.
The single rooms were plain but comfortable, with a hospital bed, a private bathroom, and a nice big window overlooking a yard and woods.

The very next day, I had my first visitor. It was Representative Jim
Ramstad, who had driven an hour and a half from his home on the
other side of Minneapolis to come see me. He showed up before my
siblings, before my lawyer, before everyone.

I walked down the hallway from the treatment wing and he was
standing there. He had tears in his eyes just like I did, but he said they
were tears of joy that I was where I needed to be getting treatment. We
sat down in a private visitors' area and just talked.

Jim wanted me to know that I did not have to be alone in this, that
he was my friend and, perhaps more important, my brother in recovery. He let me know that he was there for me, 24/7, no matter what.
He said I had to take this one day at a time, but he believed in me. He
said . . . well, he basically said almost everything that was on all those
pillows on my mom's couch that we used to snicker about when she
joined AA. But hearing them now, from this guy I didn't know well
but who said he was committed to my recovery, was a powerful experience. I'm not sure I had ever heard a man closer to my dad's age than
mine speak so openly.

We talked for about an hour and a half. And then he left me to my
therapy and said he'd be back in a week. In fact, he said he'd be back
every Saturday during my twenty-eight-day stay. And he was.

I WORKED REALLY HARD in individual sessions and the unbelievably confrontational "process group" run by Mayo's legendary therapist John Holland. I heard from lots of family and friends. One of the
most powerful outreaches I had was from my cousin Tim Shriver, with
whom I had been getting closer over the past few years. Tim was eight
years older than me and was married with five kids, so he had a much
different life from mine. But since he had moved to DC in the mid-
nineties to oversee the operations of Special Olympics—while keeping
his hand in education and his social-emotional learning project—we
came to realize we were operating in closely linked worlds. The science
of developmental disability and the science of mental illness were starting to overlap more and more as they both became part of the growth
of neuroscience and genetics. So the politics of our work was starting
to overlap as well. And we were the members of the family most actively involved in the modern iteration of what his mother and our
Uncle Jack had tried to accomplish with the 1963 Community Mental
Health Act.

Tim's brother, my cousin Anthony Shriver, had co-founded an ambitious spin-off of Special Olympics, the Best Buddies program, which
helped arrange one-on-one relationships and employment opportunities for people with developmental disabilities. My cousin Maria was
also involved with those groups, but increasingly, as their father, my
uncle Sargent Shriver, became more affected by Alzheimer's, she was
devoting more of her efforts to the growing need to support the caregivers who were on the front lines of this epidemic (along with her
work on empowering women).

But Tim and I were the ones working in the political trenches of
developmental disability and brain disease every day. We lived in the
same small town and often exchanged affectionate notes when we saw

each other on TV or in the *Post*. So I was really touched by this note he sent to me at Mayo, in a card with the famous painting by Van Gogh of his solitary chair.

Dear Patrick,

Over the last few days I have thought often of you and what must have been the maelstrom of emotions and thoughts surrounding last week's accident. While I cannot imagine how difficult it must have been, I can send you my thoughts and prayers for greater peace in the days ahead.

Surely, despite all the pressure from all sides, somewhere in a place of quiet you will find the still small voice of goodness and love that will remind you how nothing can take away all the goodness and wonder that is you. In the larger family, there are so many messages—to perform, to achieve, to be great, to be humble, to be funny, to be smart, to be more than any one person can be. Sometimes I think that each of us in our many different ways have struggled with the same realization that no matter what we do, we cannot achieve the greatness we are expected to attain. And then we've got two choices—frustration or acceptance.

For me, the athletes of Special Olympics have been great teachers of how to face such moments—great role models of self-acceptance who I can aspire to emulate. You too are a role model of this great gift—not in your achievements though they are enormous—but in your humility and honesty—in your openness not only to admit struggle but to face it directly. If each of us could muster that courage, we'd have a new family story to tell and one which could again change the world, even if only for one person at a time. . . .

All my love,
Tim

———

DURING MY FIRST WEEK at Mayo, the lawyer we had hired for my criminal case flew out to see me to discuss a possible plea agreement on my charges of driving under the influence of a drug and reckless driving. He also wanted to talk to my doctors about writing a letter to explain the drug interaction I had experienced. Over the weekend, Jim Ramstad came back. I told him I had never had an AA sponsor; while I had attended some twelve-step meetings over the years, I had never done it long enough or consistently enough to develop that kind of relationship.

I asked him if he would consider being my sponsor, and he graciously agreed, which gave me a rush of relief and hope that I still often think about. It was all new to me, but he had a lot of experience. Since committing to his own recovery in the early 1980s, he had been a sponsor to dozens of people in Minnesota and DC. While he didn't tell me this at the time, some of my staff and political friends apparently had been reaching out to him even before my accident to see if he would consider talking to me.

After agreeing to be my sponsor, he told me that besides daily twelve-step meetings he wanted to invite me to a special private weekly meeting he had been attending for years. It was at the home of Dr. Ronald Smith, who was director of psychiatry at the National Naval Medical Center and had helped in the creation of the Betty Ford Center, and included several people I already knew in the government but didn't know were in recovery. It was a powerful and generous offer, and after he left he arranged for my physician at Mayo to reach out to Ron Smith, who not only encouraged me to join his group but offered to help support me through my legal issues as a medical expert.

By agreeing to become my sponsor, Jim was taking a risk. Unlike others he had helped, I was going to have to be very public about my recovery—in a way that would run up against a lot of privacy and anonymity rules associated with traditional twelve-step programs. There was, actually, a growing group within the recovery movement, represented by the organization Faces & Voices of Recovery, which for a number of years had been trying to change that and allow those who did not want complete anonymity to feel comfortable being more open. But a lot of people in AA would find my acknowledging the identity of my sponsor—which was bound to happen—to be shocking.

We decided, however, that the shock would be worth it—because it might help the cause of parity, which desperately needed a huge boost to get it to the next level of political reality. And the story of an older Republican sponsoring a young Democrat was one that just might bring all the work we had been doing to the next level. Two weeks into recovery may have been a little soon to make such an unconventional decision. But to really make an impact against something as intractable as medical discrimination and stigma, sometimes you have to risk being a little dramatic, no matter how symptomatic you might be.

Chapter 19

As I spent more time in the small Mayo process group, where I was called out on things in a way I had never before experienced in my life, I was confronted with all kinds of ideas that had never before occurred to me. Some were profound and healing. A couple less so.

I was, of course, getting a lot of grief for being from a world of privilege and growing up in a family that had "gotten away with" things that other people with drug and alcohol and mood disorder issues did not. That was fair criticism, and honestly, nobody said anything about me that I hadn't already said, much more cruelly, to myself in my darkest hours.

But during my last weeks of treatment at Mayo, I got it into my head that there was actually a solution to this.

I needed to go to prison.

In my plea agreement negotiations, nobody on either side was suggesting I needed to be in prison. It was all my idea. I decided that I should spend a short time in jail. And since I didn't want my prison sentence to cost the taxpayers of the District of Columbia one penny, I wanted part of my plea agreement to be that I would personally pay back any and all costs of incarcerating me. That way, nobody could ever accuse me of "getting away with" anything.

My lawyer was, of course, dead set against this. He made it clear that not only wasn't I getting any preferential treatment—any Congressman would have been (and had been) treated the same way in similar circumstances—he also thought, as a practical matter, what I was suggesting would completely backfire and not only hurt my plea agreement but further hurt my reputation.

When I wouldn't let this idea go, he wrote me a long, powerful e-mail that not only challenged my strategy but, as a counterpoint to some of the hard, deeply psychological opinions I'd been hearing in group, offered one of his own. He wrote, "I suspect that in your group sessions at the Mayo Clinic, people who themselves are facing issues regarding acceptance of responsibility have challenged you or suggested, based upon their own stereotypical thinking, that you are 'getting off' in a manner that others would not. . . . I am convinced that [this] is playing directly into very deep-seated feelings you have regarding your relationships with, and the past conduct of, your mother and father. It is almost as if you subconsciously feel that by accepting responsibility for your parents' past conduct you can expiate your own problems and transgressions, simply by acting [out] what you believe will be a very public act of contrition."

He was right, of course, but I wasn't listening. On my BlackBerry, I messaged him back that I knew I was being an "obstinate SOB" but this was what I wanted. When he wouldn't do it, I actually got the number for the DC Attorney General's office and called him myself— a call that, thank goodness, went to voice mail. But the AG was informed I had called and reached out to my attorney. Ironically, they had pretty much finalized my deal earlier in the day, and when my lawyer heard I had called the AG myself from rehab, he threatened to resign. So did my chief of staff. Finally I calmed down and dropped that idea. Because of what I had done, however, I was offered a slightly less appealing plea deal, which we took.

THIS WAS ALL BEING DONE in a mad rush because my standard twenty-eight days of rehab were almost up. I could have paid to stay longer than what insurance generally covered, but politically I didn't think I could afford a longer stay without resigning from office. In retrospect, I was nowhere near ready to actually leave treatment and return to the real world—especially my real world.

Someday, I hope in the not-so-distant future, the amount of time people in my situation spend in intensive treatment will be decided not on the we'll-pay-for-twenty-eight-days standard, but with evidence-based tools informed by ways of measuring severity and information about how long a typical patient needs intensive treatment to minimize the chance of relapse. There was, honestly, no way I was ready to be released that soon. But I made that decision myself.

I also decided that rather than easing back into work, I would hit the ground running.

For the past couple years, I had been organizing a big annual conference at Brown University—which was in my congressional district—called Frontiers of Health Care. It was held in the early summer and attempted to bring together cutting-edge science and public policy in a high-profile way. It kicked off in 2004 with former Speaker of the House Newt Gingrich and I discussing one of our shared concerns: transforming healthcare using new information technology.

It just so happened that, many months before my car crash, we had scheduled the third of these Frontiers of Health Care conferences, "Imagining the Future of Behavioral Health," which was going to feature two of the nation's most powerful scientists on this subject, Dr.

Thomas Insel, director of the National Institute of Mental Health, and Dr. Nora Volkow, the director of the National Institute on Drug Abuse. They were going to discuss their own neuroscience research and the future of their fields—which were starting to overlap more than ever as new advances in neural imaging showed the similarities between how the processes of mental illness and addiction appeared in the brain.

This was breakthrough research and they certainly could have held this event without me if I canceled, which everyone involved expected me to do. Instead I decided to double down. I would not only speak to the group of over three hundred coming to Brown but would make this my first public appearance since going to rehab, and then hold my first press conference afterward.

So, I got out of rehab on the first Friday in June and went to the Cape to be with my family for the weekend.

And then I appeared at Brown on Monday, June 5, 2006, where I was love-bombed by the mental health and addiction communities with a full-page ad in the *Providence Journal*, followed by incredibly kind personal statements of support during the conference from Tom Insel and Nora Volkow.

After I finished my own talk at Brown's Salomon Center, I walked across College Green to meet reporters at Faunce House. I announced that I planned to have "the most transparent recovery that anyone's ever seen" and if my constituents expected me to come out and assure them there would be no more slipups or embarrassing incidents—well, that was a promise I was not able to make. Recovery was one day at a time.

All the press wanted to know was whether I had been drunk that night; they were obsessed by this—I think because, in our stigmatized world, it is easier to criticize a public person for a moral failing if they are drunk rather than abusing medication or struggling with mental illness. I realized then and there that I was going to have to come up with a better answer than the basic fact that I hadn't been drunk. So, this press conference—this whole day, actually—became a big turning point.

June 5, 2006, was the first day of the rest of my "comorbid" life.

IN MEDICINE, "COMORBIDITY" is a fascinating and complex term. It refers, technically, to the existence of two medical conditions simultaneously. But the inherent question comorbidity raises is the relationship between the conditions. Did one cause the other, increase the chances of the other? If one is treated will it impact the other? Or is it just a complete coincidence they appear together, a statistical truth with no unique medical recourse?

The comorbidity between mental illness and substance use disorder is one of the best known in the history of medicine. Yet the worlds of research and treatment for the two were so separate that there were three national institutes covering them: NIMH, NIDA, and NIAAA. And in the real world of diagnosis and treatment, patients and their families had clear and often very emotional feelings about how they viewed themselves comorbidly: I've met people who really prefer to be seen as mentally ill and would be embarrassed to be thought of as having a substance use disorder (because, to them, mental illness is a disease and addiction is a weakness) and others who would prefer to be seen as having an addiction because they would sooner die than admit to being "crazy"—and sadly, some die by their own hand precisely for that reason.

While this was all well-known—intellectually at least—to experts in both fields, there was, in the real world of Washington brain politics, far too little comorbidity. In fact, the conference that was being held at Brown that day was unique for that reason: Tom Insel and Nora Volkow didn't appear together all that often, because back then they were viewed as overseeing two completely different, and mutually exclusive, government research fiefdoms.

The same was true for Jim Ramstad and me. While I had been pushing primarily for mental healthcare, he had been pushing primarily for addiction care—and, in both cases, research to inform that care, and laws that fought stigma and other barriers against getting that care. It was time for both of us to focus on messaging that was comorbid and bipartisan.

So, during that press conference at Brown—at which I was only thirty-three days sober, three days out of rehab, and probably nowhere near ready to be back in public—I decided I would answer all these questions carefully and comorbidly. I would talk about mental illness and addiction together—not just because they belonged together but because, as is true for many people, they affected my life in a completely comingled way, and I was only going to survive if I addressed them both, medically and one day at a time.

I also tried to have a sense of humor about this because, too often, when experts or patients are put in front of a camera, they turn deadly earnest and, frankly, sometimes a little self-serious and boring. In private, however, I can tell you they are often hilariously funny. Part of my job was to make comorbidity accessible.

In fact, the biggest laugh I got at the press conference was with a line people say in rehab, and in inpatient psychiatric care, all the time:

"Frankly," I said, "I didn't know how miserable I was until I started feeling better."

And as word spread the next day that Jim was my sponsor in recovery—the Capitol Hill daily *Roll Call* found out somehow and we didn't deny it—there was talk not only of comorbidity but also of a unique bipartisanship. Of course, it had been bipartisanship ten years before that allowed Paul Wellstone and Pete Domenici to co-sponsor the original parity act. But they were bipartisan family members, bipartisan caregivers—which was not surprising because at that time, in the political arena at least, the people with the illnesses primarily got a voice through their parents and family members.

Jim and I were something different. We were bipartisan patients, consumers, whatever word you want to use for the people who actually struggle with the diseases and conditions. (The most recent word used is "peers.") We had what is called "lived experience."

Parents and family members tend to talk about cures and remissions. Those of us with the illnesses know that what passes for "remission" is just the times when we can hold the cravings and symptoms at bay. We aren't living for the future; we're trying to survive and actually enjoy the present.

We're also in a struggle over where to focus our anger and blame: while we can be angry at our families and at the system, just like anyone else, our best chance of remaining in recovery is to blame the real culprit here. Which is, of course, the illnesses.

We are sick because, well, we are sick.

EIGHT DAYS LATER I was appearing at district court to plead guilty to one count of driving under the influence of a prescription drug, with a supervised probation of not less than twelve months. I agreed to commit to attending regular meetings of Dr. Smith's group and other AA groups, and to submit to random urine drug screenings. I also had to do fifty hours of community service and make small contributions to the Crime Victims Fund and the Boys and Girls Clubs of Greater Washington. Jim Ramstad came to court and stood by me as his first official act as my sponsor—which he had vaguely acknowledged in the press (in stories my office had confirmed, not his), but when the judge surprised him and directly asked him in court, he told the truth.

Besides all my AA meeting commitments, I had also begun a course of cognitive therapy treatment with a psychologist in Providence, who worked in tandem with a psychiatrist in DC who oversaw my meds. So I talked to the psychologist weekly and sometimes more often than that. I spoke to the psychiatrist less frequently, but he was made aware if anything major changed. This is now a relatively common model of care, but in 2006 that was less true.

For the first time I was getting more directed, more result-oriented CBT as an outpatient. The therapist stood up to me and was quick to set limits. So when I was upset or depressed and, say, went off on one or both of my parents in therapy, my therapist talked to me about living in the present. We discussed strategies for how to avoid getting caught up in cycles of obsessing on the past and assuming that my current feelings of anxiety could be cured by somehow making sense of what happened when I was ten. And she gave me very clear and directed homework so that I knew what I was supposed to be working on between sessions and what we would plan to work on in the next session.

For example, when I was planning to go see my family at the Cape, we focused on strategies that would help me not to obsess on feeling shame for what I had done, or fall into the trap of imagining all the things my father meant or felt when he didn't directly address things or made little passing remarks. I told the therapist I was glad I had discovered mental health advocacy, because there were times when it was the only thing that made me feel useful and hopeful for the future.

Some of the goal setting was pretty basic, like getting out of bed in the morning. But when you're struggling with depression and anxiety, and still coming down from drug and alcohol addiction, fulfilling the goal of getting out of bed can actually be quite an accomplishment.

I spent the summer just trying to get through the summer. I was still pretty raw and sometimes felt overwhelmed. I remember one day in August my brother invited me to come out on the daily sail with his

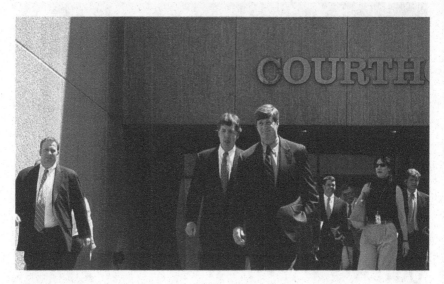

Representative Jim Ramstad and me leaving the courthouse in 2006, after I pleaded guilty to driving under the influence and Jim publicly acknowledged that he would be my twelve-step sponsor; that's my second chief of staff, Sean Richardson, at left.
(Jamie Rose/*The New York Times*/Redux)

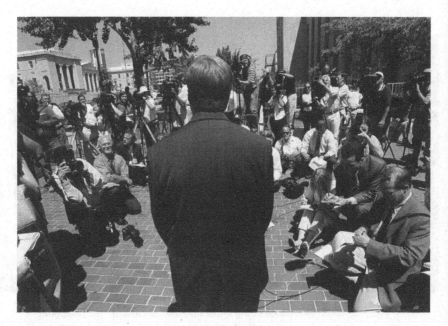

Talking to reporters outside the courtroom, June 2006.

(Copyright © Kevin Lamarque/Reuters/Corbis)

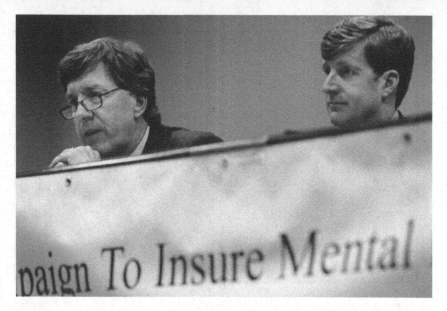

Jim Ramstad and me at the first of our fourteen parity "field hearings" to generate state and local interest for our House Mental Health Parity and Addiction Equity Act, HR 1424; this hearing was in Providence, January 2007. (Courtesy *Providence Journal*)

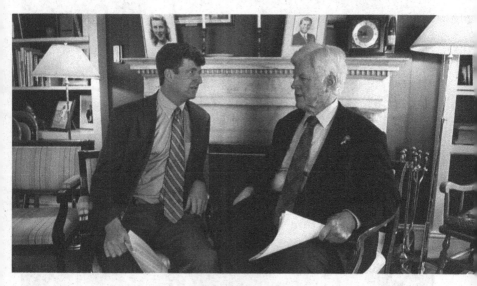

The *New York Times* photo of my father and me "discussing" our competing mental health parity bills while sitting in his Senate hideaway, March 2007.

(Doug Mills/*The New York Times*/Redux)

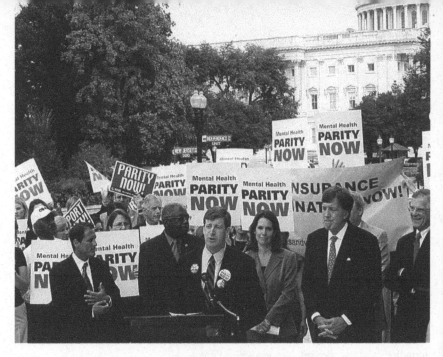

Speaking at one of our many Capitol Hill mental health parity rallies.
(Courtesy Kennedy Forum)

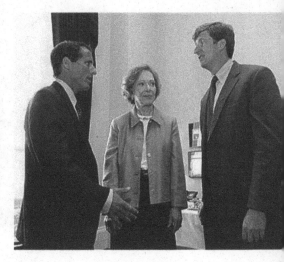

Discussing parity strategy
with David Wellstone,
the late Senator's son,
and Rosalynn Carter,
in July 2007, before the
House Education and
Labor Committee
hearing on the bill.
(Courtesy Capitol Decisions)

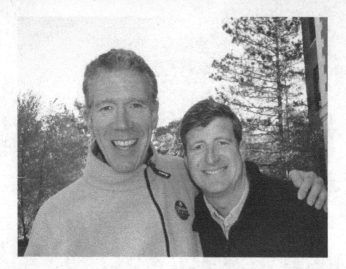

With mental health advocate Bill Emmet during the 2008 parity effort. Bill was the first person to ever speak to me about parity, when he was a local NAMI representative in Rhode Island in the late 1980s, and we worked together for many years. When I started the Kennedy Forum in 2013, he was the logical choice to be its first employee and founding executive director. (Courtesy William Emmet)

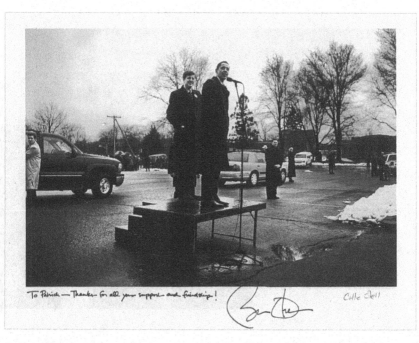

To Patrick — Thanks for all your support and friendship!

Callie Shell

Senator Barack Obama and me in Providence on March 1, 2008, in the early days of his Presidential campaign; he sent me a signed copy of this unpublished photo as a gift. (Photograph by Callie Shell)

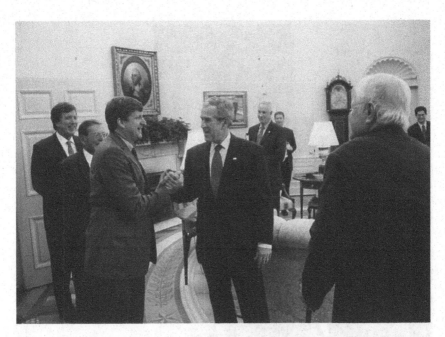

At the November 2008 White House signing ceremony for the Paul Wellstone and Pete Domenici Mental Health Parity and Addiction Equity Act, with, from left, Jim Ramstad, Senator Pete Domenici, President Bush, and foreground, my father. (Courtesy The White House)

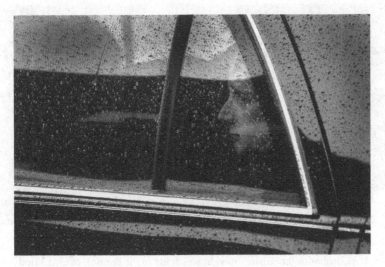

Leaving my father's funeral, August 2009. (Courtesy *Providence Journal*)

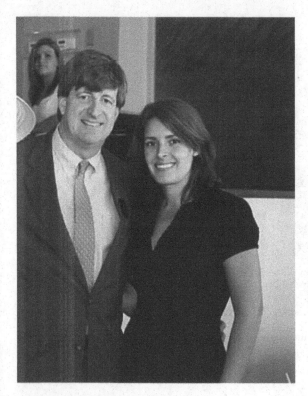

One of the first pictures taken of Amy and me when we started dating in 2010.

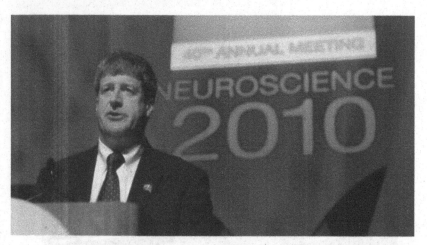

At the November 2010 Society for Neuroscience convention in San Diego, delivering the original "moonshot to innerspace" speech, which led to the creation of One Mind and much of my other post-Congress brain health advocacy. (Courtesy Society for Neuroscience)

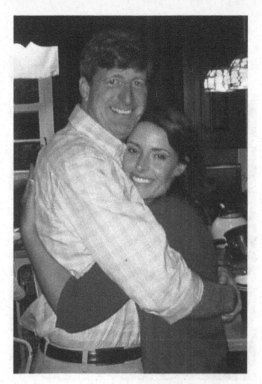

Amy and me in her parents' kitchen, after I had left rehab for a few days to be with her for Christmas—and then just decided to stay and get healthy with her and her family.

Amy, Harper, and me in her parents' living room; we lived at their house for the first year and a half we were together, and I conducted many of my "business" meetings on my cell phone from that wingback chair.

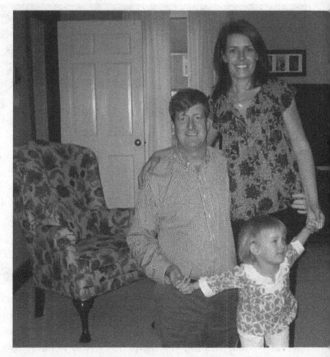

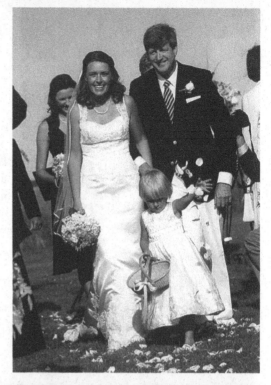

Our wedding, with Harper as flower girl, July 15, 2011.

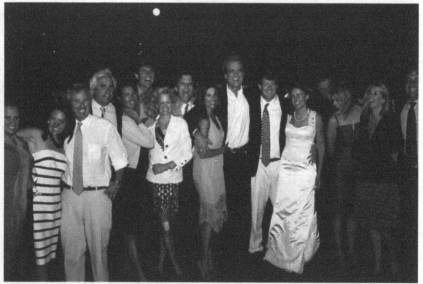

Kennedy cousins celebrate Amy and me getting married with a full moon over Hyannis Bay. From left: Kerry Kennedy, Sheila Kennedy, Chris Kennedy, Max Kennedy, Vicki Kennedy, Anthony Shriver, Linda Shriver, Tim Shriver, Malissa Shriver, Bobby Shriver, me, Amy, Bobby Kennedy Jr., Cheryl Hines, Rory Kennedy Bailey, and Mark Bailey.

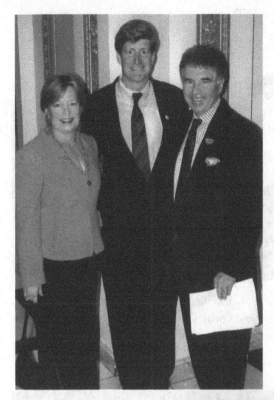

With Garen and Shari Staglin, the founders of the International Mental Health Research Organization (IMHRO), and my co-founders in One Mind. (Courtesy the Staglin family)

With Dr. Husseini Manji, the global head of neuroscience at the Janssen Pharmaceuticals division of Johnson & Johnson.

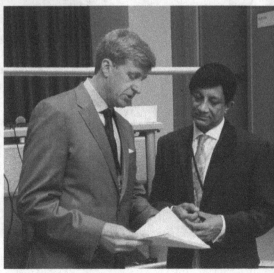

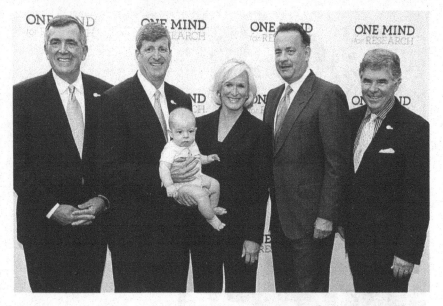

At the One Mind Los Angeles fund-raiser with, from left, General Pete Chiarelli, executive director of One Mind; me and Owen; Glenn Close, co-founder with her sister of BringChange2Mind; our emcee for the evening, Tom Hanks; and Garen Staglin. (Courtesy One Mind)

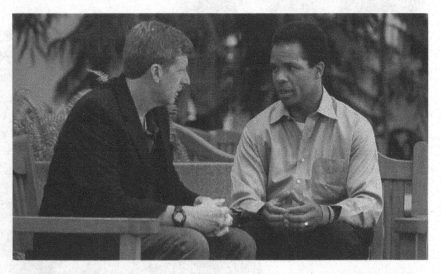

Meeting with Jesse Jackson Jr. at the Mayo Clinic in the summer of 2012, to discuss how I could help with his recovery . . . starting with talking to his dad about bipolar disorder.

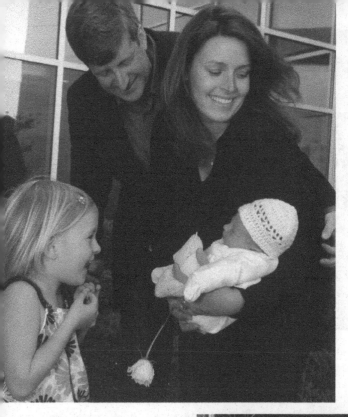

Bringing Owen home
from the hospital,
April 2012.
(AP Photo/*The Press of
Atlantic City*, Danny Drake)

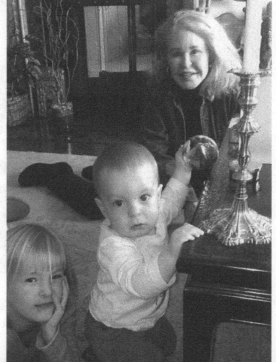

Harper and Owen
with my mom in her
apartment in Boston.

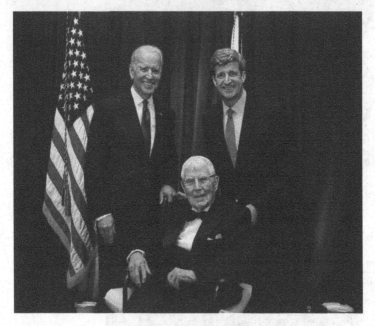

With Vice President Joe Biden and Dr. Aaron "Tim" Beck, the creator of cognitive therapy, backstage at the JFK Library during the inaugural Kennedy Forum dinner, October 2013. (Courtesy Kennedy Forum)

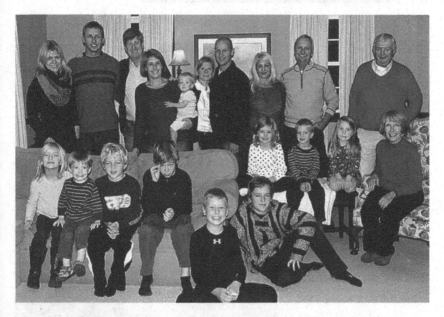

With the whole Savell family in Amy parents' living room for her birthday, 2014. Her parents, Leni and Jerry, are on the far right, in red. I have my arm around my brother-in-law Paul, and to Amy's left is her brother Chris.

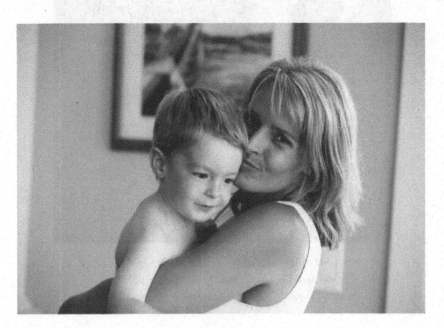

Amy and Owen.

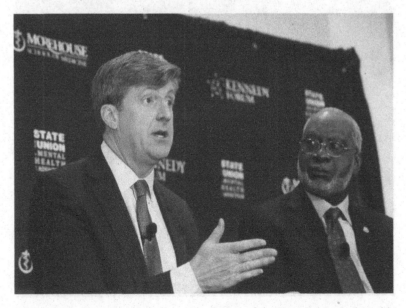

With Dr. David Satcher at the first annual State of the Union in Mental Health and Addiction at the National Press Club, February 2015. (Courtesy Kennedy Forum)

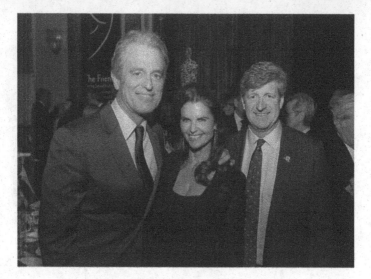

With my cousins Bobby and Maria Shriver
at the Semel Institute Great Minds Gala, April 2015.
(Courtesy Thomas Neerken/The Friends of the Semel Institute at UCLA)

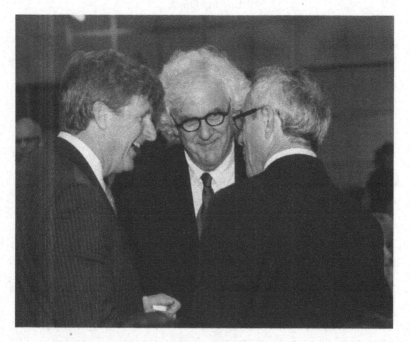

With my co-author, Stephen Fried (center), and NIMH director
Dr. Thomas Insel at the Kennedy Forum gala dinner at
the JFK Library. (Courtesy Kennedy Forum)

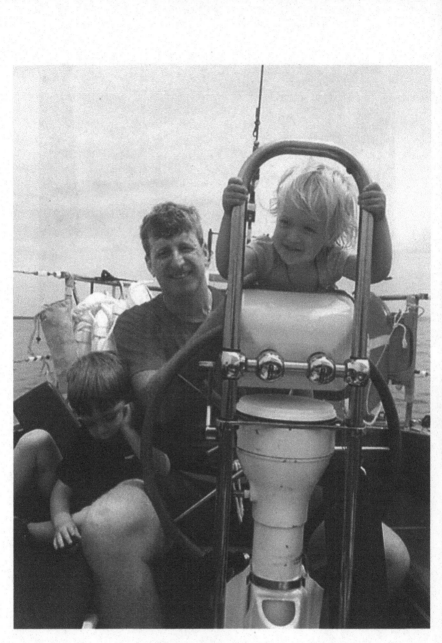

Sailing with Owen and Nora.

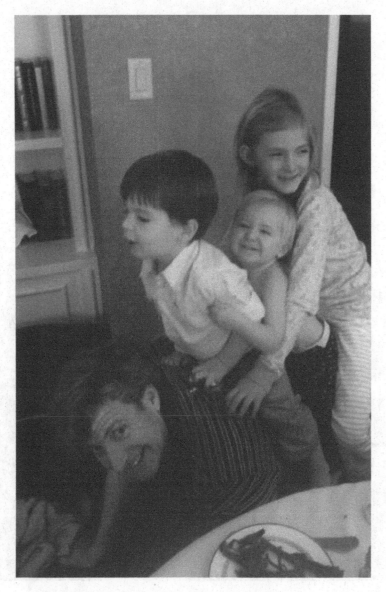

What goes on in our hotel room between speaking engagements:
Amy's picture of me and the kids.

family and some of his friends. I just couldn't deal with the big group. And then I worried that word was traveling through the family that I had turned down a chance to sail. So everyone was probably wondering what *that* meant—without anyone actually consulting me.

This is a common irritant for people with mental illness; everyone discussing how you "feel" without ever asking *you* how you feel. It's also common for us to assume our family members are having that discussion, even if we don't know for sure that they are.

POLITICAL SEASON BEGAN again after Labor Day, and Jim and I had given our big interview to the *New York Times* about our personal and political journeys and where they had led us. I was unusually frank with the reporter—being only four months sober and going to AA meetings every day will do that to you. And besides the messages we were already sending, he picked up on one I never would have brought up: that my new approach to mental health parity and addiction equity (the phrases we were developing to combine the comorbid illnesses) had to do with my own diseases, but also generational issues within my family.

Now, these were hardly generational issues unique to the Kennedys. They were true of pretty much every family in America. But, of course, my father didn't quite see it that way when the *Times* reporter called him for a comment and asked, among other things, whether or not he was still drinking. Dad described himself as being "well" over the past 15 years, a recovery he attributed to Vicki; he said he drank a glass of wine at home at night or in social settings.

My father also didn't love that I was quoted saying: "When you grow up in my family, being somebody meant having power, having status. The compensations you got were all material and superficial.

I've come to realize, in the last few months, that that life made me feel all alone."

While I'm sure I said this, it's the kind of thing people say about their families when they are recently out of rehab and not very far into recovery. I still wasn't acknowledging the illnesses as the primary culprit of my situation, or that the responsibility to change began with me alone.

The article was mostly about what had been a fairly hidden world of recovery on Capitol Hill. It was set at a regular Tuesday dinner that Jim and others had been attending for years at Morton's after their regular weekly twelve-step recovery meeting with Dr. Ron Smith—a dinner where all the drinks were soft but the revelations were often quite hard and emotional. This dinner just happened to mark my fourth month of sobriety. The article also mentioned several current and former legislators who had been part of this eclectic group, including former Senator Max Cleland—one of several members seeking twelve-step support for something other than addiction (in his case, PTSD). These meetings and dinners had become a huge part of my new life in recovery.

The story did mention that my dad and I shared a meal once a week, but even he was quoted as lauding Jim's "incredible generosity of spirit."

In the piece, Jim was quoted as saying he had come to love me "like a brother." But the reporter, who joined us for dinner, also noted the way that he told me to put my cell phone away was more like a father. I joked that I had never before taken direction from any Republican.

This piece appeared on the front page of the *Times* with a photo of Jim and me leaving the courthouse together after my guilty plea. And while our goal had been just to get our colleagues to take this legislative issue more seriously, the coverage served to accomplish something much more important: all of a sudden, the battle for mental health parity and addiction equity seemed incredibly *personal*.

THAT NOVEMBER, the Democrats finally regained control of the House, where we picked up over thirty seats and elevated Nancy Pelosi to Speaker. And I was reelected by the largest plurality of my whole congressional career, so voters seemed able to put my car crash and treatment into perspective. The Senate also came back under Democratic control, although by a much smaller margin. This allowed my father to resume chairmanship of the Senate HELP Committee, which would be the key to any legislation reaching the floor.

Yet, in the new year, my father and the leadership of the Senate threw their support behind a new mental health parity bill that was, in my opinion, far too similar to the one Pete Domenici had championed ten years earlier when the Republicans were in control. For several months, they had very quietly invited the main opponents of parity into their negotiations to make sure all stakeholders were heard from, which was fine. But they made too many compromises to keep the most powerful parties happy.

What they ended up with was the kind of legislation likely to be supported by insurance companies; large employers with many insured workers; the pharmaceutical industry; the most powerful guilds (the American Medical, American Psychiatric, and American Psychological associations); and the most powerful lobby for the very sickest mentally ill, NAMI—along with Senate Republicans, who, like many of his friends across the aisle, wanted to give Pete Domenici a well-deserved namesake bill for all his years of groundbreaking advocacy for serious mental illness.

My father's bill certainly did succeed at eliminating some discrimination in deductibles, copays, and annual and lifetime treatment limits. But it was not clear which diagnoses were covered and protected—leaving that decision largely to insurers. His bill did not mandate full parity for all mental illnesses, and it didn't include parity for substance use disorder treatment *at all*. If passed it would allow discrimination in the coverage of many brain diseases—including the ones from which Jim and I suffered—to remain completely legal.

That was far below the gold standard of parity that had already been put in place for all federal employees—including the members of the Senate and House and their families.

The bill Jim and I were writing in the House, of course, covered all mental illnesses and addictions. It was to be a full civil rights act for brain disorders—all the mental illness diagnoses in the *DSM*, and all substance use disorders. It was the kind of bill that consumers, their families, and all their caregivers and institutions of care were likely to support.

There was also one other major difference between the Senate bill and the one we were drafting, one that was fairly technical in nature but would make a huge difference. It involved how the federal bill would impact existing state parity laws. Since healthcare is basically delivered state by state—even under federal programs like Medicaid— the state laws often influence patient experiences much more than national mandates. When the 1996 federal parity act proved so ineffective, many states had passed much stronger mental health parity laws offering better coverage for more illnesses. But my father's Senate bill, in one of its most industry-friendly nods, would have legally superseded any state laws that allowed greater fairness in coverage. In our bill, if the state wanted more protection for consumers than the federal mandate, the state law prevailed.

I took the differences in the two bills really personally. How couldn't I? Theirs didn't cover parity for substance use disorders even though my mother, my brother, and I had all been treated for them—and just weeks before my father introduced his bill, my sister, Kara, who had been very curious about my inpatient experiences at Mayo, quietly checked herself in there for treatment. So now all three of us— including my much more resilient older siblings—had ended up in recovery from this family illness. Yet substance use disorders still weren't covered equitably in my father's Senate bill.

I found myself talking about parity and my relationship with my father during my cognitive therapy sessions, especially at the end of February—when there was always a celebration for my dad's birthday—and the beginning of March, when I got my AA "chip" for being ten months sober.

If I couldn't convince my father that he was not only backing the wrong bill but indulging in some strange form of legislative denial, then all I could do was try to beat him. So I decided to take a page from his own playbook. Early in his career, my father had taken an unconventional tack in his effort to pass healthcare reform: he held what were called "field hearings," all over the country. The idea was to re-create the kinds of intense, well-orchestrated, full-day hearings usually held on Capitol Hill and take them to the public, state by state, to build local support. I went along on some of them. They were great fun and often fascinating because of the chance for public testimony.

Jim and I decided we would do the same thing for parity. And since these field hearings looked and sounded official but could not be paid for out of our House member budgets, we got Mental Health America—which represented the broadest coalition of patients with the widest range of diagnoses—to fund these events and congressional supporters to host them in their home districts. That's how the Campaign to Insure Mental Health and Addiction Equity was born.

In the first three months of 2007, we did hearings in fourteen cities, starting with our home districts in Rhode Island and Minnesota, and then going on to Rockville, Maryland; Los Angeles; Vancouver, Washington; Sacramento; Palo Alto; the Denver suburb of Aurora (where, five years later, a young man with mental illness would kill twelve people and injure seventy more in a movie theater shooting); the New Jersey State House in Trenton; Elwyn, Pennsylvania, outside of Philadelphia; Dallas; Tulsa; and Pittsburgh. Eighteen members of Congress and two US Senators hosted the hearings or participated in them.

Wherever we traveled, we combined national and local elected officials, representatives of state and local care facilities and advocacy groups, and lots of "public testimony" from ordinary citizens who had been denied mental health or addiction care because it was still legal to discriminate in coverage of their illnesses. And because Jim was a hero in the recovery movement, the hearings also included people who rarely looked to the government or health insurance for their care, because they were committed to the volunteer and free support of AA and other twelve-step groups.

It was a fascinating coalition of really passionate people. And the gatherings were powerfully comorbid.

The stories we heard from patients and family members during those hearings stay with me to this day. The pain of what we heard—and, in so many cases, it was pain that could have been prevented, remedied, or reduced—was sometimes hard to comprehend. So was the hope some people were able to maintain after incredible loss.

It was important that these field hearings brought attention to state and local political leaders interested in parity—and alerted us to many regional differences in the problems of diagnosis, treatment, and insurance coverage that are hard to tease out in a half-day or full-day event in Washington. But it was the patient and family stories that haunted me the whole time, and still do.

I especially remember Steve Winter, a middle-aged man in a wheelchair who traveled to several of our hearings around the country, at his own expense. When he was growing up in Akron, Ohio, he did not realize that his mother had a mental illness. He did not understand that she had been diagnosed with schizophrenia and was taking medication—and didn't realize that when she started acting strangely, it was because she had stopped taking her medication. This happens a lot, often because when the medication works and the patient's symptoms lessen, they decide they are "cured" or "in remission" and secretly stop taking the meds. Or, in the case of Steve's mother, she had changed health insurance and there was some issue with her meds being covered under the new plan; so, since she was feeling okay, she just stopped asking for them.

One morning just after Christmas when Steve was fourteen years old, he was sitting at the breakfast table eating his cereal when he heard his mom yell. He kept eating but suddenly felt strange and, looking down, reached into his shirt and came away with a handful of blood. Then his mother stormed into the room holding a gun.

She yelled, "I shot your sister. I shot you and I'm going to shoot me so we can be in heaven together!" He was able to convince her to put the gun down and call for ambulances that came for all three of them. His sister was still alive, and while the bullet fired at him didn't hit any organs, it did hit his spinal cord and he was eventually left paralyzed from the waist down. His mother was hospitalized, not charged, and within a matter of months she was stabilized on medication.

Steve was not at these hearings for sympathy: "I'm not a professional victim," he always said. He wanted to point out just how much money his insurance company was paying for all his bills for his disability, millions and millions that wouldn't have been spent if the mental health system had been a little more proactive and had taken better care of his mom.

Steve's complaints mirrored those of many patients and family members who testified about being denied care—mostly expensive inpatient care, which was either refused altogether or withdrawn, without any real understanding of medical necessity, far before the patients were well enough to go home. Even when families had an inpatient hospitalization benefit of just thirty days, and with a high deductible, it was often hard to even get that: patients would be forced to go home after five or six days, or have their stays reviewed every two days, so instead of focusing on treatment, the families spent much of the time worrying their loved one would be prematurely discharged.

At the same time, we heard amazing stories of the value of evidence-based, gold-standard care and the importance of treating mental illnesses as truly chronic, rather than acute and episodic—practices that not only improve patients' lives but save insurers money. And we heard astonishing success stories. At our hearing in Palo Alto, we met Kevin Hines, one of the only people to ever survive jumping off the Golden Gate Bridge. To hear about what was going on in his brain the day he made that leap, and to see him years later, successfully treating his depression and engaged to be married, was so gratifying.

Stories like his highlighted the tragedy and sometimes the absurdity of impediments to care. A physician from Tulsa told us about a conversation he had with an insurance company health plan reviewer, who was trying to decide if a patient was suicidal enough to get inpatient treatment. The doctor was asked if the patient had a plan to take his own life, which of course he did or his doctor wouldn't have been trying to hospitalize him. When told that, yes, the patient reported having plans to shoot himself, the insurance reviewer then asked if the patient had a gun.

When the doctor replied that he did, the insurance reviewer actually asked this question:

"Does the patient have bullets?"

WHILE WE WERE ON THE ROAD, my dad and Pete Domenici worked behind the scenes and prepared their bill for the big day when it would have its public committee "markup"—in which committee members could ask questions, offer amendments, and, once they were through that gauntlet, take a committee vote. The markup was scheduled for Valentine's Day 2007. The night before, my father and Pete and all their aides summoned all the major advocacy groups—who had been left out of negotiations to first create consensus among insurance, employers, and the guilds—to a private meeting in a Senate conference room. They were told that, for the first time, all the major business stakeholders had agreed to a mental health parity bill, and the advocacy community was expected to support this bill and no others. Apparently they barely stopped short of asking for a blood oath. And everyone agreed.

The next day, during the actual markup, *The Diane Rehm Show*—a powerful, locally produced NPR talk show—featured the subject of mental health parity, with a panel that included a group rarely heard agreeing on much: Andrew Sperling, the top lobbyist from NAMI; the president of Cigna Behavioral Health, a major national insurer; and the vice president for health policy of the major employer group the American Benefits Council. Pete Domenici also called in during an early segment of the one-hour show. And then with just a few minutes remaining, and the guests answering calls from listeners, my father called in. In a great bit of political theater, he announced "some very good news . . . Just probably seven or eight minutes ago, we passed that bill out of our committee, eighteen to three. You're the first ones to hear about it!" He explained that with that large a majority, he felt very good about the prospects for its quick passage on the Senate floor.

He did note, however, that they were still "working with House members," explaining, "We still, um, have a few issues there that we're working on through. But that's the legislative process, and we're very hopeful and optimistic."

NOT LONG AFTER, Jim and I were summoned to a private meeting in Pete Domenici's second-floor hideaway in the Capitol. My father was there, too. This was not meant to be an amicable lunch get-together. It was meant to be one of those "You have meddled with the primal forces of nature, and *you will atone*" meetings, like in the movie *Network*.

Pete was furious that we were about to propose an alternative parity bill that would get in the way of his done deal. And when Pete was mad or frustrated he didn't just raise his voice, he threw his entire body language at you. I can still hear him like it was yesterday: "You put that stuff in there about alcohol and addicts and you're gonna *kill this bill!* That's the ultimate poison pill if you put that stuff in there!"

He also said that covering all the diagnoses in the *DSM* was ridiculous—"they have jet lag and caffeine addiction in there, for God's sake."

Now, Pete Domenici, at the age of seventy-four, was a true hero in the history of mental health politics: the first powerful politician to ever succeed in accomplishing anything to improve budgets for research and even get parity for serious mental illnesses on the agenda. And if he skewed toward the needs of those most disabled by mental illness, he came by that bias honestly: his daughter's illness, which had inspired all the advocacy he and his wife did, was much more disabling than mine.

But while I respected Pete immensely and he was a friend of my father, I also felt very strongly that he had made a bad deal. We weren't going to pull our bill just because he said we must. He claimed we were playing politics with mental health and that if we kept pushing our agenda to include addiction coverage, everyone would lose.

It was a tough meeting that didn't even end with us agreeing to disagree. He made it clear he would do everything he could to stop us.

And we made it clear we weren't going to stop.

My dad was pretty quiet through all this. This was, after all, Pete's bill, Pete's life's work, not his. He was really just standing in for his late friend Paul Wellstone. He wasn't going to intercede between me and Pete. He didn't aggressively take sides, but then he didn't have to: one reason my dad was so successful in the Senate is when he made a promise, he kept his promise. He believed that American government was based on promises made and kept.

That said, he also believed in process. And as we left this very uncomfortable meeting, he said he assumed that someday the two bills would end up in a conference committee.

"That," he said, "is democracy."

WE FINISHED UP our field hearings and finalized our bill, which we decided to name boldly by invoking the name of the late Senator Paul Wellstone. We believed that if he were still alive, he would have supported our version, because its broad coverage was what he originally wanted in 1996. So on Wednesday, March 7, we introduced the Paul Wellstone Mental Health Parity and Addiction Equity Act, which became HR 1424, on the House floor.

A week later, the Senate bill passed their budget committee. And those watching this process unfold began to realize just how personal the parity issue was becoming in the Senate and House, and within Washington lobbying and advocacy circles.

The highlight—for me, anyway; less so for my dad—was a big

Times story near the end of March under the headline "Proposals for Mental Health Parity Pit a Father's Pragmatism Against a Son's Passion." It was illustrated with a photo he grudgingly agreed to have taken, of the two of us, each gripping our respective bills, talking very forcefully in his private Senate hideaway in front of the fireplace.

Ratcheting up the personal issues even further, the article noted that not only had Jim and I named our bill for Paul Wellstone, but the Senator's two sons—especially David, who had become very active in his father's place on mental health issues—and their nonprofit had specifically asked my father and Pete Domenici *not* to include their father's name on their Senate bill, because it was not "true to Paul Wellstone's vision."

The story ended with my dad saying he was confident he and I could resolve our differences. "We will," he said, "find ways of working together."

Chapter 20

My probation ended in the middle of all these mental health and addiction politics, so no more urine tests or turning in my AA meeting sign-in sheets—but no change in my regular routines within the recovery community. And on May 5, 2007, I was greeted in my office by a handwritten, hand-delivered note from Jim Ramstad, congratulating me on finishing my first year in recovery—and the most sober twelve-month period in my life since, well, around age twelve or thirteen. We both discussed the anniversary with the media, and Jim made an interesting point I hadn't thought of—the biggest difference in my life in the past year of recovery was that "his public persona is exactly the same as his private persona."

People who are sober, he explained, don't have to put on a "game face" so much to mask their shameful secrets. You can be real; you can be yourself.

This is one of the central ideas of recovery from addiction that the mental health community could really stand to learn. Because in mental illness treatment, we are not always encouraged as much to be open—we help contribute to our own stigma sometimes through fear of being ourselves, or fear of sharing our symptoms and struggles. And our caregivers, who suffer some professional stigma themselves, often contribute to this by encouraging us to hide our illness and treatment. In fact, we need to learn to be more fearless. (I was recently at a criminal justice forum where a man with bipolar disorder was describing how he had been arrested during a psychotic episode. During his testimony, he started getting really animated and agitated, and then he paused and said, "I'm going to stop now, because I'm having racing thoughts." It was breathtaking to see that level of openness and self-awareness.)

I am one of the few people I know who shuttles back and forth between the worlds of recovery and medical mental healthcare, as a politician and a patient, with equal trust in both approaches and faith that eventually they will be integrated. Most people, unfortunately, think they are supposed to choose just one approach (and too many people, sadly, still don't choose either and just wait to "snap out of it"). In May of 2007, when I got my one-year chip, I was attending daily meetings in either DC or Providence and my weekly meeting with Dr. Ron Smith, as well as doing cognitive behavioral therapy at least once a week with my therapist in Providence (often on the phone) and speaking at least once every few weeks with the psychopharmacologist overseeing my meds. I didn't see these approaches as being mutually exclusive. Mental health parity and addiction equity isn't only about fair and equal insurance coverage. It's also about the world of mental illness treatment and the world of addiction treatment—each of which grew from what felt like a specific form of being ostracized by society—working together much more effectively.

We waste an awful lot of time trying to decide if people are mentally ill first and addicted secondarily, or the other way around. There is, at the moment anyway, no way to prove which one is primary, yet both the clinical communities and the patient communities can be amazingly judgmental of whichever approach they aren't currently embracing.

TWO MONTHS AFTER my first anniversary in recovery, I turned forty. There was a big family party for me at the Cape on a mid-July weekend. Both of my parents were there, and they both had had a few drinks. My mom never drank in public, but it was obvious when she arrived that way; my dad had substantially moderated his drinking after marrying Vicki, but still loved indulging at a summer party. It was hard seeing them both this way. It made me want to join them.

But the situation was actually even more complicated than that. I had made an interesting breakthrough in one of my group therapy sessions at Mayo. I tearfully admitted that I had always felt the most emotional connection to my father when he was drinking. When he wasn't, he seemed more intense and difficult to bond with. I also had to admit that, as I had grown older, I felt more emotionally connected to him when we drank together. And remaining sober meant figuring out how to feel more emotionally accessible without alcohol or drugs.

It took every bit of strength I had to hold my frustration and anxiety in check and not drink that day. Instead, I took more Vivarin than I should have, since caffeine was my only remaining crutch and I didn't want to be seen drinking endless Red Bulls at the party. But I was basically able to hold it together.

I had to. I had a bigger goal in sight: the first of the three House committees that had to pass our parity bill had scheduled it for markup and a vote.

Once a bill is introduced, its sponsors are completely beholden to the Speaker of the House and the chairs of the various committees and subcommittees that must pass it before it gets a chance for a vote on the House floor. We were very fortunate to have the support of Speaker Nancy Pelosi, who I know had also been told by Pete Domenici and my father that she and the House needed to get out of their way.

I will be eternally grateful that she politely ignored them and not only encouraged our bill but encouraged the three main committee chairs who would have to schedule hearings and markups—Charles Rangel of New York (chair of Ways and Means), John Dingell of Michigan (chair of Energy and Commerce), and George Miller of California (chair of Education and Labor)—and all the relevant subcommittee chairs, as well as their staffs, to make this a priority. This involves literally hundreds of people, each of whose time is scheduled out in five- and ten-minute increments, for which there is literally endless demand.

Just before my birthday weekend, the House Education and Labor subcommittee on health, employment, labor, and pensions held a hearing that was highlighted by an inspirational appearance by former First Lady Rosalynn Carter. She blew away some of the testifying national business and insurance leaders, who were there already pledged to the Senate bill and trying to punch holes in ours.

And just after the weekend, Chairman Rangel had scheduled Ways and Means—which had already held its subcommittee hearings on the bill—to do a public markup and then a vote. The markup went fine and the committee passed the bill by a vote of 33 to 9.

I tore the front page off a copy of the bill and wrote a note to Nancy Pelosi across the front of it:

> *Today, under your Speakership, this nation took another step*
> *toward fulfilling its promised ideal of equal opportunity and justice*

for all. *Thank you for both your personal and political support throughout this process.*

> *Love,*
> *Patrick*

And for the first time, all the people and organizations that were sure my father and Pete Domenici had already struck the final deal on parity realized that the discussion was just getting started.

THE DISCUSSION WAS even more complicated than it appeared. There were two competing bills mandating this thing called "parity," which was a great idea but, like "racial equality," something you couldn't just snap your congressional fingers and make happen. But, also, the dueling bills only addressed the issue by creating new rules for private medical insurance, which people got through their employers or bought themselves.

This private insurance covered about 65 percent of Americans under retirement age, and we hoped if we legislated a new standard there, it would be adopted across the board. Mostly, we hoped it would be adopted by the single largest insurer that wasn't practicing parity and still had unfairly high copays and treatment limits: CMS, the Centers for Medicare & Medicaid Services, which offered government coverage for low-income Americans, disabled Americans, older Americans, and children without private insurance. But changing the rules in CMS required different legislation, which was being pushed at the same time by our colleague Representative Pete Stark.

There was also the looming issue of mental healthcare in the military, which was starting to get more attention after the scandals about substandard care at Walter Reed Army Medical Center and the upcoming fifth anniversary of the Iraq War—which dovetailed with whispers about a dramatically rising suicide rate among recent vets. At this time we were just beginning to understand the problem that posttraumatic stress disorder and other trauma-based brain diseases were not being taken seriously enough. This was insulting to not only all the Americans who had been diagnosed with trauma-based illnesses when they were first recognized in Vietnam vets and sexual abuse victims, but now to the first "wounded warriors" from Iraq and Afghanistan. (PTSD was actually one of several illnesses that we worried would not be fully covered under the Senate bill.)

I was working to amend the Wounded Warrior Assistance Act, which was making its way through House committees, to beef up mental health provisions for veterans returning with what were starting to be called the "invisible wounds of war." While it was crucial to improve the mental healthcare within the VA, many people didn't understand how many veterans do not or cannot access mental healthcare through their veteran's benefits. A surprising number of vets rely on insurance provided by their post-service employers, which meant they needed the protections of mental health parity like everyone else.

THAT SUMMER, I decided to spend the first week in August—for which I've been with my family at the Cape pretty much every year of my life—at an intensive five-day workshop on recovery, coping skills, and spirituality at the Caron Foundation near Reading, Pennsylvania. It was a relief to be going to a rehab facility for a positive reason—I had been alcohol and drug free for exactly one year and three months—and the experiential therapy and lecture sessions were really helpful. It all reinforced something I knew intellectually but, especially in my more challenged moments, still couldn't get past.

I was, always, seeking my father's approval more than self-approval. Because I still didn't know who I was or which self I approved of.

And while it was easy enough to blame this on the pressure of living up to the Kennedy legacy, the more I was confronted in therapy, and watched others be confronted in group therapy, the more I had to admit that my family issues were not unique at all. Fathers and sons, worrying about expectations and legacies, speaking but not really talking. Families trying to ignore mental illness and addiction. These are common problems, really common.

And the way to treat them was also common: hard work, commitment to recovery and medical treatment, humility, building more connections to others who knew my real self, living in the present, and not making every little thing said—and unsaid—a referendum on the past.

So I made a deal with myself that I wasn't going to seek anything from my father anymore. Easier said than done, of course, but I was going to try. And if I couldn't handle being in big group settings with everyone at Hyannis that year, it would be okay. I felt a little guilty not being there as much, assuming people would be talking about sulky Patrick avoiding the family. But I was just trying to break some endless cycles I felt were challenging my ability to remain sober, and remain committed to the medication and psychotherapy for my bipolar disorder. And you can't ask everyone around you at the shore not to drink, you just can't.

As Congress got back to work after Labor Day, the parity fight got more intense and, if possible, more personal.

I had strongly suggested to the leading lobbyist in Washington for addiction care, my friend Carol McDaid—who was in recovery herself—that she try to organize every group that felt left out of the form of parity proposed by the Senate bill. So she brought together over two hundred organizations from across the country to create the Parity Now Coalition, which went to Capitol Hill battle with the more establishment Coalition for Fairness in Mental Illness Coverage. (The only major group straddling both coalitions was Mental Health America.)

Then on September 17, Jim Ramstad announced that he wasn't going to run for reelection in 2008. So, more than ever, the mental health and addiction equity bill was going to be his legacy.

The very next day, the full Senate approved the parity bill sponsored by my father and Pete Domenici. The day after that, our bill was approved by the House Ways and Means health subcommittee, which meant it would be sent to the full committee.

And then two weeks later, Pete Domenici stunned Washington by announcing that he wasn't going to run for reelection and then disclosing the reason why: he had been diagnosed with a serious neurological condition, frontotemporal lobar degeneration. By the time he left office, we were heartened by the news that his diagnosis had changed somewhat. The cognitive impairments that had led to his original diagnosis appeared to plateau rather than worsening quickly as predicted, so his prognosis improved considerably. But his announcement in early October of 2007 just reinforced what we already knew—that he considered his version of the mental health bill to be his legacy.

EVEN THOUGH this was the toughest political battle I had ever experienced, something else was going on behind the scenes that I found equally remarkable. There was an outpouring of sympathy, empathy, and openness that I had never imagined possible in Washington. People were frequently taking me aside to share stories of their own mental illness and addiction, or that of a spouse, parent, child, or close friend. They wanted advice on treatment options—figuring that by now I had tried every inpatient facility and outpatient treatment, and had consulted (either personally or professionally during a hearing) with every major government, academic, and private expert there was.

These outreaches were, honestly, the most bipartisan phenomenon I had ever seen on Capitol Hill. I associated them not only with my openness about my illness and our legislation, and the fact that I was attending AA meetings, but something else I had never expected to be part of my Washington life. As the search for spirituality became a larger part of my recovery, I decided to attend some Capitol Hill prayer meetings, which included many of my colleagues who were also prominent members of the Christian Coalition.

Now, coming from a liberal and Catholic family background, I knew little about the Christian Coalition except that they sometimes supported legislative positions that didn't seem all that "Christian" to me. But in these prayer meetings I had with members, I must say, there was some serious soul searching. These guys would lay it all out! There was as much or more being put on the table as there was in our process groups at Mayo.

Each week someone was assigned to read a portion of the Bible, comment on it, and tell their story. It was a fascinating bonding experience, and afterward when you passed each other in the hallway at the Capitol you knew you'd shared a level of intimacy and understood something about what made each other tick—and it could be profound.

I started realizing this when I first went to Mayo and I got more heartfelt get-well cards from Republicans than Democrats to a tune of, maybe, eight to one, which blew my mind. I had been the chair of the DCCC, pummeling the Republicans relentlessly. This was just so unexpected, and so reassuring.

That said, they didn't all vote with me. I had many experiences with colleagues who came up to me after meetings and shared that

their spouses had tried to commit suicide, or their friends were struggling with mental illness or addiction, and then they voted against the
parity bill.

I do wonder today how some of them feel about that, especially
now that there is more openness in society about mental illness and
addiction as illnesses rather than moral failings.

As we headed into the fall of 2007, the supporters of the Senate
bill started panicking. They were afraid that if there were no compromise on parity before the presidential campaign got into full swing, we
would miss our chance. The loudest voice in the advocacy community
for this position was NAMI's national office in Washington, which
was pledged to the Senate bill. But they also knew that, at the grassroots level, a lot of their state chapters and local members supported
what we were doing. It was a confusing political time.

Privately, of course, I kept getting more messages that Jim and I
were on the right path, and that we couldn't let mental health parity
be passed without attaching it to equity for substance use disorder
treatment.

In my own family, while I was struggling to stay sober and healthy,
my sister, Kara, had a slip and decided to go back into rehab just
before Thanksgiving at Father Martin's Ashley in Havre de Grace,
Maryland. She sent me a card from there that I treasure, not only because of the moving sentiment of her note but because I took the card
with me to a meeting where I had a real breakthrough in my understanding of all I had to keep balanced to stay well. I actually used the
inside of the envelope the card came in to take notes: drawing a cir-
cle with four quadrants, one for my physical challenges, one for my
mental challenges, one for my emotional challenges, and one for my
spiritual challenges.

My mother was also going through a rough time that fall and winter. She decided that the root of her depression was not mental illness but the "jail" of her guardianship by us, and that she should go away for long-term treatment somewhere far from Boston. This is a pretty common dynamic in medical guardianships and an extreme version of the challenges of any consumer/caregiver relationship: out of sheer frustration over not feeling better, it is easy to blame the treatment rather than the illness. And there is, in twelve-step recovery and other modes of treatment, an ingrained fear of patients overbelieving in what has classically been referred to as "the geographical cure"—the old-fashioned notion that there is nothing wrong with you that a "change of scenery" couldn't fix. Still, there was nothing wrong with the idea that she might benefit from a restful wellness retreat where she could also be monitored, and she chose Canyon Ranch in Arizona.

While she got good care there and we were pleased she was being aggressive about trying something different, her letters home made me a little concerned. They seemed to suggest that she was blaming her shame, especially her "public shame," for her alcoholism and depression, rather than the illnesses themselves. She also blamed the guardianship itself for her symptoms, saying that it had made her sicker and more depressed than she had ever been before.

In one note she apologized to me for her drinking and said she admired my sobriety. "I want what you have," she wrote. "Will you share some of your strength with me?"

DURING THE HOLIDAY RECESS in late 2007, I was with Senator Arlen Specter on a trip to Israel, Syria, and Pakistan. As representatives of the Senate and House appropriations committees, we went first to Jerusalem, where we met with Prime Minister Ehud Olmert and Defense Minister Ehud Barak, and then to Islamabad.

It was an intriguing trip with a number of very long plane rides, where Senator Specter and I had a lot of time together, just the two of us. We talked about a lot of things and I even asked him what it was like to be on the Warren Commission investigating my Uncle Jack's assassination. He said he just remembered the whole thing being rushed, in a way that nobody could really understand—because it was such an unprecedented situation and they were aware they had to balance the search for the truth with their fear of the country falling apart if they took too much more time. But he knew they hadn't had a chance to pursue all the leads he would have liked. This didn't shock me at all; in fact, it made me understand the situation better. It was also ironic that we discussed it, considering what happened next.

In Pakistan we met first with President Musharraf and then with Afghanistan's President Karzai. That evening, we were scheduled to meet with Benazir Bhutto, the former prime minister of Pakistan and opposition leader who was considered crucial to the country's future and any peace process. She had a long-standing relationship with my family, as had her father, starting from when she had been educated at Harvard. I had first met her in 1989, when I was in my early twenties, at a dinner my father hosted for her at the JFK Presidential Library. We weren't close, but we had been crossing paths for a long time in international politics.

I was just leaving my room at the Serena Hotel to go meet her at her home for dinner when someone who was traveling with us called out and said I should see what was being reported on television—the horrifying news that Benazir Bhutto had been attacked. The first news stories made us fear the worst, but we initially received word through the US embassy that the media might be exaggerating the story and they had heard her wounds were superficial. Which made it all the more stunning when, an hour later, we heard she was dead, at the age of fifty-four.

It was hard to know what exactly we should do. Senator Specter and I decided it would be too dangerous to go to her house and try to pay our respects, so instead we went to the headquarters of her party, the Pakistan Peoples Party, and laid a wreath under a large poster of her outside the building. A photo was taken of us, flanking the poster with looks of complete shock on our faces, as Pakistanis surrounded us, placing flowers all over.

That night, we watched from our hotel as the city went up in flames. I remember thinking that this must have been what it felt like all over America the day Dr. King was killed—her death, like his, dashed the hopes of so many. The situation was so unstable our military attaché felt we needed to get out of there as soon as possible. They flew us out very early the next morning.

Chapter 21

B y the time our parity bill finally approached a vote on the House floor in early March of 2008, there had been a seismic shift in Washington. The American economy had begun its free fall, with the Dow diving and subprime loan specialist Countrywide Financial collapsing. In the aftermath of the Iowa caucuses, several prominent Democrats, including our friend Chris Dodd, dropped out of the presidential race. Then my cousin Caroline, followed by my father, proceeded to stun the party by endorsing Barack Obama. After her op-ed in the *Times* and his announcement, the three of us appeared with Senator Obama at a rally at American University to drive home the strong Kennedy family endorsement.

On March 5, the day the bill was scheduled for a vote, we held a big lunchtime rally outside of the Capitol, attended by all our congressional supporters, led by Nancy Pelosi, Paul Wellstone's son David, and perhaps our most resonant ally, Rosalynn Carter. Jim and I met her when her limo pulled into the horseshoe in front of the Rayburn building, and there was a ton of press, all sticking microphones in her face. Somebody yelled out, "Mrs. Carter, do you have a position on who

you'll support, Senator Clinton or Senator Obama?" Jim and I immediately thought we were doomed, because whatever she said would
steal all the thunder from the parity bill.

Mrs. Carter paused for a second and then, with a big smile, said, "I
support . . . Patrick Kennedy for President!" The media were perplexed,
but it was a brilliant dodge of the question.

We were sure we had the necessary votes and in normal times that
would have been enough. But these weren't normal times. The economy was imploding; New York brokerage house Bear Stearns was just
days from announcing that it was almost out of money. On the eve of
the fifth anniversary of the war in Iraq, remaining support for American involvement there was cratering. And the presidential primaries
just made everything a lot louder.

OUR FLOOR DEBATE in the House began at one fifty-seven P.M.
While there were many speeches in favor, there was also a lot of very
specific opposition. One of the more vocal opponents was Pete Domenici's colleague from New Mexico Heather Wilson, who entered into
the record the names of the hundreds of organizations supporting the
Senate bill, as if they all opposed our bill (which of course many didn't,
since Rosalynn Carter's Mental Health Program was on the list).

Pete Domenici was still very much battling us. When asked that
day for comment on our bill, he told a reporter, "To me this is an absolute disaster." Besides the opposition from insurers and employers, even
President Bush came out against us: the day of the vote the White House
Office of Management and Budget announced our bill would "have
a negative effect on the accessibility and affordability of employer-
provided health benefits and would undermine the uniform administration of employee benefit plans."

After nearly two and a half hours of debate, there was a break for a procedural matter on another bill. At 4:28 we began again, and as we did a buzz began on the floor and from the gallery. I was sitting up front so I didn't initially see what was causing the commotion, but then I turned and saw.

It was my father, walking toward me.

Now, I had grown up watching my father on the Senate floor, and even after being elected to Congress, I sometimes went over just to see him in action. But my father rarely came over to the House to watch me; it had happened maybe twice in thirteen years.

I was stunned. He came up to where I was, put his arm around my shoulder, gave me a squeeze, and then sat down next to me.

I felt empowered and eight years old at the same time. And I was very conscious of just how many people on the floor and in the observation areas realized how big a deal this was—to me, and to mental health parity. It was like we were all watching a movie, and in their minds, everyone was saying "ahhh" the way they do when the couple finally kisses, the lost dog returns, or the estranged father and son finally break down and hug. And as I caught myself looking at it from the outside, as I always did, I focused on being there, in that moment. It was a moment I had been waiting for as long as I could remember.

He sat there with me for a long time, and I'll never forget the way he kept patting me on my knee when people mentioned my work on behalf of the bill—and since there is so much pro forma praise members get if their bill actually reaches this point, that was a lot of knee patting. He was whispering to me in what my siblings and I called "Dad-speak," cryptic half sentences whose meaning was always somehow crystal clear.

"This is big, this is big," he kept saying. "You've really got something here."

And then after another member spoke, he would say, "Keep it up, keep it up, we'll work it out."

Because my father was there, New Jersey Congressman Frank Pallone yielded me time so I could give my speech. I began a little nervously, trying to keep to my prepared remarks and conscious of my dad's presence. And then I just put all that aside and spoke.

It was one of the best days of my life, even before they took the vote. And the final tally was 268 to 148, with 47 Republican members crossing the aisle to join 221 Democrats.

The next morning, I got this handwritten note from my cousin Tim Shriver:

> *Congratulations on the tremendous victory on the mental health parity bill. There is no question but that it would never have passed if not for you. I'm only sorry we didn't have these provisions when we were kids!*
>
> *I hope you are well and proud. I've always believed that one of the toughest things to express in our family is a sense of pride and achievement and satisfaction. You deserve them all.*

AND HERE'S A PERFECT EXAMPLE of what it's like to have a mood disorder: instead of feeling well and proud, I quickly went from the greatest day of my adult life to a feeling that everything was starting to fall apart with no warning, rhyme, or reason. Four days after that historic House vote, I was telling my therapist that I felt unanchored and depressed, and feared slipping more than I had at any time since my accident.

This change in mood was likely exacerbated by a piece of shocking news—my former chief of staff, Tony Marcella, who had been battling ALS, had a heart attack and, at the age of forty-three, was on a ventilator and not expected to live. But what I know about bipolar disorder is that I could have just as easily felt this way without that outside trigger.

The truth is, we sometimes rely on these potential triggers as ways of explaining our mood disorders to those who don't have the illnesses: it's easier for them to understand the disease if breakthrough symptoms are triggered by something external, something that makes sense to them. And the illnesses would be much easier to live with if the mechanism by which debilitating anxieties and depressions rise and fall were that predictable.

I did my best to struggle through this depression, tried to go to as many meetings as I could and, when I felt the urge to drink, tried to sleep instead. It was a challenging few weeks, especially because I was starting to realize that I had stopped moving forward in my recovery, and I wasn't as comfortable relying on my sponsor and telling him everything that was going on. At the time I blamed this on the fact that he was so much older than me, and I felt embarrassed about being as open with him as I was with my therapist on some issues; in retrospect it might also have been that I knew Jim was leaving Congress soon, and it's not exactly breaking news that I had a big issue with father-figure abandonment.

However, anyone who has been in long-term recovery would say I was stuck between the fourth and fifth steps—with Jim, and with myself. In the fourth step we're supposed to aggressively inventory every issue in our lives with other people—all the things we have done wrong that affected others and all the wrongs and injuries done to us. In the fifth step, we're supposed to share that list with God through prayer, and then with our sponsor, who is trained to help us see our responsibility in situations where we might try to blame others. And for situations where we were blameless—such as sexual abuse or other violence done to us—we're helped to understand that these were not our fault. The person responsible for these injuries was also ill, and being angry at them is a way to keep giving them power.

It's a very challenging process, so you have to be all in. The process doesn't make all the resentments just disappear—any more than doing the proper medical treatment makes all your mental illness symptoms disappear—but it helps you find a way to see all these insults more objectively. And by better understanding how your own actions played a part in them, you become more accountable.

In both the psychotherapy and twelve-step approaches, the hard-won goal is "insight" into your illness, which is what helps you through the challenges to come and the cyclical return of symptoms, because the diseases don't just go away. My cognitive therapist was trying to accomplish some of the same goals with me. There are aspects of twelve-step and CBT that are very similar, although accomplished in different settings: if you can afford the cost in time and, in the case of therapy, in money, I can say from experience that each has its value. The biggest issue in either is your own commitment to the process and to yourself as a well person.

Instead of admitting to Jim that I wasn't being rigorously honest with him, I started telling my therapist that maybe I needed a new sponsor. When something changes in your recovery process from addiction, or in your mood disorder symptoms, it is often easier to blame someone else's actions rather than just admit that the illnesses can be moving targets and sometimes they just get worse. But I was nowhere close to having that kind of insight.

I was coming to better understand the dilemma of that recovery phrase I heard so much, "fake it 'til you make it." It generally refers to your ability to put on a good face and function until you actually feel better. My problem, ultimately, is that I was way too good at faking it and somehow being able to function at a pretty high level—or have my staff make sure that collectively we functioned at a pretty high level.

And as I was completing my second year of sobriety, I was beginning to understand the difference between abstinence and real recovery.

FIVE DAYS AFTER I got my two-year chip in early May, I smashed my hand trying to break a board at a karate exhibition to raise money for cancer in Rhode Island. When I got back to DC, it was still really hurting, so I went over to Bethesda Naval Hospital to have it X-rayed. I asked my office manager Terri Alford to come in the car with me. Terri had been with me longer than any other member on my small staff—when she started I was in my mid-twenties and she was in her early forties—and besides doing her job flawlessly, she had always served as an emotional rock for me.

My hand was broken and after splinting it they, of course, gave me two Percocets, which I immediately took without thinking. And, since I was taking naltrexone at the time—which counteracts any of the euphoric feelings of opioids—I didn't really feel anything but pain relief. But they also handed me a prescription for a bottle of sixty more, with three refills. I was already planning in my mind to stop the naltrexone so I could feel the effects of them.

While Terri went to get the car, I had the prescription filled. When she got back, the nurse told her where I was, and when she realized what the prescription was for, she told the nurse I wasn't supposed to have it. "You've seen his records," she said, "he cannot have narcotics." But the nurse, and then the doctor, said they knew nothing about that, and it wasn't on my charts at all.

So we got into the backseat of the car, and I was clutching the bag. She said, "I don't want you to have those." But I held on to them, and during the entire thirty-minute ride back to DC, all I could think about was how I was going to get her to let me keep them. She asked me for them again, and I just held on to them and ignored her.

It was like the height of the Cold War, nobody was sure who would blink first. Oh my God, the tension. I mean, I *loved* Terri. She was like a second mother to me. She was my protector. I would be jeopardizing that entire relationship if I defied her. In all the years I knew her, she had seen me really ill and knew a lot about my health, but had never been in a situation to actually confront me, try to stop me.

And her timing was perfect—I was really struggling, even though I had literally just celebrated my second full year of sobriety a few days earlier.

So I knew that this represented an ultimate challenge of trust.

When the car got to the apartment, I got out and she followed me in. She said, "I'm not leaving until you give them to me." We stood there for what seemed like a long time. And, finally, I just told her, "No, you take the bag."

And she said, "Oh, Patrick, that means so much to me." We hugged each other. She started crying, I started crying. I'm crying right now just thinking about it. Because I can still remember how much I craved those pills, how much one part of my brain wanted the drug, and the other part of my brain was telling me it wasn't a good idea. And I'm still amazed at how much courage it took for Terri to confront me, and how many acts of emotional bravery, large and small, it really takes to care about someone with these illnesses.

AND THEN, A WEEK LATER, the phone rang and everything changed again.

My father was on a helicopter being airlifted from Hyannis Port to Mass General. He had suffered a grand mal seizure, and nobody knew why.

My brother, sister, and I immediately flew to Boston to be with him. So we were all together with him and Vicki when they got the news: the seizure was caused by advanced brain cancer, a malignant glioma of the left parietal lobe. While he actually felt pretty good, he needed dramatic treatment. And just as he had marshaled the country's experts on healthcare challenges in the past—both for public policy and for our health—he looked for someone who might be able to save him or buy him some time.

He found that in a neurosurgeon at Duke, Dr. Allan Friedman, who was able to remove most of the tumor. He gave my father an extra year of life. And he gave all of us who loved Dad an extra year as well.

MEANWHILE THE STAFFS from the House and Senate were still "conferencing"—which is a euphemism for political hand-to-hand combat—over the two versions of the parity bill. The Senate staff, led by my father's energetic longtime assistant on the Senate HELP Committee, Connie Garner, was still holding out for their bill to triumph. I'm sure they were upset that we had been able to bring our alternative bill this far—not only because of all the hard work Connie and her staff had put into it, but because the Senate always sees itself as more important than the House. Also, Connie had known me since I was a kid.

But our staff had something going for us that they didn't: the 2008 elections were coming, and it appeared the Democrats might do even better in Congress than they had in 2006 and could retake the White House. We felt that, if anything, if we had to hold our parity bill until the next Congress we might do even better. And their bill, as written, was unlikely to stand in a new, Democratically controlled Senate.

Eventually, the negotiation turned on our softening our stance concerning the role of the *DSM* in what would be covered—which the Senate side would later use to suggest we'd blinked first. But the truth is, we never thought our bill was going to codify the medical necessity of insurance coverage for everything listed in the *DSM*. That's not what the *DSM* is for. It's just the most up-to-date book of diagnostic codes and descriptions, an encyclopedia of what to call all the things that might be wrong with your brain or mind, and a resource for how to differentiate between them when making a diagnosis.

We had been using the idea of covering every single diagnosis in the DSM—admittedly, an extreme concept—as a way of counterbalancing the extreme way many insurance companies interpreted the idea of "medical necessity" to their own economic advantage. We were trying to make sure that our bill mandated a standard driven more by evidence, clinical common sense, and long-term outcomes; basically we wanted whatever was clinically indicated to be covered for the brain, like it would be for any other organ.

We also wanted a bill that banned not only "quantitative treatment limits"—obvious caps on numbers of visits or treatment days—but the trickier, and sometimes more damaging, "non-quantitative treatment limits" or NQTLs. For insurers, NQTLs allowed care to be restricted through burdensome pre-authorization procedures and obstructive medical management that sometimes prevented the most important medical "step-downs" in treatment. These included extra days in the hospital, or reimbursement for intermediate care in day programs and other partial hospitalization, which were so important for a successful transition back into healthy daily life. Ultimately we conceded that covering the whole *DSM* would not fully address those problems, even symbolically. And we admitted it would take years of interpreting and triaging the new law before it really worked the way we wanted on NQTLs. So we let the provision go.

In exchange for this, the Senate gave us two things we felt were much more significant—the bill extended parity in mental health and addiction coverage to out-of-network services as well as in-network, and allowed the states to keep and even improve their own parity laws if they offered consumers more protections. The compromise allowed individual plans to file for a one-year exemption to parity if they could prove it cost them more than 2 percent more in the first year, or 1 percent more in any other year—but the requirements for filing were so onerous that nobody was ever really going to do it.

Jim and I felt really good about the deal. Certainly, there were still some thorny issues that would have to be decided during the rule-making that is often done after a bill becomes law. In most major bills like this, it is the rules that the government devises for the law that make the difference, followed by the legal challenges to the bill and the rules. But we felt comfortable that most of what we had held out for made its way into the bill.

In Washington, people often talk about not letting "the perfect be the enemy of the good." We felt that mission had been accomplished.

The last arguments were over the name of the bill. There was a small debate about whether "mental health" or "addiction" should be first, and whether we should use just one word for both—"parity" or "equity"—or let each have its own word. The big fights, of course, were about whose name went on the bill and in what order. The Senate wanted Pete Domenici's name first and of course we insisted Paul Wellstone be first. There were some people who just wanted one name on the bill—those most interested in honoring Pete wanted his, those most concerned about memorializing Paul wanted his. I remember getting into one argument about this issue that ended with me telling a very powerful legislator, "With all due respect, we're talking about a bill that will save the lives of millions of people. Who the hell cares whose name is on it?"

When he first became ill, my father was concerned that his illness could stall the process of the bill becoming law. So he had asked one of his best friends in the Senate, Chris Dodd, to step in for him on parity.

And now that the conferencing was done, Chris took a bill that everyone in Washington already viewed very personally and did everything he could to make sure that any obstacles were overcome.

MY FATHER CAME BACK to Washington for the first time in July, to be there to cast the deciding vote to stop the Republican filibuster of a Medicare bill to reverse cuts in payments to doctors that the Republicans had made. I was there to escort him into the chamber, along with the others he had chosen to be with him: Chris Dodd, his fellow Massachusetts Senator John Kerry, and Senator Barack Obama.

My father waited in Harry Reid's office, which was right off the Senate floor, and then the five of us stood in the cloakroom outside the Senate chamber, about to make our surprise appearance. We pushed open the very heavy wooden swinging doors onto the Senate floor and strained a bit to hold them so Dad could make his entrance. And as he walked in we did everything we could to help him manage without appearing as if he needed much management, to show him at his best.

When we entered, the whole Senate stopped what it was doing—they were in the middle of a roll-call vote—and suddenly every major big-ego player was transfixed by him. It was like an emotional depth charge had been dropped in the Senate; everybody turned to watch it explode. The thing I was struck by is that, in a nanosecond, all these Senators just became *people*; nobody was a legislator anymore but suddenly it was just Chris and John and Carl and all of his colleagues and his enemies were just his buddies, Republican and Democrat. They were just all people whose hearts went out to him. It was magical.

He was walking through, saying "Thank you" and "Good to see you," and when they're doing a roll call, no matter where they are in the alphabet, if a member comes in who wasn't present when his name was called, they call him. So they yelled out, "Mr. Kennedy," and he walked to the table near the front, banged on it—which was also a way to steady himself—and yelled out, "Aye!"

His vote broke the deadlock on the filibuster, after which nine Republicans switched and voted with him.

MANY IN WASHINGTON assumed that might be the last time they would ever see my father again in public life, especially after news circulated a few days later that he had suffered a seizure not long after his Senate appearance. But seizures were not that uncommon so soon after serious brain surgery, and he was otherwise making good progress. He fully expected to be at the Democratic National Convention and at Obama's inauguration in January. And then he hoped to get back to work—because he was convinced that Obama would be the President who finally passed the sweeping healthcare reform he had worked for his entire career.

By this point in midsummer, the conference committee on the parity bill had finished, and the Paul Wellstone and Pete Domenici Mental Health Parity and Addiction Equity Act was ready. All that was left was to attach it to a bill that could be used to offset some of its costs, which had been estimated at over $3.4 billion over ten years. Nobody thought it was a good idea to try passing it as a stand-alone, because now that the bill was more ambitious than the one all the business groups had promised to support, there was no guarantee they would fully support it. (In Washington, the default position is always to say no until something looks absolutely inevitable, and even after you get to yes, businesses will still be looking for ways to get closer to no in conference committee or in rule-making after passage.) There was discussion of attaching parity to a tax extender bill. But there was still no clear path to getting the bill to a vote in the House and Senate and onto the President's desk to sign. In the meantime, the economy kept getting worse, the Iraq War casualties mounted, the presidential campaign kept getting more brutal, and on a personal and political level, it felt like time was running out.

On Sunday, August 24, my father flew into Denver with Vicki, hoping he would be able to address the Democratic National Convention the next evening. He had such severe abdominal pain on the flight that they went directly from the airport to a hospital—where he was diagnosed with kidney stones, a common side effect of chemotherapy. Once they knew what was wrong—and that it was something he could tough out—he was even more committed to appearing at the convention. His staff worked with him to cut the original twenty-minute speech he prepared in half, but he refused to let them cut it further. He wasn't going to just give a three-sentence speech and wave. But he knew he was going to walk onstage in excruciating pain and still at risk for a seizure.

I remember standing in the wings with my father and Vicki and my siblings—there were a number of us back there, although some family members chose to watch from the audience. And, as we waited, I was having this interesting and incredibly random conversation with the guy who was in charge of the teleprompter. His company had been in charge of the teleprompters for a lot of previous conventions, and he was telling my father and me how proud he was to have done this for so many Kennedys over the years. And just before my father was ready to go out, the teleprompter guy said, "I appreciate your work on mental health." People affected by this truly are everywhere.

My father was still incredibly strong, but his symptoms were unpredictable. During every second of that very long standing ovation when he came in, and when he started speaking, every time the audience burst into applause, I worried how long he could hold up. But then I realized that he was using those applause breaks to regather his energy and get focused on the next page coming up on the prompter.

He was magnificent, inspirational, resilient. Even with all that medication in his system, he was on fire out there. He was really sparkling and in his moment.

He didn't make it look easy; that wasn't what my father was about. He was always the hardest-working senator in Washington, and that's who he was that night, doing his job for his family, for his country.

Of all the things I was ever honored to watch him do, I was most honored to be near him on that stage as he spoke these words:

When John Kennedy thought of going to the moon, he didn't say, "It's too far to get there, we shouldn't even try." Our people answered his call and rose to the challenge. And today an American flag still marks the surface of the moon.

Yes, we are all Americans. This is what we do. We reach the moon. We scale the heights. I know it. I've seen it. I've lived it. And we can do it again!

There is a new wave of change all around us. And if we set our compass true, we will reach our destination. Not merely victory for our party, but renewal for our nation. And this November, the torch will be passed again to a new generation of Americans. . . .

The work begins anew.

The hope rises again.

And the dream lives on.

Chapter 22

Ten days after my father's speech at the convention—and exactly two years, four months, and one day since my last drink—I had a beer on a Thursday night after work. And the next Monday after work, I went out to a bar and got drunk. Scared by what I had done, I immediately went to meet with Jim Ramstad and Dr. Ron Smith to try to get my bearings. I was starting to feel anxious all the time and often bursting into tears about my father. I felt sore all over but honestly couldn't tell if I was in pain or just wanted pain meds.

I seriously considered going back into inpatient care immediately, but we were at a very fragile moment in the parity bill process. The legislation had the full support of the Senate and the full support of the House, and we had just held another big rally in front of the Capitol to get it passed. But every time congressional leaders tried to tie it to another bill, something went wrong.

Every day that this dragged on, I became a little more unglued. Those lobbyists and advocates who were also in treatment or recovery probably knew. But they didn't feel comfortable saying anything to me. The mental health advocates assumed I was having breakthrough symptoms of my bipolar disorder, because that was their medical worldview. The addiction-care advocates assumed I was drinking or abusing drugs again, because that was their recovery worldview.

They were both right, but here's the larger issue: everybody knew that I was a train wreck except me. Everybody around me was walking on eggshells. I was, at this time, really upset with my stepmother, Vicki, because I thought she was limiting my time with my dad for no reason—and like a lot of children of divorce, I was still jealous of the new family my father had made with her and her kids.

In reality, Vicki was probably doing my father and me a favor. I realize that now because I remember a very specific moment early that fall, when I saw her at some Capitol Hill healthcare function where she was substituting for my father. I remember the look on Vicki's face when she saw me for the first time in a couple weeks. Without saying anything, she let me know: "You're not healthy, you're uncomfortable to be with." There was a little moment of clarity in the way she looked at me, and I remember that startling me.

When I asked about seeing Dad she basically used the legitimate excuses she was using on everyone—"He needs time alone," "It's too much," "I'll let you know when it's better"—but to me this was all a kind of euphemism for "I can't bear to have your father see you like this."

THE CLOCK WAS TICKING ON parity and what was left of my sobriety. I was able to come to work each day and basically function, and I did sneak away to a quick weekend at the Caron Foundation near Reading to see if that would help. But I was still drinking at night, and using too much caffeine and Adderall during the day to stay awake.

Politically, the economy was sinking deeper and deeper into distress. Both the House and Senate were deeply conflicted about the idea of passing a massive bailout bill, the Troubled Asset Relief Program (TARP), which could cost up to $700 billion. We had, up until that point, been looking to attach the parity legislation to a bill that absolutely had to be passed—a spending bill, a tax bill. As the days of the session dwindled, we were beginning to realize that the continued debate over TARP was going to destroy our chance to pass parity—which, ironically, had already been approved solidly by the House and Senate.

I remember just calling everybody, desperate for some solution, some action. Finally I called my father, who was living at the house in Hyannis Port with Vicki and, generally, reaching out when he felt able. Since his illness, it was harder to just call up and get him on the phone, but this time I did talk to him.

"This is the last chance we're going to have for parity," I said. "Is there anything you can do to help?" He said he would call Chris Dodd and see what they could do. And Chris, who was not only filling in for my father on the HELP Committee but was also chair of the banking committee, came up with a brilliant Hail Mary solution.

What if the toxic TARP bill was actually attached as a rider to the beloved parity legislation, instead of the other way around?

What if the Paul Wellstone and Pete Domenici Mental Health Parity and Addiction Equity Act became *too big to fail*?

There were a handful of people who had to get on board—especially Nancy Pelosi and Harry Reid. And, then, suddenly, it was a done deal. The parity bill, HR 1424, had the TARP attached to it, in a way that could guarantee quick passage on the very last day of the legislative session.

Who was going to care that mental health parity could cost $3.4 billion over ten years? It was delivering a bill that, depending on how many other financial institutions failed, could cost $700 billion in ten *months*.

I still cannot believe the confluence of events that made this happen. If any of this had taken place during ordinary times with a normal calendar and the opportunity for people to dig in and mess everything up, it probably never would have passed. I can't take credit for the various iterations and twists and turns; you could never have organized or ordained the way this happened. For anyone to claim credit for this would be an insult to the fates.

It was a miracle. An incredibly quiet, deft Washington miracle, with the power to improve, or in some cases save, millions of American lives.

Chapter 23

I just barely survived the year after the signing of the parity act. Four weeks after the bill became law, Barack Obama was elected president in one of America's most historic campaigns. I was reelected in a campaign I barely participated in—but the voters in my district, thank goodness, felt I had been doing a good job for them and took my obvious problems (my hand was now visibly shaking during public appearances) as a sign of my justifiable reaction to my father's illness. As soon as the election was over, I quietly checked back into the Mayo Clinic for help with benzodiazepines, alcohol, and Adderall.

Among all the other issues that came up in group, there was one I had been discussing privately with my therapist since the parity bill got signed. When I felt really depressed, there was a question that haunted me, something I had never had the guts to ask my father before he became ill. And now it was probably too late.

Did he realize that one of the families that this bill was supposed to help destigmatize was *ours*? Did he know that making sure that the bill wasn't only about mental illness but about alcoholism and drug addiction was about us, too? He never, ever described it to me that way, and whenever I had tried to broach that subject before he got ill, he would always tack in a different direction. I was never going to know for sure.

I ended up leaving rehab early because of something my dad's office arranged. For some time, my father and I had been complaining that the parity act never got the deserved presidential attention because of the drama of the TARP and the upcoming election. Now that that was over, and both Domenici and Ramstad were retiring, we agreed it would be nice if the President did something to commemorate the parity act.

My father reached out to the President's staff and let them know he would be interested in coming back to Washington if the President would agree to a commemorative signing ceremony. And on November 21, the Friday before Thanksgiving, we met in the Oval Office. My father came in walking with a cane that he explained had been used by his father. President Bush was sitting behind what he reminded us was the most famous desk any president had ever used, because it was the one JFK sat at, the one that John Jr. had famously crawled out from under. We talked for a long time—about politics, about baseball—and then the President signed a copy of the bill. At a typical signing, he would have used several pens so each of us could have one. But since this was ceremonial, he announced he was going to use just one pen—which, because of all the history the bill represented, he said he wanted for his presidential library. And then, at the last minute, he gave the pen to my dad anyway.

During the course of the ceremony, my father couldn't help making a little joke at my expense. He teasingly said to the President, "Don't you think these young people should have some respect for their elders?"

I turned to President Bush and gave him a look that only a second-generation national politician could possibly understand, like we would always just be the kids, full of existential fears of being loved and living up to expectations. The President had these issues with his dad as a young man. And, of course, my dad had those issues with his own father. It was political déjà vu all over again.

I said to the President, "You know, it's pretty tough to follow your father in public life."

"Boy," he said, "don't I know it!"

I HAD A NICE THANKSGIVING with my father and my family in Hyannis. And three weeks later I was back at the Mayo Clinic again. I had hoped to be finished there before Christmas, because we knew every family holiday was likely to be the last, but when the day came I was nowhere near ready to leave treatment. I got a day pass to spend Christmas at Jim Ramstad's house. It was really hard, and when the anxiety reached a level I couldn't stand, I did something I knew I wasn't supposed to do. During my first couple days at Mayo, I had pocketed two pills of the tranquilizer Librium instead of taking them like I was supposed to. I took them at Jim's house.

When I got back to Mayo several hours later, I admitted I had taken them. So they wanted to give me a drug screen—in rehab!

I left Mayo in early January and was invited to live in an apartment that Dr. Ron Smith has at his house, where many others have stayed during difficult periods. I was still staying there when Inauguration Day arrived—a very special day, because my father had sworn he would be with Barack Obama when he was administered the oath of office, and I was going to accompany him on the dais. Because of my father's health, he had to be in a chair with arms on it and they put him very close to the President. So I'm in every major picture of the swearing in—it's my Forrest Gump moment.

After the swearing in I walked back up with my father, who needed some help on the stairs. We went into the old House chamber, where the luncheon was going to be, and he collapsed. He was saying, "I'm cold, I'm cold," and then he had a seizure.

After so many years of making sure that my father was never, ever seen in a vulnerable position in public, here he was having a seizure in front of the entire nation's leadership, who were already being seated for the lunch. I remember looking up and seeing the shocked face of Orrin Hatch, who was watching his friend and main political rival for all these years lying on the floor. It must have been a startling experience for him. Luckily, one of President Obama's best friends, Dr. Eric Whitaker from the University of Chicago, was a guest at the lunch, so he helped us until we could get my father into an ambulance.

I rode with him, and since I had never seen anyone have a seizure before, it was terrifying until he started coming around. He was still a little confused, but when we explained what had happened, he said, "I caahn't *believe* it!" That was one of his go-to lines, "I can't believe it," and it was often associated with something that was bad, but he managed to say it in a way that made it sound like we got caught doing something mischievous. He had a great sense of the absurd and surprising in life, because he had seen so much of it.

And then we looked out the window to see where we were. The ambulance was making great time to the hospital because it was going down the cleared path of the inaugural parade that was about to begin. And given everything that had and hadn't happened in my father's political life, that seemed even more surreal, more worthy of another, "I can't believe it."

BY VALENTINE'S DAY I WAS back at Mayo again for a week. Besides all the things I had been talking about in rehab for years, and the obvious issues brought up by my father's illness, there were two new ideas starting to occur to me.

First, I wondered if I was ever going to have a real life: if I would ever really fall in love, have a family, have what really matters. And, second, I wondered if I should leave politics—because while everyone around me assumed that politics was the only thing keeping me going, I wondered if being in elected office was, in fact, a big part of what was killing me. Or was causing me to kill myself.

That Mayo visit—and my ongoing consultations with my doctors there over the next months—helped me stay focused on my recovery and on making sure my remaining interactions with my dad were positive, not regressive. Not long after one rehab stay, I spent the weekend with my dad, Vicki, my sister, Kara, and some of my cousins as we went sailing on the *Mya*. Back at the house, my father made some time for us to speak privately—which we hadn't done in a while—and while much of the conversation was about politics and legacy, it was warm and moving. I sent him a long letter afterward, thanking him for letting me come, letting him know I would always have his back, reinforcing that he had always been my "emotional sustenance," and saying, "There is no one I know who could have endured more emotional heartache than you have in your life and yet you've managed to keep *living and loving your family.*"

What I didn't mention, but continued to pray for privately, was my hope that one day someone might say all that about me.

I DOUBT THAT IT WILL come as any great surprise to my House colleagues or staff, or my family, to learn how much I was struggling during my last term in Congress. In the spring of 2009, as my father's condition worsened and I was clearly losing control, both Vicki—on behalf of my dad—and Jim Ramstad were begging me to go back into rehab. One day, I took a water bottle to work that was filled with vodka. I was growing afraid to leave the house in fear I would screw up in public. I had my car put in storage so I couldn't drive it. Between April and June, I missed more than half of my House votes, but I was still up and down enough that I had plenty of days I could get work done.

Then, on Thursday, June 4, I was on the floor of the House in the early evening and the last vote had been finished. The session remained open for members to make speeches on the record, and I was planning to get up soon and speak. I had taken a handful of Ativans—I don't know how many, but by then my tolerance was pretty high—and clearly people recognized that I was starting to become impaired. They decided they needed to get me out of there before I did something really stupid live on C-SPAN. A call was made to the congressional physician's office, which reached out to one of my doctors to report that I was "stuporous—not walking in a straight line." My office was contacted.

First, one of the pages handed me a note, which read, "Your office on four"—so I went out to the cloakroom, booth four, and it was one of my young staffers on the phone from the office, asking, "Do you still want to give that speech?" I thought this was odd, and he said, "You don't have to give it, you can go home right now." And I said no, I wanted to give it and went back out on the floor.

Then the Democratic Clerk, Barry Sullivan, a Tip O'Neill appointee from Boston, took me aside and said, "Terri wants to see you. Now."

Back in the cloakroom, I was met by one of the Navy physicians on call for members of Congress; I was taken to his office where Terri, my administrative assistant and protector, was waiting for me.

She said, "You are going to George Washington University Hospital right now." She and the doctor walked me down a back stairway and into a car that was already running with someone behind the wheel.

We drove to GWU, where we pulled up to a rear exit door. I was put in a wheelchair and rolled down an empty hallway and into a single private room, where they immediately laid me down on the bed and a nurse came by to take my blood pressure and put in an IV. No checking in, no showing my insurance card. Terri said, "I'll see you in the morning. We're going to get some help for you, *tomorrow*," and then she left.

My mind was spinning that all this could be pulled off. Actually, my mind was just spinning, because all the pills I had taken were finally reaching their full impact. I blacked out and didn't wake up until the next morning.

By then, Terri and Dr. Ron Smith had arranged to drive with me to Father Martin's Ashley, the secluded rehab retreat on Chesapeake Bay. I slept the whole way there, I was so out of it.

When I realized where we were, I said to Ron, "I can't stay here, my career will be ruined if I do."

He looked at me and said, "Patrick, your career will be ruined if you *don't* stay here."

Once I was settled, my office issued a statement that I had decided to "temporarily step aside from my normal routine to ensure that I am being as vigilant as possible in my recovery. I hope that in some small way my decision to be proactive and public in my effort to remain healthy can help remove the stigma that has served as a barrier for many Americans reluctant to get the help they need." We didn't specify how long I would stay.

FATHER MARTIN'S ASHLEY was different from Mayo. It focused more on spirituality, and the group therapy sessions weren't as aggressive as the Mayo process groups. I liked the enhanced spiritual component but sort of missed the in-your-face confrontations. I needed them both.

Perhaps because I had really scared myself with the Ativan incident in the House, I found myself being unusually honest at Father Martin's. The worksheets I filled out by hand on the first day contained more hard truth than most of what I had shared with Jim Ramstad when he was my sponsor. They asked very detailed questions about situations of "powerlessness" and "unmanageability" and I did a very harsh accounting in which, for the first time, I blamed only myself for these situations.

I stayed there for a month, leaving just before July Fourth weekend, and then went up to the Cape to spend time with my father. He spoke less than usual, and when he did he occasionally came up with incorrect words because of his deteriorating condition.

I was actually touched that a couple times during that visit, when he called out to me he referred to me as "Splash," not Patrick. Splash was the name of his absolute most beloved dog. I joked with my brother afterward about this, saying that if I was going to be in the doghouse with the family, I was glad to be associated with the favorite dog.

But he could still tell stories and ask me to retell stories, which is what we loved to do. Sometimes we would sit on the front porch and look out over the ocean, but mostly he would sit in the piano room. If there were a couple of visitors someone would play the piano and we would get out the old song sheets and have a sing-along. The last time he and I sang together that summer, we did a duet of "You Are My Sunshine," and then he and Vicki sang "Just a Closer Walk with Thee."

He was still working, or at least work was being done with his input and approval. In mid-July, his HELP Committee staff completed the first draft of his version of a healthcare reform bill, beating out the other Senate committees drafting theirs. On August 4, he was one of twenty-six senators who signed a letter to the Secretary of Labor, the Secretary of the Treasury, and the Secretary of the Department of Health and Human Services, demanding that they promptly issue regulations that would allow the Mental Health Parity Act to be properly implemented by clarifying the law's scope of services and medical management requirements. And he was still working on his memoir, which Vicki would read aloud to him.

One of the things he still was able to do was go visit his sister, my Aunt Eunice. Now in her late eighties, Eunice had had several medical setbacks, including a series of small strokes over the past two years, from which she continued to miraculously come back. She was there at the house with my uncle Sarge Shriver, who had been suffering from Alzheimer's for some time. My dad was taken over to her house almost every day, and the two of them would sit out on the back patio overlooking Nantucket Sound.

I was, by this time, starting to make a lot of notes about what I would say at my father's memorial service. My rehab at Father Martin's was the first one where I wasn't drafting letters to my father about all the things I thought he should know, the things we still needed to discuss. Instead, on whatever paper I had lying around—the backs of mental healthcare policy memos, my American Express bill—I was writing about what he had done, what we had shared, what it had meant to me.

It was also interesting to be doing this as, just down the road, I knew my cousins were doing the same thing for Aunt Eunice. And as I thought about my own life and what I might do next, the idea that I wouldn't run for my seat again was becoming very present in my mind.

I had recently spoken about this, very briefly, to my dad—on the back of a big motorboat owned by his friend and local physician Larry Ronan from Mass General. Each time he boarded the boat, and he had to take my shoulder to steady himself to get on, I took it as some form of what could be our last hug. And then we would just cruise around the bay. We were sitting there talking about politics, leaning with our heads close so we could hear over the wind and the sound of the engine, when out of nowhere he said, "You know, you don't have to run for public office anymore. You can do what makes you happy."

I was so stunned I didn't know what to say, and so upset that the first thing I did after we got off the boat was ask Dr. Ronan if he'd write me a prescription for Adderall. I claimed I couldn't get ahold of my regular doctor. He just looked at me with a smile that let me know he wasn't falling for that excuse. And then he said, "No." I spent the rest of the day worrying he would tell Vicki what I had done, and consumed with anxiety that I still couldn't handle my own feelings without a pill or a drink.

But, regardless of my anxiety attack, what my father said made a huge impact. He was giving me his blessing to think about what would make me happiest and healthiest.

What would I do? I felt like two family legacies were staring me in the face.

There was my father's life in the public eye in the Senate, with a guiding hand and resonant voice in so many different kinds of decisions and emergencies and issues. And there was my Aunt Eunice's life, focused on one set of issues, one set of disenfranchised Americans, trying to address their needs from inside the system and outside, and when necessary even instigating the creation of new systems; she was one of the first to see the need for what we now call "public-private partnerships," which acknowledge that government funding can only be part of the solution.

While a lot of people knew what my father had done, many did not appreciate just how much Aunt Eunice had accomplished and what was still being done in her name for neonatal care, children's health, and developmental disabilities.

I had spent my entire life trying to live up to my father's expectations. Once he was gone, was I going to keep aspiring to be my father? Or should I actually aspire to be a version of my Aunt Eunice on the issues of brain disease that mattered to me the most?

This all assumed, of course, that I would be able to get some sustained control over my illnesses and start building an actual life for myself.

Because if I didn't, I might not live long enough to aspire to either.

———

IN EARLY AUGUST, Aunt Eunice had a major stroke, and my Shriver cousins came rushing to the Cape to see her in the hospital. She died early in the morning on August 11 at the age of eighty-eight, and that evening the family held a private Mass at their home. My father was there for the prayer service, which was a wonderful surprise for the extended family. For many, it was the last time they would see him.

Two weeks later, it was our turn to say good-bye to our father, who had spent the last few days before his death watching old James Bond movies and finally letting go of his fierce grip on life. Sadly, I wasn't there when he died.

By this point, I was appearing on my father's behalf at events he couldn't attend. I was scheduled to go to Northern California to do an appearance with United Farm Workers president Arturo Rodriguez. My father was close to Rodriguez, just as he had been with his predecessor Cesar Chavez, a relationship that spanned the years from farmworkers' rights to immigration reform.

I was with Rodriguez outside a farmworkers' hall in Santa Rosa, a very rudimentary building with an aluminum roof, and it was jammed with farmworkers at the end of their day. Just before we went in, I got a call from Vicki, who said that my father was very close to death—but that I shouldn't drop everything to fly back because I would never make it in time, and my leaving a public event abruptly could trigger a lot of media attention when we just wanted him to pass peacefully.

So I hung up my cell phone and went in. When Arturo introduced me as "*el hijo de* Ted Kennedy," the workers immediately rose and chanted, "*Viva* Kennedy! *Viva* Kennedy!"

In my broken Spanish, I started, "*Yo soy el hijo de* Ted Kennedy," and there was applause. I did my best to hold back my tears and get through my remarks, and when I was finished they chanted again,

"*Viva* Kennedy!" They presented me with an album of all the pictures of my dad with farmworker leaders, back to the 1960s. And then several people told stories to reinforce the importance of immigration reform, these heartrending stories, about family separations, fear, intimidation, and exploitation. But they all came back around to how my father and my family had stood with them. They were so warm and loving, saying, "Please tell your father we love him and we are praying for him."

As we walked outside and were getting in the car, my phone rang again. It was Vicki, who told me my father had just died, with family members surrounding him. And I realized that he had passed at exactly the time that all these people in a big hut in the valley surrounded by vineyards were yelling, "*Viva* Kennedy!"

I flew home in tears. And when I got to Hyannis, I realized that everyone had already been told what their responsibilities would be over the next few days of events, starting with a vigil with the casket in the house and ending with a funeral Mass in Boston, which would be broadcast on national television because President Obama had agreed to deliver a eulogy and three past presidents would be in attendance.

I had assumed all along that both Teddy and I would give eulogies—I had been drafting mine for weeks—and Kara, who was much more private, would read a prayer. Instead, I was informed that there was only time for Teddy to give a eulogy. I would be reading a prayer.

While nobody said this out loud, they clearly were afraid that it would be too risky to let me speak on live television, especially right before the President. They may have had some reasons to be concerned, and for me one of the hardest parts of being in recovery has been owning up to that and letting go of it. But, I can still vividly recall my seething anger and outrage at being told there just wasn't going to be time for me to eulogize my father, that I had been deemed not worthy to pay tribute to him because I had an illness that could be embarassing or inconvenient. Hearing this triggered every issue I ever had with my dad during my entire life, making me feel like I was going to be in permanent emotional exile from my family if I backed down and accepted this. So I made it very clear to Paul Kirk—then executor of my dad's estate, and the messenger of this news—that I was going to deliver a eulogy after my brother and before the President whether they liked it or not.

My father's casket was brought to the house in Hyannis, draped with an American flag, and placed in the sunroom, where most members of the family, young and old, took turns standing vigil. I then rode in the front seat of the hearse as the casket was brought to the JFK Presidential Library for a two-day public viewing.

There were so, so many people lined up outside the library for the viewing each day. It was an awesome tribute to our father but also pretty daunting, because Teddy, Kara, and I felt that at least two of us should be there in the receiving line at any given time. And that was a lot of receiving.

At the end of the first day, Kara had already gone back to the hotel and Teddy and I were still shaking hands and accepting warm condolences when a woman came up who we hadn't seen in years. She had been one my father's secretaries in Washington decades earlier, before he had married Vicki. She approached us and handed us a sealed envelope, which had our three names written on it and the words "To be opened after my death."

Teddy and I were shaking; we didn't know what to do. So when the receiving line finished we went up to the seventh floor of the library, the Family Room, and we shut the door and called Kara. We told her we didn't need to open the letter right away, we could bring it back to the hotel and do it later, when we were all together. And she said we should open it immediately, so we did, and we read it aloud to her over the cell phone on speaker. We were all in tears, sobbing.

It was a beautiful letter, so moving, full of all the things you'd ever want to hear from your father. It had been written during the 1980s, and one of the things he said—which I so needed to hear at that very moment—was that he hoped that, if we felt comfortable doing it, we would speak at his funeral.

I took this as a sign directly from heaven that I had made the right decision to fight for my right to eulogize him.

The next evening there was an invitation-only memorial service at the library, where mostly his Senate colleagues spoke—they told wonderful stories—followed by my cousin Caroline. And the next morning we were all at the funeral Mass at Our Lady of Perpetual Help Basilica in Boston.

My sister, Kara, my step-siblings, Curran and Caroline, and a number of our young nieces, nephews, and cousins read prayers or quotes. My brother, Teddy, gave a really wonderful eulogy. He delivered his last lines, "I will try to live up to the high standard he set for all of us when he said, 'The work goes on, the cause endures, the hope still lives, and the dream shall never die.' I love you, Dad, I always will, and I miss you already." And then I quickly got up from my place on the front pew, squeezed past Kara and Vicki, and met Teddy as he walked past the casket for a long embrace. I walked to the podium, almost forgetting to kneel and cross myself, and pulled out my eulogy.

My voice was shaky, my brain was shaky, and I was trying hard to stick to what I had written.

"When I was a kid, I couldn't breathe," I began, and I talked about how my early health struggles had a silver lining, because they had led my busy father to spend more time with me. Most of my eulogy was about my childhood with him because, honestly, most of what happened after then was still too raw for me. I didn't talk a lot about politics, except about what an honor it was to serve with him. But I did want to say one thing about the last thing we had done together as legislators, the Mental Health Parity and Addiction Equity Act.

"This bill represented not only a legal victory for fifty-four million Americans with mental illness who are being denied equal health insurance—but as one of those fifty-four million Americans, I felt he was also fighting for me to help ease the burden of stigma and shame that accompanies treatment."

When I talked about how he would be remembered, I made a point to include all the children he had helped raise. "Most Americans will remember Dad as a good and decent hard-charging senator," I said. "But to Teddy, Curran, Caroline, Kara, and I, we will always remember him as a loving and devoted father."

"I love you, Dad," I finished, "and you will always live in my heart forever."

When I came down off the podium, President Obama, waiting to go up, gave me a warm embrace, and Vicki gave me the most relieved hug and kiss ever.

We flew with his casket to Washington that afternoon, and he was buried in the same spacious plot as his brothers in Arlington National Cemetery.

WHEN I RETURNED to the office, there was, among all the condolences, a very kind note from Al Franken, who had just taken Paul Wellstone's seat in the Senate. He said he wished he had been able to serve with my father (although he did fondly remember attending a Democratic Caucus retreat where my dad called the square dance one night). He complimented my brother and me for our eulogies. And then he said something intriguingly honest.

"I've decided that your vulnerability is a gift to the nation," he wrote. "I mean that in the most heartfelt way. You are a courageous man."

I prayed he was right.

Chapter 24

I n the weeks leading up to my father's death, when my moods were getting really unstable and I was relapsing in my recovery, I called my physician at the Mayo Clinic for advice on what I should try next. When he asked what substances I had used, I thought for a minute and then just said, "Everything."

As I tried to adjust to life after my father's funeral, the same could be said for my treatment regime. What was I trying?

Everything. A lot of everything.

Unlike an inpatient setting—where you are often given different kinds of therapeutic interventions but someone is supposed to be monitoring all of them and making sure there are no interactions, multiple treatments for the same thing, or just flat-out mistakes—out in the real world, patients still basically direct our own care. We get appointments with the caregivers we call, we get answers to the questions we ask, we get the drugs prescribed by whoever is allowed to prescribe them to us—and their knowledge of what other drugs we are taking comes, all too often, from what we tell them. Then we either take the drugs, or don't take them, without any real monitoring.

In all my decades of outpatient care with many top doctors, I have never—except for the year when the court ordered it—been given a blood or urine test to see if I was misusing drugs or drinking alcohol. And I have rarely been tested, outside of a hospital setting, to see if my psychiatric meds are at a therapeutic level in my bloodstream. This is a major blind spot in our medical system.

I had now been through enough different types of treatments—and had advocated for them politically as well—to know what I was choosing from. It wasn't that there were all that many new treatments, but a lot of the ones that had been around were being used in new, more aggressive ways.

There was still traditional inpatient care covering bipolar disorder and addiction—for which I was lucky enough to have excellent federal employee coverage and could afford to pay out of pocket for anything not covered. This inpatient treatment could include a variety of medications, a variety of supportive psychotherapies, the new low-dose courses of ECT (which I have never tried), and education in everything from nutrition and exercise to spirituality. Once discharged, we were placed back in the care of our private doctors and encouraged to connect with the lifesaving all-peer twelve-step meetings of AA, NA, and other affiliated and unaffiliated groups around the country.

However, just as many surgical procedures had gone from requiring a hospital stay to becoming basically an outpatient procedure, people like me who were pretty functional and also pretty ill—and were trying to balance the two without losing their jobs—were using more day programs and outpatient rehab. There had also been a big increase in the use of medical addiction psychiatry and medication-assisted treatment, and more patients were being tried on the drugs designed to take all the relief (and the fun) out of addictive behavior. These drugs were being recommended more often than ever before—sometimes by private physicians, sometimes by one of the nation's 2,900 "drug courts," which can legally mandate treatment.

While these were all advances in different aspects of care, they also represented a lot of uncoordinated systems that still weren't that hard to manipulate. In fact, some people hired "life coaches" just to try to keep themselves from gaming the system. I hadn't really done anything like that since my parents had hired someone for me when I was in high school. But I had met a yoga teacher and clinician at Mayo who I liked, and I had hired her to come east and act as my coach for yoga and mindfulness, and hold and dole out my medications. Some of those people treating me thought having her in the mix was a good idea; others would have preferred someone with more medical training.

Two days after my father's funeral, I went to the congressional physician's office in the morning to get my monthly shot of Vivitrol. It was a huge horse needle you got in your butt once a month, which was so painful that the prescription for it came with a shot site rotation chart.

Vivitrol was the latest of the many medicines I was taking. It was a relatively new monthly injection form of the drug naltrexone, which had previously been available only in pill form. I got my first shot of it while I was an inpatient at Father Martin's Ashley and associated it with my positive experience there. So I decided to try it as an outpatient.

Before you can get the monthly shot, you have to have a urine test. I failed. I tested positive for stimulants—specifically Adderall which had become my primary drug of dependence. I had convinced myself this was okay because the pills helped me remain focused on my job. And I had doctors in DC and New England who would write me prescriptions.

I also tested positive for opiates, which I couldn't understand because I didn't recall taking any. I had been fighting a cold and had been given an antibiotic and cough medicine, which I didn't think contained an opiate, so I was pretty sure this was a false positive. I was so sure that I urged them to give me the shot anyway, knowing that if I did have opiates in my system, the shot would immediately trigger withdrawal symptoms. After a phone consult with my doctor at Mayo, they gave me the shot. The congressional physician was also monitoring my prescription for Antabuse and gave me my next pills.

That afternoon, I went to a new prominent psychiatrist in Washington for a second opinion. (Actually, considering how many doctors were already in the mix for my care, this might have qualified as a ninth opinion.) He wanted to make some changes in the eight different medications I was taking for my mental illness and addictions: he wanted to get me off of Adderall and onto something less abuseable, and off my antidepressant, Wellbutrin, in part because of its small seizure risk.

Later that same day, the congressional physician called my doctor at Mayo to point out that the antibiotic I had been given can sometimes create a false positive for opiates in a urine test.

I realize these are a lot of treatment details, but I list them to note that this was just one day in my life as a person with bipolar disorder and addiction. Every question raised by every doctor was a reasonable one, and every one of these physicians was trying to do his or her best for me. But that is a lot of moving parts for one sick patient's care—and that doesn't even take into consideration the new emotional issues of bereavement and how they would play into diagnosis and treatment.

This gives an idea of how ridiculously complex care can become and how many cracks there are to fall into, or hide in. It makes you wonder if this really is the best way to be treating illnesses, especially illnesses that can cause changes in perception and judgment.

THAT FALL WAS THE BATTLE of the Affordable Care Act (ACA). The biggest thing I could have contributed to Obamacare had already been accomplished. The various forces we had brought together to push through the Mental Health Parity and Addiction Equity Act were able to remain focused and engaged during the much more difficult fight for the ACA, to make sure that the two things that mattered most to us were included: a complete ban on refusing coverage because of preexisting conditions, and inclusion of mental illness and addiction as one of the "ten essential benefits."

While I suspect that the preexisting condition ban would have been part of any healthcare plan from either party, I have no doubt that if we hadn't already passed the parity act in the last Congress, it would have been impossible to gather the political muscle needed to force it into a broader healthcare reform package. Especially without my father and Pete Domenici available to call in a career's worth of political favors. Even with parity passed, it wasn't easy to lock in mental health and substance use disorder as essential health benefits, and I worked hard with colleagues like Senator Debbie Stabenow of Michigan to try to get that done.

This made me feel much better as I watched a good bit of the work of healthcare reform from a distance. The night in September when President Obama announced the initiative to a joint session of Congress, I was sitting in the gallery with Vicki, Teddy, Kara, Curran, Caroline, and other family members, so we could be photographed together when the President invoked my late father and his lifelong mission of healthcare for all. I spent many of my weekends trying to make progress in inpatient or outpatient treatment, or recovering from binges, and did my best to control my agitation and anxiety around the office and on the House floor.

I also spent a good bit of my private time—at home and in rehab—reading and wrestling with my father's memoir, *True Compass*, my last chance to hear his voice. I sent out copies of the book to everyone in politics I thought would appreciate getting one from the family. But mostly I just read it, marking up passages in pen and Magic Marker and wondering what they should mean to me.

On Saturday, November 7, the morning of the House vote on our version of healthcare reform, I was in rehab at Father Martin's Ashley. Nancy Pelosi called and said she really hoped I could come back and vote. So my staff quickly arranged for a car and driver to come get me in Havre de Grace, Maryland, and I made the two-hour trip back to DC and to my apartment to get changed so I could be there by eight P.M. for the vote and completely shock the Republicans who thought they had it won.

The driver dropped me off at the Capitol, I was checked in with the caucus whip, and I waited for about an hour. I walked onto the House floor, voted, and then Nancy Pelosi came over to me, took me aside, and said, "Thank you sweetheart, now you go right back to treatment," and I walked out of the Capitol, back into the car, and back to rehab.

AMAZINGLY, BECAUSE OF the focus and determination of my staff—and my ability, which frankly was beginning to frighten me, to function just well enough in public when I wasn't anywhere near well—not only did the office keep running smoothly, but that fall, I missed the fewest votes of almost any session of my career: I cast all but four of my 246 votes from October to December.

But the longer this continued, the more I came to realize I really needed to make a major change in my life—to leave elected office. I talked it over with a number of people, all of whom were far more concerned about my health than my political career. While I had first broached the subject in therapy over a year before, the first time I said it out loud to someone in political life was to my father's former chief of staff Dr. Larry Horowitz, who reached out to me several months after Dad's funeral to see how I was holding up. While he encouraged me to make and to really *own* my decision, he didn't dissuade me from making this change—and he also made it clear that even if I was thinking about it, I needed to discuss it with Nancy Pelosi right away. This was something she could not hear about secondhand from the wrong person, and I would need all of her support to make such a transition go smoothly for me, both personally and politically. We talked about how I could discuss this with her—and, knowing Larry, he probably quietly reached out to her to minimize her surprise.

When I came to see Nancy, she was unbelievably supportive, gracious, and maternal, not only encouraging me personally but helping me with the practical politics of the situation. I wasn't doing this because I was trying to get ahead of a scandal, I was doing it to save my own life and prevent another scandal. But if I started fund-raising in February—like all Congressmen do in an election year—and then I later announced I wasn't running, that would be its own scandal. So Speaker Pelosi did me one in a long line of favors—she told my staff that she needed me for some work during the February break, a CODEL of some sort, and I wouldn't be available for fund-raising. That way, there would be no cause for speculation or rumor when I abruptly canceled political fund-raising because the Speaker "needed me to do something for her."

We quietly bought airtime on local stations in Rhode Island for an ad, which David Axelrod helped us with, and on a Friday in mid-February, word began to leak that I had taped an ad and given an embargoed interview to *Rhode Island Monthly*. On Saturday, February 13, 2010, I confirmed that I would not run again for my congressional seat and would retire from elected office at the end of the year.

This was all happening in the middle of the frenzy over the Affordable Care Act, which got hung up in the Senate partly because Republican Scott Brown won a special election for my father's seat and the Democrats lost their majority. When Senate Democrats wanted to compromise, it was Nancy Pelosi and the leadership of the House who held out for a stronger bill, and I was honored to be part of that process. On Sunday, March 21, we passed the bill and it was sent to the President for his signature. At the White House signing ceremony two days later, Vicki and I were both wearing "Tedstrong" rubber bracelets. After the President finished signing, I presented him with a gift: a copy of my father's very first national health insurance bill from 1970.

But, for me, the more important act of closure had come earlier. The morning after the bill had passed, I went to Arlington before it was open to the public, so I could have some time alone at my father's grave. While sitting there, on the grass next to his gravestone—not far from where his brothers Jack and Bobby were buried, and the marker for their brother Joe—I took out a piece of the note-sized congressional stationery I always carried in my suit pocket and a blue marker.

I wrote, "Dad, the unfinished business is done." And I placed the note to the left of his gravestone.

Chapter 25

A week later, I found myself in Atlantic City giving a speech at a $125-a-plate fund-raising dinner at Caesars. It was for an organization called The Arc of Atlantic County, a regional branch of the national charity for developmental disabilities that actually predated my Aunt Eunice's work in this field. (The Arc began in 1950 as the National Association for Retarded Children.) I had agreed to do the speech at the request of my House colleagues from New Jersey, Frank Pallone and Rob Andrews, who had both been very helpful during the parity fight.

I had no idea how my life would change that night at the Caesars Palladium Ballroom.

After the speech and dinner, which raised $95,000, I was mobbed by people who wanted to talk to me. Among them was a beautiful, athletic thirty-year-old junior high school history teacher from nearby Absecon. Her name was Amy Savell, and she said she had come to the dinner as a last-minute replacement for her father, Jerry, a retired special-ed teacher and longtime local Democratic politician who was home with a bad cold. What she didn't say was that she had just become a single mom, and this dinner was the first time she had gone out dressed up since her separation.

Amy asked me for an autograph for her dad. As subtly as possible—which, for me, isn't very subtle at all—I hit on her. In the note to her father, I wrote, "Sorry I missed you, but it was a pleasure meeting your beautiful daughter." She beamed at me and headed back into the throng.

Since I am pretty bad at hiding my emotions, I did my best not to appear overly interested as I watched her return to table 123. I had to play it cool. I couldn't beeline right over to her or they'd all say, "There goes that Kennedy, after the pretty girls." So I had to strategically shake hands with dozens of different people at different tables without appearing to be working my way toward her.

When I finally got to Amy's table, I diplomatically struck up a conversation first with her mom, Leni, also a retired schoolteacher. But it was pretty clear why I was there.

I told Amy that if she ever wanted to, you know, bring her class to Washington, I was still in Congress for a few more months yet and would be more than happy to show them around. I insisted on giving her my card. As I handed it to her, I said something that surprised both of us.

"Please call me," I said. "But pretend I called you first."

EVEN THOUGH HER DAD WAS, like many older Democrats, a longtime Kennedy buff, Amy wasn't exactly sure who I was. She ended up Googling me to figure it out.

About three weeks after we met, she did call. We talked for a while and agreed to get together. I took the train from Union Station in DC to Philadelphia, and then had a car drive me to Atlantic City—where a friend had instructed me to make a reservation at the Knife and Fork

Inn, a well-known restaurant. We had dinner together and then went to a club where Amy, who wasn't sure how this evening was going to work out, had arranged for us to meet up with one of her brothers, as well as her best friend with her husband, both fellow teachers.

The evening was fun and comfortable. I stayed overnight at Caesars, and the next night we went to a prizefight at Harrah's, where I had arranged for ringside seats for us and Amy's friends. It was one of the bloodiest fights ever, and Amy's friend's husband was wearing a white dress shirt that got splattered with blood. He took it off and we had the winning fighter sign it.

The weekend was a tentative success, and I kept coming back. Since I wasn't running for reelection for the first time in sixteen years, I could actually take the weekends off. I stayed at a smaller, noncasino hotel, the Seaview, where I felt more comfortable. Only my close aides knew how often I was taking the train to Philly and a car to Atlantic City.

Our courtship was as therapeutic as it was romantic. I was very tired and very emotional. Amy realized I was still trying to process my father's death and everything unresolved between us, I wasn't sleeping well, and I wasn't in great condition physically. Even when I came for the weekend to visit, there would be days when I hid in my hotel room at the Seaview and couldn't get out of bed. This was far from normal dating. Luckily, Amy saw me as basically openhearted and kind, and different from other men she had known, who hadn't been that open about their feelings. So, while other people might have found me insecure and whiny—I know I sometimes found myself that way—she enjoyed being around someone so willing to admit his fears.

Amy also had family members who had struggled with mental illness and substance use—including a middle-aged cousin with schizophrenia she was close to and a grandmother who had died from alcoholism before Amy was born. As a schoolteacher she had dealt with students being treated with psychiatric medications and therapy, as well as their families. And she recently had been attending meetings of Al-Anon at a church near her parents' house. A teacher friend had recommended Al-Anon as a good tool kit for her around the time when we met, and she kept going as a way of being supportive of me. She also stopped drinking completely, and the few times I ordered a drink at dinner when we were first dating it was very noticeable.

At that time, I was not going to AA meetings as regularly anymore. Ever since my sponsor Jim Ramstad had left Congress the year before, I had been going less and less.

It was a young, long-distance relationship—and a secret to the press, who were increasingly interested in covering my last months in office as the end of the Kennedy era in Washington. We would meet in Philly for a weekend at the Four Seasons, or in New York. We were both still a little gun-shy, especially about me spending much time with her adorable three-year-old daughter, Harper, until we knew where this might be going.

As THE SUMMER WAS ABOUT to begin in earnest—the first summer since losing my father—I decided that instead of being with my family for July Fourth, I would join a congressional CODEL that was going to Liberia, Kenya, and several other African nations. Because of the large Liberian community in Providence, I had always wanted to visit there. This was going to be my last chance to go as an elected official.

My staff was completely against this, because they knew I was not well. But unlike several years before, when I was trying to put the trip together myself, this was a journey organized by my colleague Representative David Price, the chairman of the House Democracy Assistance Commission, and already included Representatives David Dreier, Donald Payne, Allyson Schwartz, Keith Ellison, Mike Conaway, and Vern Buchanan. A significant group of staffers would be on the trip, including congressional doctors who already knew they had to keep an eye on me.

By this time, I had dispensed with the medicines that prevented me from using opiates and was taking OxyContin pretty regularly. I thought I had enough pills for the entire weeklong, five-country trip. And I was doing fine when we were in Liberia. In fact, I gave an impromptu speech supporting the country's current leader, President Ellen Sirleaf, who I greatly admired (and the next year would win a Nobel Prize), and loudly railing against the possible return of the regime of Charles Taylor, the former president who was awaiting trial for war crimes. The speech was controversial in a positive way, and a perfect example of why I had always wanted to visit Liberia.

Unfortunately, not long after that speech, I finished all the Oxy-Contin I had brought, and with several more days of travel ahead, I began to detox when we arrived in Kenya. I was sweating profusely, doubled over in pain. The congressional physician with us was kind enough to suggest that perhaps I had contracted malaria and needed to go home early—although I think a number of people involved with the trip knew that was a lie. The physician contacted my staff back in DC and told them exactly what was going on and that my physical condition was beyond their ability to treat me in Africa. And I left the trip, suddenly quite relieved that there was no American press coverage of the CODEL.

I was flown home through London, where my staff had arranged for someone to meet me and fly with me the rest of the way home. I told them I didn't need help, but they thought otherwise, and there was someone already accompanying a senator over who was available to fly back with me. But any time a legislator is walking through the airport like that on a trip, the embassy in London is alerted. So the US Ambassador, Louis Susman, who knew my family, was informed of my situation, and word quickly got back to my brother and Vicki—who were now facing their first-ever "Patrick crisis" without my father or his staff (and since I had announced I was leaving, much of my own staff had already moved on, too). They had every reason to believe that this might be the beginning of what my life after Congress could be like. They were worried about me and angry with me.

And then I proceeded to make the situation worse. This fiasco had so completely exposed me, despite all my best efforts to disguise what I was doing. It laid me bare and vulnerable and I was very resentful and bitter and defensive. So, after I had been home a few days and had survived the worst of the detox, I had my assistant schedule a call with the Ambassador—so I could, of course, blame the whole thing on him.

The minute he got on the call I started yelling, "I don't know what school of diplomacy *you* went to, but you should know better than to be talking about such private things . . . ," and I dropped a few f-bombs in the process. He was stunned and didn't say anything, although I'm sure this just confirmed every image he had of what was happening during my trip back from Kenya.

Luckily, this was never covered—because by this time, with the end of my term in sight, I was desperately trying to finish my congressional career without any more scandals. All I wanted to do was make it to December alive and reasonably intact, so I might still have some chance to go into a long-term rehab after I was finished and possibly retain the chance to reinvent myself.

WHILE I WAS IN AFRICA, Amy was getting to know me in a way I hadn't planned. I told her she was welcome to use my house in Rhode

Island, which I was getting ready to sell, for a vacation while I was away. She decided to go up there for a week with a friend, partly to relax, partly to help me start getting "organized."

They were having a nice time, but after a day or two Amy could no longer deal with what a mess the place was. I had been living there, alone, without any major relationships, for several years. So her vacation gave way to a pretty major cleaning. She hoped something like this would help me get a fresh start when I returned, but she also just couldn't help herself, because the place was so dirty and disorganized.

She told me she wasn't surprised by anything she found of mine— the mess, the decades of worn and stained clothes that needed to go, even the handful of stashed porn magazines. She considered that all fairly predictable. She was a little freaked out, however, to discover a stock of Uncrustables—the premade peanut-butter-and-jelly sandwich pockets she never allowed her daughter to eat—in the freezer. That did make her wonder a bit.

After I recovered from the detox after Africa, which Amy knew all about, we had a terrific summer. I spent a lot of my weekends with her. Mostly, we stayed in and around Atlantic City, where, after a while, she started feeling comfortable letting me get to know her family, especially her daughter, Harper (whose custody she shared with her ex-husband).

I spent my first-ever Jersey Shore summer with them, hanging out on Brigantine Beach and eating pizza on the boardwalk in Ocean City. We would take Harper out to pick blueberries, or to visit Storybook Land, a kiddie amusement park. It was great, something I had never really experienced before, being at the shore with a small, low-profile family who were reasonably careful with each other's hearts.

It felt like something I'd heard about in the endless nautical metaphors of my family but had never really experienced myself:

Safe harbor.

The more I was around Amy and Harper and their family, the more they felt like home.

WE SPENT MORE TIME TOGETHER in New Jersey and at my shockingly clean house in Rhode Island. But, mostly, we just got to know each other. I was still pretty raw, and there were times when she wanted me to come join her for a walk on a beautiful day, or to visit somewhere and I just didn't have the strength to do it. But I think she knew that I wanted to do it and just couldn't. I was in terrible shape emotionally and physically, weighing a lot more than I ever had in my life.

At the same time, I still had this burning political and advocacy ambition, especially when it came to the diseases that were doing their best to try to destroy me. And not only because of the work we had already done and the political coalition we had built to pass the parity law (which was still fighting over the language in the federal regulations written after passage). There was, unfortunately, an entirely new front opening up in our war on inadequate treatment and medical discrimination: a new generation of veterans with a new generation of brain diseases.

It was becoming alarmingly clear that veterans were facing an unprecedented problem with suicides. Some vets were suffering from primary mental illness—mood disorders, psychotic disorders, anxiety disorders, trauma-induced disorders. Some vets were suffering from mental illness secondary to traumatic brain injury, or TBI, the new signature wound of war.

And as had always been true of war, the medical challenges among our soldiers and veterans held the most hope for advancements in medicine and public health, because they were the only patients for whom we could generally find money in federal budgets. It was a medical trickle-down effect hardwired into the American experience. It went back to the Revolutionary War, when young Dr. Benjamin Rush wrote in the nation's first text on war medicine, "Fatal experience has taught the people of America that a greater proportion of men have perished with sickness in our armies than have fallen by the sword," and prescribed some of the earliest forms of preventive care, including one of the first mass vaccinations for smallpox. It continued through the development of better limb amputation techniques in the Civil War; expanded use of transfusions, X-rays, and broken-bone setting in World War I; the government-sponsored mass production of the first true antibiotics to fight infection in World War II; and advances in trauma surgery and helicopter medical evacuation during the Korean and Vietnam Wars.

And now, our first twenty-first-century war was insisting we finally focus on brain disease. And what seemed like very specific "invisible wounds of war" actually had broad connotations for those who were not veterans. New interest in the diagnosis and treatment of battlefield traumatic brain injuries could also call attention to the stateside issue of concussions from car accidents, sports, and other causes. New interest in suicide prevention for veterans could lead to more diagnoses and treatment for all Americans attempting to take their own lives. New interest in other mental illnesses among veterans (some of whom were ill before they enlisted) and the challenges of treating those diseases within their families could lead to better early diagnosis, individual treatment, and family treatment.

This was the cause I thought I should devote my energies to after leaving Congress. If I could only get control of the diseases in my own brain.

DURING THE FALL, I kept visiting Amy at the shore. I was becoming well-known to the management of the Seaview Hotel. It was my hideaway from life in Washington, which was becoming increasingly frantic. I had hired a doctor to work with me as a medical coach and pretty much separated from the psychiatrists I had been seeing for years. I was finding it easier to hide from everyone who was concerned about my care, including my staff, who were desperately reaching out to my late father's former aide Dr. Larry Horowitz and to the physicians at the Capitol. I was cutting back on my psychiatric meds, and becoming more and more manic.

My mania had a good focus—I was really getting energized about connecting the dots between the mental health community, the addiction treatment community, the neurology community, the brain research community, and the military. But it was still mania. Everything you do when manic is not necessarily bad. It's just that the way you do it will, eventually, be bad for you, because mania never stops when you want it to. You can win a big race, but you can't get your foot off the accelerator, full-throttle, until you and the car run out of gas, crash into a wall, fall to pieces, or all three.

A lot of people were scared for me, and I was scared, too. But somehow Amy wasn't scared. That's partly because I was able to put on my best face for her, and in a long-distance relationship she was spared some of my day-to-day challenges in Washington. And we were taking things slow. But we were also falling in love—and she was seeing something I could be, with her, that I had never been myself. For me, that was a little scary, too.

I remember taking her to talk with the person in the family who I felt had the most perspective on addiction and recovery—my cousin Chris Lawford. He had been sober for a long time—he credited my mom with taking him to his first AA meeting in the early eighties—and had written a bestselling book about his own and other people's recoveries. Chris had always been very supportive of me and knew a lot of things that I would never share with others. For that reason, he also had only the most exceedingly cautious optimism. When Amy and I went to talk to him, he didn't sugarcoat anything.

"Tell her what I'm dealing with," I said, "tell her the dirty dark truth, that we can go off the edge at any time."

And he said—I'll never forget this—"I have never seen a case worse than you, Patrick. You've been at this for so long, and the fact that you've survived and you're still doing it almost makes you more dangerous. You're able to manage it, just like your father managed it. And that's what should scare anyone who falls in love with you."

He told Amy, "If he doesn't stick with recovery, you should run as far away from him as you can get!"

He said he knew that at any given moment, I could say I wanted to go off to Australia with all my money and drink and drug myself to death. What he didn't know, and neither did Amy, was that I had considered such a plan. After I announced I wouldn't run for Congress and knew I would be inheriting money from my father's estate, I had actually asked my financial adviser if there would be a way to transfer all my holdings to Australia so I could just disappear there. I always remembered that Nevil Shute novel I read in high school, *On the Beach*, about people going to Australia to wait for the coming apocalypse. Whenever I worried I would never be able to dig out of all the angst and depression and negativity, I imagined being Down Under, waiting out the end with whatever offered me even temporary relief.

IF YOU WANT AN INDICATION of just how manic I was at this time, in the middle of all this, in early October of 2010, I was negotiating to write a "sobriety memoir" with a publisher and a collaboration agreement with a reporter I knew. Fortunately, both Amy and my brother eventually convinced me that signing these agreements, at this point in my "sobriety," would be an act of singular self-destruction.

During this time, Amy sold the house where she and Harper had been living after her divorce and moved back temporarily into her childhood home with her parents. So I decided to prove my commitment to the relationship, during this very challenging time, by buying us a house in nearby Brigantine on the water. I started looking and found a place, but Amy was nervous about this: it all seemed too soon. We were in love with each other but I still didn't have enough love for myself to commit fully to her, to her daughter, to my health, to anything. I was reliable only in small bursts. The rest was chaos.

I was so torn. I had this bright-eyed, beautiful woman who said she really liked me and I knew she was good people—in my *bones* I knew she was good people. And I was still saying to myself, should I do this or should I not? Should I have a chance at a real life or not? Should I continue to *live* or not?

It shouldn't even have been a close call and yet it *was* a close call. Here's how close:

When Amy and I were apart during the week, I would still sometimes connect with women I had dated before. Basically, this was just me being an idiot guy who had made it to his early forties and still had no idea how to be in love and commit to a relationship. Amy had some understanding of this—we had not been going out for that long, and she knew I was trying to adjust to a lot of things that were normal for most people and not, so far, for me. She was patient and, generally, unshockable. Even when we sometimes spent hours together with me sitting in the bathtub almost catatonic, and her sitting on the closed toilet asking me what it would take for me to commit to my health and my life and, presumably, to her, she believed in me and believed I was trying.

In early November, we spent a leafy fall weekend together at my house in Providence. On Sunday, I had to leave early to make an appearance with my mom and my brother to commemorate the fiftieth anniversary of JFK's election; we appeared on the steps of Providence City Hall, where JFK had spoken the night before he was elected. Amy was going to close up my house and drive back to New Jersey herself. But, as she was packing her stuff, she came across some evidence that I was still in touch with other women—the phone at the house kept ringing, someone left a message. And she decided she was done. With me.

When she called, I was on the platform in the Providence train station waiting for the Acela to New York, where I was scheduled to appear on the *Today* show the next morning. She was crying and packing. She said she couldn't believe I was doing this to us. She had believed I was sincere about our relationship and had put up with a lot based on that belief, but now she realized I wasn't capable of being all in.

"You're not serious about this," she said. "It's over."

And then she hung up.

At that moment, I felt like the bottom dropped out of my life—and there had been very little holding it in place to begin with. I also felt that maybe it was just as well Amy had discovered that I wasn't worthy of her love and support anyway. This was her way out, and she should take it.

And as I stood there on the platform, my last chance to save myself lost, I imagined myself jumping in front of the Acela as it came into the station. I could see it. I could do it.

While most suicide attempts are long considered, which is why so many are preventable, there are some that are wildly impulsive, of the moment—based as much on depression as timing and access to the means. The Acela was approaching the station, and I had just ruined my life, my last chance.

When I look back at all the other things I did impulsively during that time, I'm terrified that the thought of jumping crossed my mind. There was very little distance back then between what I thought and what I did.

The impulse passed, I got on the train, and went to New York. And at seven forty-five the next morning I was on the *Today* show with Meredith Vieira, who wanted to talk about the end of my congressional career—and the last days of the more than sixty years when there was a Kennedy serving in Washington.

Instead of answering her opening question, I was able to pivot and talk about what I hoped might be my professional future—something I had been discussing for the past year behind the scenes in Washington but hadn't really shared much in public. It was a new brain research initiative that would be tied to the anniversary of JFK's "moon shot" speech and would, for the first time, include mental illness and substance use disorders as brain diseases. I was scheduled to give a special guest lecture at the Society for Neuroscience international meeting in San Diego on this subject in a week and had been working with a top speechwriter on how to bring these complex ideas across. I was using the show as a way of trying out some of our new ideas.

The first answer sounded pretty good—sometimes you don't know until you hear yourself say something out loud if it works—and so, from that point on, almost every question she asked me, I brought back around to issues of the brain: mental illness, veterans with PTSD and traumatic brain injuries.

While I was visibly grimacing during the entire interview—and, each time, catching myself and forcing a forlorn smile—those five minutes and six seconds of airtime made a real impact on my life. It felt like I had caught a second wind.

Maybe I didn't have to be this lonely pitiful loser. Maybe I wasn't completely damaged goods yet.

I didn't call Amy right away, because I didn't think I deserved another chance, and it would be too self-serving of me and disrespectful to her to ask for one. I thought I should just put everyone out of my misery.

But a couple days later, she called me.

"Let me get this straight," she yelled, "you're not even going to *try*?"

She was incredulous and angry at me for accepting her word as the last word. I told her, very honestly, that I didn't realize that "trying" was even a possibility because I had never been in such a place in a relationship before, didn't really understand all that "women are from Mars" stuff. We talked for a long time and I was deeply relieved when we decided to try to keep moving forward.

It just so happened that the day after this conversation, the bid I had made on that house on the water in Brigantine was accepted, and the deal was quickly closed by a lawyer in New Jersey. The house needed a lot of work and was not habitable but it was there—either a great sign of our future together or, as Amy still occasionally worried, a place where I might still move after our relationship was over and I was finished in Congress.

I BOUGHT THE HOUSE on a Friday, and that Monday I was in San Diego to give the speech that I hoped might launch my post-congressional career. I was speaking to well over ten thousand neuroscientists from around the world and trying to turn their esoteric scientific meeting into a political rally. My talk—scheduled up against nanosymposia with titles like "Postnatal Neurogenesis" and "Visceral Nociception: Bidirectional Interaction Between the Viscera and Brain"—was something a little bit different: "A Neuroscience 'Moonshot': Rallying a New Global Race for Brain Research."

I got up onstage, and between the unflattering lighting in the San Diego Convention Center ballroom and the fact that I was in a deep agitated depression, I looked like I was suffering from all of the illnesses I was there to discuss. The only good thing about this situation, as I continually wiped sweat off my face, was that I felt so utterly horrible that I was too nervous to deviate at all from the speech.

I was there to dare them. I talked about the upcoming fiftieth anniversary of my Uncle Jack's seminal "moon shot" speech, in which he dared the nation's disparate scientific communities to come together for a goal that would seem beyond impossible only until they achieved it: the goal of sending an American to the moon and back. I announced it was time for an even more ambitious journey to a newer frontier: the inner space of the brain. That's where all the diseases they researched lived. That's where all the diseases I advocated for lived. We only have one brain. And it was time for us to commit to being of *one mind* for brain research.

If we really wanted to succeed, we needed to look to the Manhattan Project, we needed to look to NASA, we needed to look not just to science, but to *political* science. And in political science, there's a simple equation that always works: we are stronger together than we are divided. In all my years on the House Appropriations Committee, I had heard so many different smart, committed, powerful people ask for money for their priority, and their priority only—with seemingly no idea of their common goals, their common enemies, their common purposes. Many of them offered almost the same exact basic information about what needed to be done, even the same explanations about how stigma and prejudice had kept it from being done, and then offered completely competing conclusions about why their thing needed to be done first. Yet the moral of every story they told was that we needed to develop a common language and a united front for making a concerted impact on the global burden of brain disease.

And I explained that the tipping point for all this—and it was a tragic one—was that our military was also figuring this out, the hard way, from all the returning veterans dying from the signature wounds of war: brain injuries on the outside and on the inside, TBI and PTSD. Just as NASA and the Manhattan Project had been driven by the politics of national defense, so would our effort.

I finished up by saying that when I looked out in the convention center, I saw a room filled with modern-day astronauts in our race to inner space. After the talk, Steve Hyman, the provost of Harvard and former head of the NIMH, bounded toward me and demanded to know where he could sign up. He was followed by Tom Insel, the current head of NIMH and a much more laid-back person, who looked at me and said, "I *like* being called an astronaut."

All that was left to do was figure out a way to plan and fund this neuroscience revolution. We needed to be thinking really big—like maybe war bonds big.

I BROUGHT AMY HOME for Thanksgiving to meet my whole family. That was an important step forward for us, but the next few moves I needed to make on my own. I needed to finish out my term in Congress, say good-bye to Washington, and then go away and do something I had never done—not just retreat to an inpatient facility, but stay thirty, sixty, ninety days, however long it took until I was actually well enough to begin a new life.

I made my rounds in DC early and did all the interviews about what would come next without letting on a thing about what had actually been happening in my life during my last term. I had an emotional good-bye with Dr. Ron Smith's Tuesday night twelve-step meeting and dinner group, who had not been seeing all that much of me over the past months.

Nobody seemed to pay attention when I started packing up my office with two weeks left to go in the session and then missed my last week of votes. If they did notice, I'm guessing more of them were praying for me than upset with me. Because, even for many of those closest to me, the only thing they feared more than me being in Congress was me *not* being in Congress.

I went directly from my last day as a Congressman to my first day in the roughest detox I had ever experienced: at Virginia Beach Psychiatric Center, arranged by the concierge medical adviser I was still working with. After a seven-day detox there, I was going, for as long as it took, to a retreat-style rehab on the Outer Banks of North Carolina, Two Dreams. It was run by Dr. Andrea Barthwell, who I knew a little bit from politics: she had served President Bush as Deputy Director for Demand Reduction in the Office of National Drug Control Policy from 2002 to 2004.

For patients, advocates, and professionals, mental illness and addiction is a small world.

Two Dreams was exactly what I wanted—on the water, excellent staff and facilities. But after a few days, with Christmas approaching, the first Christmas of my new life, I just couldn't do it. I called Amy, who I'm sure was shocked and scared when I told her I was leaving rehab and coming to be with her and her family for the holidays.

I flew from the Outer Banks to the Jersey Shore, and was driven from the airport to Absecon where we passed the Wawa market and the American Legion post and the family pizzeria where Amy had once waitressed, and then made a left onto the tree-lined street where her parents lived. When I showed up at the front door of their two-story colonial house, Amy hugged and kissed me like I was home. Sick, sad, and depressed, with a nervous twitch in my hand I was hoping was from medication and would go away sometime, but home.

I had planned to stay for just a couple days and return to my room at Two Dreams. A couple days extended to New Year's, and then beyond, and I just never left. Harper was sleeping in Amy's old bedroom. Amy and I stayed in her brother's much smaller old bedroom, which her parents had turned into an office—so whenever her dad needed to use the computer, I had to finally get up out of bed, or at least scooch over.

It was like some odd mental illness sitcom. But it felt like the safest place for me to be.

Chapter 26

When the holidays ended, Amy returned to teaching, Harper returned to day care, and Amy's parents, both retired teachers, just went about their business. Except for breakfast—which they called me for but I almost never came—and dinner with the family, they pretty much left me alone.

I was still talking about maybe going back into treatment—there were local people I could hire to be my health life coach—but I actually liked the idea of starting over completely. So with the help of a local caregiver, I tapered myself off all my psychiatric medications. This was a risky thing to do, and while I understood the risk and had access to medical help if needed, I would caution anyone else against taking this route without complete family and medical support—and an understanding that while you may be tired of certain side effects, nobody can predict how you will feel without the meds at all. Too many people stop their meds haphazardly, and sometimes hide that fact from caregivers and family. They risk not only the return of symptoms but sometimes the medical effects of halting a drug improperly, because many medications require a slow titration down to stop taking them safely. People can make themselves sicker just by the way they abruptly stop taking medication.

What I did was experimental and I had someone around me all the time (even if it was just Amy's mom asking if I was ever going to pick up my clothes in the bedroom). I was careful, but this was a gamble. It was one of the many gambles Amy and I decided to take, knowing full well the risks, for our future.

As I came down off the medications—the hardest one to give up was Adderall, because quick-acting stimulants were my last addiction—I came to better understand my feelings and my symptoms without any pharmacologic intervention. I found that I was even more quickly choked up and tearful than ever before. I could also get very agitated very quickly, and felt the need to either leave certain situations right away or confront my agitation with whoever I was talking to, rather than just waiting for it to pass. I recognized these as symptoms of my mental illness. I also recognized that accepting them as symptoms and dealing with them without medication was something I wanted to try. I was getting in better shape, running forty-five minutes a day, often to blow off agitation or depression.

I was also occasionally attending a twelve-step meeting at a church down the street where Amy's grandparents had once belonged. I was doing my best to use this temporary family cocoon as a way of getting healthier.

Two months after I showed up on her parents' doorstep, the anniversary of my father's birthday, February 22, was approaching. Amy and I talked about this—actually the best part of what was happening was that Amy and I talked about *everything*, fearlessly. While I had always intended not to drink again after returning from treatment, we were realistic about the challenges to my sobriety on occasions like my father's birthday. But, instead, that morning, I got up, went to my seven thirty A.M. meeting at the church, and went for a run. I did the same thing the next day, and the day after that. And when February 22 had come and gone without a slip, I decided I was going to be fully committed to my recovery and use that as my sobriety date. (I am, as of this writing, four and a half years sober.) But I didn't discuss this with Amy at first, and she didn't immediately bring it up. She just noticed something had changed and waited for me to say something, which I did after about a week of feeling more sober than I ever had in my life.

We talked it over, and I decided that I would focus all my energy into traditional twelve-step recovery, to see how that made me feel. I was not against using psychiatric medication again and was not in a twelve-step group that would frown on that if I did. Over all my years of sampling medication—prescribed and otherwise—I realized that the anticonvulsant Lamictal (lamotrigine) seemed to give me the most relief. It was now a popular mood stabilizer, used for patients with bipolar disorder. I no longer wanted to take multiple meds to address the same issue, which some called "cocktails" and others "polypharmacy."

So Amy and I agreed that if it seemed I really needed medication again, I would ask our local physician for a prescription for Lamictal. He could consult with an addiction psychiatrist I had recently started seeing in New Jersey. But I didn't want to go back to psychotherapy or psychiatric meds: if you have comorbid mental illness and addiction, I think you have to be sober first to treat either illness successfully. I wanted to work the program of recovery as my baseline and see where that took me. One day at a time.

And that was, really, when Amy and I finally found one another.

AS WE WERE WORKING through all this, I was co-founding a new nonprofit and planning a huge international conference—which was going to happen in May whether I was ready for it or not, because I had already reserved the JFK Presidential Library.

When I had first decided to use the "moon shot" imagery to organize the disparate stakeholders in the world of brain science, I had asked my cousin Caroline if we could use her father's presidential library on May 25, the fiftieth anniversary of my uncle's famous speech to Congress that called for America to land a man on the moon. Since I had booked the library, I wasn't going to let any health or life struggles get in the way of this event.

My partner in this whole project was Garen Staglin, a Bay Area financier turned winemaker who, with his wife, Shari, had quietly become one of the most aggressive and successful philanthropic forces in the world of mental health. Their journey began in 1990 when their brilliant teenage son, Brandon, was diagnosed with schizophrenia. They spent the first several years focusing primarily on helping Brandon get proper care and rebuild his life—he was fortunate to be diagnosed just when Clozaril revolutionized care, and has steadily improved ever since, so he finished college, married, and works in the family business and in multiple advocacy roles. In 1995, they decided to hold a fund-raising concert and wine dinner at the Staglin Family Vineyard and use the funds for mental health research. That dinner grew and grew each year—better-known musicians, bigger supporters from the worlds of science and society—until they had raised over $100 million for what they had always referred to as "mental health" but now were talking about rebranding as "brain health." Garen and Shari had originally given most of the money they raised to one of the first major mental illness research charities, NARSAD (which is now called the Brain and Behavior Research Foundation), but later decided to fund research and academic chairs themselves by creating a new nonprofit, the International Mental Health Research Organization (IMHRO).

Besides giving millions, Garen and Shari were very knowledgeable and demanding about where their donations went: they were ahead of the curve on financing research into the possible prevention of mental illness, starting with learning more about what is called the "prodromal" period in schizophrenia, which some believe is a period when the disease, or at least its severity, can be thwarted with very early treatment. They had also financed an incredibly forward-thinking anti-stigma effort with actress Glenn Close and her family members suffering from mental illness, the Bring Change 2 Mind campaign, which had amazing TV public service announcements.

Another thing I really appreciated about the Staglins is that they were very "out" about their work. Brandon spoke openly and eloquently about his illness, and Garen and Shari about their family situation and their mental health politics. That still wasn't very common: many of the top funders of mental illness research remained pretty quiet about it. Even in philanthropy, there was a stigma.

The Staglins had been very supportive of me for the past five years—in fact, we had been planning their first fund-raising event for my work in Congress on mental health in 2006 when I had my Capitol car crash, and I had to call them from rehab to ask if it would be okay if we postponed. They were great about it—people who have been through mental illness and addiction in their own families learn to be amazingly kind, patient, and forgiving. Garen and Shari, as they often joked, had a high tolerance for behavior that was not "straight down the middle" and gave people a lot of room. They were people who really meant it when they said, "These are brain disorders."

So Garen was as patient as he could be with me, as we were both trying to start a new nonprofit called One Mind and planning an unbelievably ambitious three-day international conference in Boston around the moon shot anniversary—a sort of Woodstock for brain research, mental illness, substance use disorders, veterans' brain care, pharmaceutical discovery, and concussion research. We were also funding a ten-year plan for the neurosciences, all using the emerging model of public/private partnerships for everything.

Garen was probably the only one who realized that when I was calling the President or Vice President to appear, and trying to round up all the scientific, political, and business dignitaries involved, I was calling not from a new, post-congressional office complex, but from a wing-back chair in the very cozy living room of Amy's parents' house or from our tiny bedroom. I would do most of my calls in between my twelve-step meetings and my daily runs. The "Offices of Patrick Kennedy" from which people got e-mail confirmation was a very nice young woman in a nearby South Jersey town who was working from her house.

At the end of March, I decided I wanted to propose to Amy. During a visit to DC I went to a jewelry store and bought a ring—a diamond with pink sapphires on either side. And then I had to figure out how to ask for her parents' blessing first without Amy's finding out—since, of course, we were all living in the same house and Amy's mom is not a great secret keeper. So, on a Thursday morning—when Amy was at school and Harper at day care—I asked her parents, Leni and Jerry, if they could join me in their living room.

A couple days before this, Amy and I had a disagreement during dinner with her parents that escalated in the living room afterward into a little family feud. Amy and I had actually already talked it through—the best thing about our relationship was that we talked through everything—and we were fine. But I don't think her parents knew that. So when I asked to speak to them, they thought I was going to tell them I needed to get some distance from their family for the sake of my fragile sobriety. They were tearfully relieved to find out

I wanted to marry Amy and double down on the life I was making with her.

In fact, I explained, that was why I was so sure I wanted to do this so soon: if Amy and I could be so committed to working through a confrontation like that instead of isolating from each other, what we had was real.

Amy and I left for Providence directly after school on Friday so her mom wouldn't have the chance to slip. The ring was burning a hole in the pocket of my khakis, but I wasn't sure when to ask her. We had a nice dinner Friday night but that seemed too obvious. And on Saturday we were going through some of my stuff so that I could begin packing to move permanently to New Jersey. We were in the little apartment over the garage of my house, which overlooked a beautiful orchard. We were knee-deep in my messy life, not the most romantic moment in the world, but it felt right.

I said, "I want to talk to you about something."

And before she could respond she blurted out, "Oh, look!" and pointed out the window: right in front of us, less than twenty yards away, was a pair of huge deer, standing frozen in place in the orchard. And for a second, we just stared at them and they stared back.

"I guess this is the sign," I said. "Amy, I want to be with you. . . ."

I fished the ring out of my pocket, shoved a couple boxes out of the way so I could get down on one knee, and asked if she would marry me.

When Amy and I announced our engagement, we expected mostly cautious optimism. But people were enormously happy for us, and even more enormously hopeful. I was, of course, well aware over the next weeks that all the people we were bringing together to celebrate our engagement and all the people we were bringing together for One Mind were probably thinking the same thing: they were wondering what the chances were that I could hold it together. And so was I. Amy and I both were. But we were in love, we wanted to be married, and we wanted to help raise her daughter together and have kids of our own. I was turning forty-four and had never been married before. I didn't want to wait another second.

IN LATE MAY OF 2011, we held the first One Mind conference in Boston. There were three days of who's-who talks at the Westin Copley Place hotel. Cutting-edge scientists and business leaders from around the country gathered to hear Dr. Francis Collins—formerly of the Human Genome Project, then director of the National Institutes of Health—as well as the directors of the NIMH, NIDA, NIAAA, and FDA, and leading researchers on veterans' brain injuries. In the evenings there were special presentations: the nation's leading researchers on concussions spoke in a big private box at Fenway Park, and actor Martin Sheen and former Senator Max Cleland came to present a searing new documentary they had worked on called *Halfway Home* about the visible and invisible wounds of war.

Steve Hyman presented a ten-year plan for the neurosciences, which he had orchestrated with the directors of all the brain-related institutes in NIH, the Society for Neuroscience, and the Institute of Medicine. Dr. Husseini Manji, the global head of neuroscience at the Janssen Pharmaceuticals division of Johnson & Johnson—our earliest corporate supporter and the biggest player in pharma brain research— gave a stirring, hopeful talk about how drug companies could be more innovative and collaborative and transparent with their current research, and more open to sharing information gathered in the past.

On the last day, Vice President Biden gave an astonishingly moving keynote at the JFK Presidential Library, invoking his own experiences with neurosurgery and the searing saga of a close friend of his from college whose son was suffering greatly from a mental illness—and he didn't know what to do. He described to Biden his feeling that his son was at the end of a string, out there in space, and said, "I'm so goddamned afraid that if I tug too hard on that string it will break, and I will lose him forever."

But the most exciting part of the meeting was the electric interactions during breaks and meals among people who were usually at separate meetings, strategizing about how to compete against each other. People were imagining how they could build things together, research things together, solve the unsolvable together. After all, sitting in the same room were the people who had cracked the genetic code of DNA; the people who turned the deadliest epidemic of our lifetime, AIDS, into a treatable illness; and so many other brilliant people capable of taking us to inner space. An incredible array of talents and passions to all be of one mind.

FOR ME, HOWEVER, the highlight of the One Mind event was family—because for the first time in my life, I was appearing in public as a man no longer alone. Amy and Harper were there for many of the events, and it was joyful to share all this with them.

My brother and his wife were there. My cousin Caroline came and spoke—just after appearing at the JFK Presidential Library to give the annual Profiles in Courage awards. And, perhaps most amazing, on the last day of the One Mind meeting, my mother came.

It was only the second time she had appeared in public in years (the other was my father's funeral). Even though she had spoken about her challenges decades ago, in recent years she had been too ill to ever be part of the work we did on mental health and addiction parity. So, on the last day of the three-day meeting, before I gave the closing talk and the call to action, I was so moved to see her enter the side door of the

Westin hotel conference room. She had told me ahead of time that it was okay for me to speak in public about her struggle if it would help people get treatment. But I wasn't sure she would actually come—she was, by then, getting pretty frail and would often need to cancel engagements at the last minute because she wasn't feeling well.

She walked very slowly and deliberately, with tiny steps, so she could remain steady. She was wearing a lovely teal suit and her blond hair was long and beautiful. She sat down in the front row. And as I went through the list of people I needed to thank for this conference, I couldn't wait to get to her.

I talked about what it was like when my brother was diagnosed with cancer and the whole world turned in sympathy to my family—in part because we had no problem saying out loud that a family member of ours was suffering from a disease that needed to be treated with the utmost urgency. But I also remembered being struck from a very young age with the difference between how people talked about my brother's illness and my mother's illness. She had the double challenge of not only confronting an illness, but confronting the prejudice and stigma of being someone who society felt didn't deserve the same medical care and sympathy as her son with cancer.

"My mother has been such an example to me," I said. "And I want to tell you today, my mother is my profile in courage for all that she's done to stand up to this stigma."

And I walked down off the stage to give her a hug and kiss while everyone in the room rose to give her a standing ovation.

Chapter 27

Amy and I didn't want to wait long to get married, so we arranged to have the ceremony at Gramma's house in Hyannis Port in mid-July, a time when most of the family was down there and could be with us. She and I went to Paris for a week before the wedding, as a sort of pre-honeymoon. And when everyone got to the Cape, instead of a bachelor party—which we all agreed would be a really bad idea— my brother Teddy took the family sailing the day before, and spent most of the ride teasing me and asking Amy, every way he could think of, if she realized what she was getting herself into. In reality, Amy understood that better than Teddy did—and probably better than I did. The weather that Friday afternoon for the wedding was absolutely perfect, so we could do the ceremony out on the lawn, overlooking the ocean. I just remember looking out and seeing all the chairs lined up out there and thinking this was a fairy tale, because I never thought this was going to happen for me.

Harper was our flower girl, of course. Our Justice of the Peace was Supreme Court Justice Stephen Breyer, a longtime family friend. During the reception the sun set, and as a very full moon began rising over the harbor, Vicki treated us to an incredibly thoughtful, nostalgic gift. She had hired the company my dad had used for fireworks during my birthday when I was a kid, and they put on a breathtaking display.

After the round of rockets exploded in the air, some sparks hit the dune grass at the end of the lawn, and I was worried about a fire. But the fire department was already there, prepared. And when I asked the chief if we should stop, he said, "Are you kidding me? You see that pump boat out in the water there, you see this fire engine? Your dad helped us raise the money for all of these. You're having your fireworks!"

Our wedding was the last event scheduled at the house before it shifted from family control to the control of the institute my father set up before his death. And I was going to end up owning the only part of my grandparents' house remaining in private hands.

The house had a separate garage building in the rear of the property, which had a small apartment above it where I often stayed during visits to the Cape. In his will, my dad left me that little building, and left the rest of the historic home and grounds to the nonprofit (which would also run his Edward M. Kennedy Institute for the US Senate, adjacent to the JFK Presidential Library). It was a sweet little apartment and was nearby President Kennedy's old house, which my brother had bought. For Amy and I, who already lived on another shore where we planned to raise our family, the apartment would be a wonderful little place among the big family homes.

AMY AND I WANTED TO have a baby right away, and wanted Harper to have a sibling. Amy got pregnant shortly after the wedding, but we kept it quiet for a couple months. In mid-September, we decided we would start telling family, beginning with my sister, Kara—who was the first family member Amy had met, and among those family members most overjoyed I had finally found a true mate.

Kara had largely stayed out of the public eye, working behind the scenes in film and TV in Boston before moving to Washington to raise her kids. She had worked on videos for Very Special Arts, the group founded by my Aunt Jean as part of the Kennedy Center to provide arts education for children with disabilities, and she was on the boards of several organizations, including the National Organization on Fetal Alcohol Syndrome. She had beaten lung cancer in her forties, but at a price—the strong treatment had affected her heart.

Amy and I were planning to tell Kara over the weekend, and I had gone down to Washington a day early to appear at a political rally. I was in my hotel room at the Four Seasons, preparing my speech, when I got a call from Sean Richardson, my former chief of staff, who was still the one in Washington who people reached out to when they wanted to quickly track me down. He said he had just received a call from Kelly O'Donnell from NBC News with a terrible, unconfirmed report concerning my sister. He said "they found her" in the steam bath of her health club, just after she had finished swimming laps, which she did almost every day. For a second it just didn't compute what "found her" meant.

Finally he said, "I don't know how to tell you this . . ." and then it just clicked that she had died. I couldn't believe it. She was fifty-one.

I immediately canceled my speech, called Amy to let her know, and then called my brother, who couldn't get there until the next morning. But we agreed I needed to go be with Kara's teenage kids, Grace and Max, immediately, so they would first hear the news from me. I called one of Kara's closest friends, who the kids knew well, to go over with me. We got to my sister's house late in the afternoon. The kids were home—Max was fourteen, and Grace was about to turn seventeen in a few days—and we all went into the living room. I spoke first, and while I'm sure what I said is vivid in their minds, the whole moment for me was and still is a blur. I could still barely conceive of this thing myself, and I just thank God I was able to be there with them and tell them, and that I was able to do that sober. I do remember telling them over and over that they were her *everything*—nothing was more important to Kara than Grace and Max. I also told them some stories I wasn't sure they knew about their mom's life as the oldest child, and the only girl, growing up in my family.

I had this profound sense that I had to honor Kara in the way I acted during those first twelve hours. And I just kept thinking: *I've got to be present for them and tell them the truth. I can't do what was often done with us—talk about other things and ignore all the elephants in the room.*

I stayed up with them late into the night, just trying to be whatever they needed me to be. It was, in a strange way, one of the most fatherly acts of my life. Not that I was their father, but I was doing what my father would have done—be strong and comforting at a time of loss.

OUR SON OWEN PATRICK KENNEDY was born the next spring, and I was immediately a father in a way I could never have prepared for. The feelings of love and protectiveness were overwhelming.

By then, we had been living with Amy's parents together for over a year. They were so helpful during Amy's pregnancy and after she gave birth—and I was on the road all the time, giving speeches about mental health and brain science issues, as well as human rights and labor issues. Since we'd decided that the new house I had bought needed more than work—it needed a do-over—we rented a house on the other side of Brigantine Island from it, just a block from the beach, and made that the place Owen would have his first experiences. (Including being taken care of by me and my coauthor when Amy used the opportunity of our early interviews to get out of the house.)

I was, at that time, involved in the planning for the second One Mind conference, this one set in Los Angeles at UCLA. And we had just hired our dream leader for the organization: retired four-star General Pete Chiarelli. As Vice Chief of Staff for the US Army, Pete had been the Defense Department's loudest voice, for years, on traumatic brain injury, post-traumatic stress, and the rising epidemic of suicide in the military. I had dealt with him many times during the appropriations process, and he was clearly the face of the defense establishment finally taking neurological and psychiatric conditions seriously. He also was leaving the Army after forty years, at the age of sixty-two.

Pete was a perfect choice for One Mind, and after the May 2012 meeting in Los Angeles, it was time for Garen and I to let our fledgling nonprofit begin to grow under its new leader. Pete felt strongly that what the group could best contribute, besides being a convener for great neurological minds to share ideas, was to focus on the things he had realized were holding progress back when he was in the military: lack of transparency in research, failure to find and wrestle with really big medical and scientific data sets, and lack of support for research and treatment for the trauma-based brain diseases that had become the invisible wounds of war. He did not come from the worlds of mental illness and addiction, and while he recognized both of them as a big part of the veteran suicide problem, he also had different ideas about how to fight the stigma against diagnosis and treatment than those of us who grew up in mental health advocacy.

For example, his very practical solution to the problem of stigma was to stop calling illnesses "disorders," because that was stigmatizing. In fact, he was part of a group that was trying to get the APA, in its upcoming version of the *DSM*, to change the name of post-traumatic stress disorder to post-traumatic stress injury or just post-traumatic stress.

Pete and I were on the same side on most issues of brain disease, and I was thrilled with where he was taking One Mind. But I had originally envisioned the group as bringing together everyone's science and advocacy when it came to anything concerning the brain. And I could see that One Mind's mission had become the bright future of brain research, big data, and transparent, cooperative neuroscience. One Mind was also becoming more international, our original idea of a NASA of inner space expanded to more of an International Space Station, making sure brain researchers in Europe and Asia all used common language and protocols so the science could be replicated and more quickly lead to meaningful results.

It was amazingly ambitious and forward-looking, and already making a difference. But I could see One Mind was going to focus on brain research for the future—and I felt that we needed to simultaneously be working to improve American mental health and addiction care *today*. That would mean pressing the case for the implementation of the parity act and making sure that discrimination in healthcare coverage was ended.

So, after the second One Mind meeting, I started putting together another group. This new effort would use a different President Kennedy milestone as its rallying point: the upcoming fiftieth anniversary of the signing of the Community Mental Health Act, the cornerstone of much that had gone right (and wrong) in the care of brain diseases. So, at the end of the summer of 2012, I invited a small planning group to Hyannis Port for a Kennedy-infused planning meeting, one of the first to be held at Gramma's house since it was being run by my father's institute.

The group included Steve Hyman, who was now running the Stanley Center for Psychiatric Research at the Broad Institute of MIT and Harvard; Richard Frank, who had emerged as the country's leading expert on mental healthcare economics and delivery, at Health and

Human Services and at Harvard; health law advocates Paul Samuels, the director of the medical public interest group Legal Action Center in New York, and Matt Selig, my father's former assistant chief counsel for healthcare, now executive director of Health Law Advocates; Linda Rosenberg from the National Council for Behavioral Health; Andrew Sperling, still the top lobbyist for NAMI; and two representatives from industry: Dr. Ian Shaffer, medical director of a number of top behavioral health insurance companies, and former Pennsylvania State Senator Joe Rocks, who now managed a network of behavioral health centers.

While this was a pretty high-powered group, everyone was dressed very casually, in short-sleeve shirts and shorts or khakis; hardly anyone wore socks because we were hoping to sail in the afternoon. We spent all morning discussing the Community Mental Health Act and how it had changed the world, how it had completely *failed* to change the world, and what might be done to mark its anniversary and restart the conversation it had once provoked.

While this was pretty hard-core policy talk, the conversation was occasionally brought back to earth by the cooing or laughter of my infant son, Owen, who was sitting with Amy just next to me until it was my turn to hold the little man. My mother also joined us for a while to talk a bit about her interest in the subject—and her willingness to be more outspoken about her struggles with alcoholism if it would help. And I couldn't resist pointing out to the group, during a brief lull in the dialogue, that the girl in the bathing suit walking down the path to the docks was singer Taylor Swift, who was then dating my cousin (and probably already composing the song about their breakup).

After several hours of conversation, we, too, headed to the docks, and a launch took us out to where my dad's boat, the *Mya*, was moored. My brother, Ted, now owned and took care of the gorgeous teak sailboat, but he let us use it. On board, our dialogue continued right where it left off—except that when the wind picked up, everyone had to yell a little louder to be heard. There were rants about limited insurance coverage, FDA regulation, nonquantitative treatment limitations, cutbacks in pharmaceutical R & D for psychoactive drugs, cutbacks in federal funding for basic science research, the problems with the upcoming new *DSM*.

And, every so often, the rants were interrupted by requests for cans of soda or bottled water, or the sound of Owen (in the baby seat Amy was clutching for dear life) squealing with delight when we went over a wave.

By THE END of that windy August afternoon, I had decided to create another group, to honor the fiftieth anniversary of JFK's Community Mental Health Act—and make sure that this time, the changes being made to help those with mental illness *actually helped them*.

Our goal was nothing less than launching a new civil rights movement, to finally force medical equality for diseases of the brain. To do that we would vigorously defend the legal protections and requirements of the Mental Health Parity and Addiction Equity Act. We would define and demand the level of coordinated and proactive care that is required to treat these illnesses properly. And we would create a true community of mental health. We would help Americans understand that the community of mental health is "all of us" and not "them."

By achieving these goals, we could ensure more effective diagnosis for mental illness, addictions, intellectual disablities, and cognitive impairments. We would make a "checkup from the neck up" as regular as taking blood pressure. We would demand these diseases be treated as early as possible, not only when it's almost too late—well before their final stages or, "B4Stage4" (using a smart phrase coined by our friends at Mental Health America). We would insist that all public servants—

including police officers and schoolteachers—be trained in "mental health first aid." We would attack prejudice against people with brain diseases. We would confront the "don't ask, don't tell" attitudes between doctors and patients that keep both from engaging on questions of mental illness and addiction. And we would promote strategies for better understanding and prevention of suicide, the ultimate avoidable tragedy of all these brain diseases.

These were not goals that could be achieved overnight. They required creating a new process, a new meeting place for the community of mental health as defined as broadly as possible, so all the stakeholders were at the table and the common enemies were the problems, not each other. The effort needed to be bipartisan not only politically, but in the spirit of give-and-take. Patients and families and caregivers couldn't always be right; insurance companies and pharmaceutical manufacturers couldn't always be wrong. The idea was to pick the things that everyone agreed needed to be done and could only be done cooperatively, and to make that our mission.

We decided to call this mental health leadership initiative the Kennedy Forum.

One Mind is where we want to go. The Kennedy Forum is where we live.

OVER THE NEXT YEAR, we worked on developing both One Mind and the Kennedy Forum, and in between I gave dozens and dozens of speeches on brain disease and healthcare issues. But I always did it in a way that respected my recovery, my marriage, and my family—the only things in my life that I can't afford to lose.

I did actually set up a functioning office with a couple of assistants, and set up my schedule so I could attend a twelve-step meeting wherever I was on the road, and made sure I had enough time at home to recharge with my family and my local twelve-step group and sponsor. Being in recovery is an everyday challenge, and although I do not have any "One day at a time" pillows like my mother, I get those same phrases and reminders delivered to my smartphone several times a day by texts from twelve-step apps and my fellows in recovery.

While I am committed to recovery as my lifeline, I kept my promise to myself and to Amy that if I needed to go back on some psychiatric medication, I would. And after several years of sobriety, I decided to add a daily dose of the anticonvulsant Lamictal to my regimen of twelve-step meetings and exercise.

Taking an anticonvulsant has made a real difference in helping control my moods and especially my agitation, which also helps me maintain my sobriety and my commitment to recovery. Interestingly, after I started taking Lamictal again, I found out it was one of the medications my father had taken, at a higher dose than what's used for mood disorders, to control seizures after his brain surgery. When you take the medication for seizures, of course, there's no stigma at all. When I take it for my mood disorder, there's stigma because I have the mood disorder, and some stigma from old-school recovery folks who think that if I was really working the steps I wouldn't need any medication. Luckily, I have a more enlightened sponsor who is more open-minded about medical treatment. But I am still amazed at all the ways that just taking a medication you need to treat an illness can be controversial.

THE POLITICS OF DRUGS took a different turn for me in early 2013 when I decided to help Dr. Kevin Sabet, a former Obama administration senior adviser in the White House Office of National Drug Control Policy, found a group called Project SAM, Smart Approaches to Marijuana, which questions the medical and scientific wisdom of legalizing pot without any medical policy in place to treat those users in whom it is likely to trigger or exacerbate brain changes—including, in some cases, anything from psychosis to functional dependence.

I favor decriminalizing marijuana possession so you only pay a fine. And I also want to see a system in place where people are screened for mental illness and drug dependency—*not* by the criminal justice system, but by the healthcare system.

I know this can be a hard sell for some liberal Democrats. But even before I had kids, I noticed that a lot of parents my age—even those of us who smoked pot—were worried about the mass legalization of high-potency marijuana and products that include the ingredient in pot believed to make people feel high, THC.

They should be worried. The kind of legalization that we've seen in Colorado and Washington state is opening the door to complete commercialization of these products, creating the next Big Tobacco. It is also exposing people, especially young people, to sometimes absurdly high doses of THC in products they can eat like candy and drink like soda because they are candy (edibles) and soda (elixirs) and they don't make you high right away. In the handful of states where they are legal, THC edibles have become a leading cause for emergency room visits, especially for children and teens unaware of just how high the doses really are.

And besides all these new THC products, smoked and "vaped" pot is much more powerful than what we ever had, and being used at increasingly younger ages when the brain is even more unformed.

The moment I knew this idea was getting some traction is when Stephen Colbert had me on *The Colbert Report* to talk about it, and seemed ready to just set me up for a big punch line. But then I described to him how THC-laced cookies, drinks, and gummy bears were proliferating in Colorado, with free samples being given away on ski lifts. I think as a parent he finally got that this issue is much more complicated than it seems.

I WAS AT JOHN KERRY's swearing in as Secretary of State when I looked across the Benjamin Franklin State Dining Room at the State Department during the reception and saw him: Louis Susman, the US Ambassador to the UK. I hadn't spoken to him in nearly three years, since that day I cursed him out for telling my family I was detoxing in a London airport.

The old me would have ducked and dived and made a beeline for the door. But I was trying really hard not to be the old me. So I walked right over to him. I needed to make amends.

In recovery, this is one of the most powerful and spiritual aspects of the journey, and it's the kind of transformational moment that doesn't come naturally. You just have to do it. You have to make right what you made wrong. In the program, we say we have a physical allergy, a mental obsession, and a spiritual malady. A lot of people don't like the medical disease concept of addiction because it can lead people to hide behind their diagnosis instead of taking responsibility. The difference was that now I was taking responsibility.

"Mr. Ambassador, the last time we spoke I was very rude to you," I said. "It was uncalled for, and I am deeply apologetic for having yelled at you. I was being very defensive because I was sick and I didn't want anyone to know about it. I was mad you had told Vicki and the reason I yelled at you was because I was so ashamed of the situation and was angry at myself. I took it out on you, and I wanted to say I'm sorry."

He looked me in the eye and said, "As of this moment, I've forgotten all about it. I appreciate you saying this, and it's behind us."

I really had a cathartic feeling, like I had done something that would make me a stronger person. About five minutes later, a woman came up to me and introduced herself as Ambassador Susman's wife. She said she had been reading about my new life and my wife and new family, and wondered if we would come visit them sometime. And she added, "Of course, we loved your dad." And in that moment I realized something about the implications of my behavior over all those years, that it was more far-reaching than I could have realized. Because a lot of people loved my father and my family, my self-destructive behavior wasn't just affecting me.

After that, I started making amends to others in my life. I apologized to Terri Alford, my former office manager, for all the times I put her in unfair positions. And then I apologized to my mother. It was Christmastime and my mother had been very ill. We were at her apartment—I was in her bedroom with her, and Amy and the kids were in her living room. I told my mom that now that I was a father, and committed to the health and well-being of my children forever, I had a profound appreciation for how my illness must have affected her. I told her I now understood how difficult it was for her to see me not well and to worry about me like she must have.

And without missing a beat, my mom came alive, her eyes lit up, and she said, "Thank you, Patrick. It means a lot to me that you said that. You know how much I love you."

MUCH TO MY UTTER ASTONISHMENT, we were well into the fifth year since the Mental Health Parity Act had been passed, and there was still no end in sight in the battle to get the government to issue final rules. They had issued interim rules in early 2010, which offered less clarity than confusion and even a little fear—laws are in the details, and since the conference committee on the bill had left a number of issues unresolved, we were increasingly worried that consumers could lose in the interpretation.

The lobbying for the final rules had grown so intense that Jim Ramstad and I decided to ratchet up the volume by going out on the road again to do some field hearings. We arranged to kick off this effort at the National Press Club with members of the Parity Implementation Coalition, a lobbying group made up of many players who had been with us through the parity fight before.

The field hearings were, again, to remind communities that the issue of parity was basically state and local—it was about holding their local private health insurance providers accountable using either the federal law or their state law, whichever was stronger, and accessing the enforcement power of state insurance commissioners and state attorneys general.

We were actually learning a lot about this from a relatively new player in our midst, an Israeli lawyer from Los Angeles named Meiram Bendat. He had recently started a practice called Psych-Appeal that only took cases of medical insurance discrimination for mental illness and addiction. He was very smart and aggressive, and was working in various states to win cases that would both help his clients and also bring to light more information about how care approval and reimbursement decisions were made by insurers. In order to get to the point where we could advocate for best practices, we had to know more about all the practices.

And, in defense of the insurance companies, without final rules on mental health parity from the federal government, there was no easy way to know what was a violation of the new law.

In the midst of the Kennedy/Ramstad reunion parity tour, two of my closest allies in mental health politics got into a damaging dispute in the pages of the *New York Times*—about something they actually didn't even disagree about. And the public got a glimpse of how challenging it can be to keep leading experts in our field rowing together.

The headline read "Psychiatry's New Guide Falls Short, Experts Say," and the story was stunning: Tom Insel had written in his NIMH director's blog that the new *DSM*, about to be published by the American Psychiatric Association, suffered from a "lack of validity" and that "patients with mental disorders deserve better." And, of course, that set off my friend Dr. Jeffrey Lieberman, the schizophrenia researcher who is chief of psychiatry at Columbia's medical school and was, at the moment, serving as president of the APA (where I did some consulting). Insel's blog post was primarily a chance to draw attention to his fascinating new program Research Domain Criteria (RDoC), which was meant to push brain research beyond the existing diagnostic categories—which are reductionist but, at the moment, the best we have—by expanding the rules for NIMH studies so proposals no longer had to follow DSM categories but could explore across them as well.

Insel believed this would, one day, revolutionize diagnosis and treatment, incorporating more genetics, imaging, and cognitive science. And so did Jeff Lieberman and I, and anyone else who cared about the future of brain health. The problem was, the head of the NIMH can be disappointed by the progress in the field and in the new *DSM*, but to suggest that the whole diagnostic system "lacks validity"—because it isn't good enough yet—is to suggest that every patient and clinician involved in treatment in this current system is involved in something scientifically invalid. Nobody but anti-psychiatry haters believes that.

Lieberman did his best when the *Times* reporter called for comment. And after the story sent shock waves through the mental health community, Insel and Lieberman, who have known each other forever, immediately issued a joint statement explaining that *DSM* "represents the best information currently available for clinical diagnosis of mental disorders. Patients, families, and insurers can be confident that effective treatments are available and that the *DSM* is the key resource for delivering the best available care. The National Institute of Mental Health (NIMH) has not changed its position on *DSM-5*." The statement went on to explain the RDoC initiative, which is extremely important for the future of neuroscience. But hardly anyone ever saw that statement, which just went out as a press release from the NIMH and APA. And it got no coverage, no correction in the *Times*.

Some of this was about money, of course: Insel was looking for more funding for NIMH for RDoC and Lieberman was also protecting *DSM*, which is an important diagnostic reference and the cornerstone of APA's budget. But the leaders of the NIMH and APA have to be on the same page, always, about the importance and validity of mental health treatment.

As Jim and I were doing our last parity field hearings, we got word that the White House was calling a special meeting on mental health, and everyone had to be there. Unlike the conclave that the Clintons and the Gores had in 1999, which was years in the planning (if you included the Surgeon General's report), this one came pretty much out of nowhere. Many of us were invited, literally, a week or two before the event, and were told nothing about the agenda. We were appreciative of the mental health protections in the Affordable Care Act—and also understood how he had to juggle our needs with those of the powerful insurance companies whose support was needed to pass the landmark bill. But a lot of us were concerned the administration had not been focused enough on the epidemic of suicides, overdoses, and addiction, and that it was dragging its feet on full implementation of mental health parity.

President Obama gave a very stirring speech to start the White

House meeting. And he was very kind to give me and the parity act a big shout-out during his remarks.

> There are . . . people who are leading by example [like] my great friend Patrick Kennedy. When he was running for reelection back in 2006, he could have avoided talking about his struggles with bipolar disorder and addiction. Let's face it, he's a Kennedy. . . . His seat was pretty safe. Everybody loved him. And yet, Patrick used his experience as a way to connect and to lift up these issues, not hide from them.
>
> And one day, a woman came up to Patrick at a senior center and told him she was afraid to tell her friends she was taking medication for a mental illness because she was worried they might treat her differently. She told Patrick, "You're the only one who knows aside from my son."
>
> And so Patrick started realizing how much power there could be for people to speak out on these issues. And Patrick carried these stories back with him to Washington, where he worked with a bipartisan group of lawmakers, including his dad, to make sure the mental health services you get through your insurance plan at work are covered the same way that physical health services are—a huge victory.
>
> So because of Patrick's efforts and the colleagues who worked with him, it's easier for millions of people to join him on the road to recovery, which brings me to a second point. It's not enough to help more Americans seek treatment—we also have to make sure that the treatment is there when they're ready to seek it.

I was grateful for his acknowledgment, but the White House conference came and went, offering no real funding for anything new and no real political action of note. There wasn't a hint about when they would finish the final rules for the parity act or, perhaps more important, extend parity from the private insurance companies covered in our act to Medicaid so almost all Americans would have parity.

BY THE FALL OF 2013, my quiet post-congressional life was exploding. I was making all my recovery meetings and taking good care of myself physically, but my travel schedule was incredibly challenging. I was glad so many organizations and companies wanted to hear me talk about healthcare and parity, but I was spending too much time in planes, trains, and cabs.

Amy was pregnant again and Owen was starting to get an inkling that he wasn't going to be getting all the youngest-kid attention anymore, just as Harper had realized when her brother was born. Construction on our new house had been delayed so many times that we were now wondering if we might actually have to head back to Amy's parents' house for a bit.

At the same time, we were just weeks away from the inaugural Kennedy Forum meeting at the JFK Presidential Library. And things weren't going quite as smoothly as I might have hoped.

I was sure, in my heart, that the Kennedy Forum was something long overdue—the broad community of mental health desperately needed a convening forum, a meeting place, a way of identifying a handful of common goals all the stakeholders could never address individually. I believed that if we built it, they would come. Yet, in early October, less than three weeks before the event was supposed to take place—an event to which we had already committed a budget of a million dollars—we were hundreds of thousands of dollars short in our fund-raising. And we still didn't have a commitment from the White House that Vice President Biden and Health and Human Services Secretary Kathleen Sebelius—whose department was still holding the parity act hostage by not issuing final rules—would be there to give the keynotes.

We had also assumed, incorrectly, that the federal government would never have allowed the five-year anniversary of the parity act— five *years*—to pass without issuing the final rules. That anniversary was October 3, so we had felt pretty confident that the Kennedy Forum event on the twenty-fourth would be a chance to celebrate the final rules. Instead, the anniversary passed, and there were still no rules in sight.

The Vice President and Secretary Sebelius did have a pretty good excuse—the Web page for the Affordable Care Act had gone live on October 1, and they were a little busy triaging that disaster. But as the HealthCare.gov situation got worse, our time was running out.

We had an opening speaker lined up for the dinner, NFL star Brandon Marshall, who had recently gone public with his own psychiatric illness. Dr. Aaron Beck, the ninety-one-year-old inventor of cognitive behavioral therapy, had agreed to be there so we could honor him with our first Kennedy Forum Community Health Award. And we had already secured an amazing array of people to appear at sessions the next day—every panel was packed with the kinds of seriously opposing points of view that you never see at a conference. Chelsea Clinton had agreed to run a panel on the future of mental healthcare in the community (JFK's original idea, which still wasn't really being practiced). Dr. Rhonda Robinson Beale, a brave medical director from one of the nation's top health insurers, agreed to speak openly about the concerns of industry. We would have appearances from former Surgeon General Dr. David Satcher; Pamela Hyde, the director of SAMHSA; top mental health educator Dr. Mary Jane England, and many others.

But we still had no keynote for the opening-night event. We still didn't have enough money for all the planned Forum events. And there was still no final rules for parity. We had built it, but they were really taking their good old time coming.

It wasn't until less than a week before the event that the White House announced that Vice President Joe Biden would appear—and, perhaps more bravely, so would Secretary Sebelius.

And, suddenly, a lot of people and organizations wanted to be at the Kennedy Forum. And a lot of people offered to step up and help us build and support the organization, from my dad's former staffer, lawyer Allan Fox, to leaders I had never met in business and science from around the world. The event turned out to be twenty-four amazing hours of politics and policy. And all anyone wanted to know was what this new community could accomplish together.

A WEEK LATER, I got a call from the staff of the Senate Judiciary Committee saying that Senator Richard Blumenthal from Connecticut wanted to hold hearings on the absurdly long delays in issuing federal rules. Blumenthal had appeared at the parity field hearing we did in Hartford, Connecticut, the year before, and he was a big supporter of the legislation. He invited me and Cathy Morelli, a Connecticut mother who had also appeared at our hearing, telling an achingly painful story about her fourteen-year-old daughter, who suffered from an eating disorder, anxiety, and depression and had made multiple suicide attempts but was repeatedly refused inpatient care—or discharged prematurely—by her health insurer.

The morning of the actual hearing, November 7, I was sitting in Senator Blumenthal's office making some last notes on my testimony when we received word that the final rules likely would be released the next day. So, before the hearing began, its goal had already been achieved. A very Washington result. And that was fine.

Because what we already knew was that the final rules would not be the final word. The final parity rules laid out the initial definitions of a lot of terms, and included some rulings that favored insurers and others that favored patients and caregivers. But it was going to be many years, many court challenges, many efforts of advocacy and brinksmanship, before we knew their real impact.

They could finally lead the country to realize my Uncle Jack's vision of America where those with mental illnesses, addictions, and developmental disabilities would "no longer be alien to our affections or beyond the help of our communities." Or they could be an unenforceable disaster.

We had our work cut out for us.

BUT FIRST, I needed some long-awaited family time. Only days after the final rules were published, Amy gave birth to our daughter, Nora Kara Kennedy, six pounds, eleven ounces. And we moved into our new house—built from scratch on the lot where the house I bought us in a panic three years before had stood—just in time for Nora to come home to it. It wasn't quite ready for Thanksgiving dinner, but we were able to have the first of many family Christmases there.

As I maintained my sobriety, my health continued to improve until, out of nowhere, in the fall of 2014, I developed a bad case of shingles, which was really painful. Doctors wanted to give me painkillers—which I, of course, wouldn't take (but was tempted). Then they offered another kind of pain medication, Neurontin (gabapentin), which is used for seizures and mood stabilizing but also deadens nerve pain.

It worked; I felt better on it. It not only relieved the pain from shingles but a lot of the pain from anxiety—a psychic pain. In fact, when I decided to talk to my doctor about staying on it—since it did many of the same things as Lamictal—I wondered if the fact that I liked it was a bad thing. That's how paranoid I am about abusing medication, because I know I have an absurdly high propensity for abusing anything. So I started asking everyone I knew who might have an informed opinion on this issue, which is a pretty large group.

I was mostly asking around because I'd heard a rumor that some people considered Neurontin a drug of dependence. It isn't. In fact, when I finally decided that perhaps I would stay on it, I told my primary care doctor in New Jersey about how difficult the decision had been. He had a medical resident with him that day, and the resident said he had recently read a study in *JAMA Internal Medicine* about this very subject. Neurontin had been studied as a treatment for the cravings of alcoholism and had shown a significant benefit in increasing rates of abstinence in a long-term, single-site trial at the Scripps Research Institute in La Jolla, California. He quickly ran to the computer to get me the citation, wrote it out on a piece of paper, and handed it to me.

Interestingly, my primary care doctor said he would not be comfortable writing me another prescription without a consult from a specialist, so I went back to the addiction medicine specialist I had seen when I first moved to South Jersey—my backup psychiatrist, in case I needed one—and he wrote it. The drug seems to address more of my symptoms more effectively than the Lamictal, and for the time being, I'm staying on it.

Reading this might make some hard-core abstinence folks in recovery a little squeamish. But the future of care for mental illness and addiction is a new level of collaborative care, so physicians, psychotherapists, counselors, nurses, and lay support groups work together, not against each other, to make the best group effort for each individual patient. Every treatment we get needs to be more evidence based than it is now, every caregiver needs to understand and support the combinations of treatments that can be successful, and every patient needs to view their treatment and recovery as an integrated medical process.

Patients should have choices, and as long as those choices are evidence based, our medical insurance should cover them—just as it covers prescription drug remedies, surgical remedies, lifestyle remedies, preventive remedies, and combinations of these for every other disease.

It's the only way.

Chapter 28

Very early on a perfect August Sunday morning in Hyannis Port, I met my cousin Tim Shriver at Gramma's house for coffee. It was the only time, when the whole family was at the Cape for a summer weekend, that we could actually speak calmly and quietly, before everyone's kids woke up and took over.

Tim was finishing up his inspiring book, *Fully Alive: Discovering What Matters Most*, and I was working on mine and on building the Kennedy Forum, so it was a great time to be reflecting on the legacy of our parents, and their families, in the world of medical care and advocacy. He had also been exploring his mother's correspondence, especially on the subject of our Aunt Rosemary, just as I had been exploring the history of JFK's Community Mental Health Act and the family's involvement in brain disease reform. We were both looking for ways to make a difference for families with intellectual disabilities, mental illness, and addiction. Families like ours.

We were also talking about family secrets. I told Tim my story about lying to my therapist as a teenager until I browsed the "Kennedy section" of a bookstore and saw how many of the things I was trying to keep secret had been published in books.

He laughed. "The family pathology, which everybody in the family does have, is *secrecy*," he said. "And that *is* pathology."

We talked about how differently the worlds of intellectual disability and mental illness in America had grown over the years, as we grew up and watched our parents handle the politics and advocacy, and now that we were both involved in that full-time ourselves. I admitted to being envious of the destigmatizing power of Special Olympics, the way its programs fostered inclusion. I wondered how I might help encourage something equally transformative for mental illness and addiction. And we talked about the challenges that would face both of our fields in the future.

While our conversation was mostly about America, we also discussed the problems in the rest of the world. The World Health Organization recently had pronounced untreated mental disorders the leading cause of disability on the planet, accounting for 13 percent of the entire global burden of disease. WHO also claimed that no matter how stunning the "treatment gap" was in America and other high-income countries—where over 35 percent of people with severe mental illness got no treatment at all—the problem was more than twice as bad in less developed countries, where the percentage of untreated people could reach 85 percent. And there had been recent media coverage about many foreign countries that were just beginning to address the issues of warehousing of patients—with no real accurate diagnosis or treatment—that the US had begun confronting in the 1950s. In some places there was no care at all.

In a lot of these countries, Tim said, most people still didn't understand the difference between intellectual disabilities and mental illness, and didn't believe in a biological or medical basis for either. They just saw certain young people as cursed. In fact he vividly recalled a conversation with a woman from a village in Tanzania who had a son with an intellectual disability. When asked how her son was doing, she explained that she was proud that he was never "tied."

I asked what that meant. Tim said the mother told him that young people in her village who couldn't function well enough to be brought with their mothers to work in the field had to be left in the home all day, tied in a closet or in the yard.

This was such a common occurrence that these children were referred to as "the tied" or "the chained." We just sat there for a moment, looking out over the lawn and Hyannis Harbor, taking in that concept.

As family members started stirring in the homes surrounding Gramma's, I saw Amy walking over with the baby to join us for coffee. Tim and I agreed that with the improvements in neuroscience and the new protections of mental health parity and the Affordable Care Act, we had—for the first time since the early 1960s—reached a moment in history where great change, great improvement of health and life, were possible. And sitting on the porch where his mother and our uncle had discussed, debated, and argued about the nation's first laws to reform the care of mental illness and intellectual disability, we realized just how many challenges were ahead of us.

NOT LONG AGO, we had a Kennedy Forum meeting of top experts on different aspects of parity from all over the country, to begin refining our new agenda. Instead of holding it in a conference room in Washington, DC, or Boston, or out on the Cape, we decided it was time to start establishing our new home and our South Jersey community as a meeting point.

The closer I am to home, and the more I am able to spend time with my wife and our kids, the more mentally healthy I am. And even though I still push myself too hard in several-day bursts away from Brigantine, what keeps me centered is that in my mind, I am always with Amy.

Now that our family has grown so quickly, Amy has decided to leave teaching for a while to focus on a new mental health initiative for schools. She has also become a really effective public policy advocate for everything from neuroscience funding to social and emotional learning programs for the classroom.

We held our meeting on the third floor of our house, where I have my office and a study with a balcony that overlooks the bay. That view of the water was a good reminder that we could not solve every problem, or, as politicians and management consultants like to say, you "can't boil the ocean."

So we talked about just five major priorities, five pillars. We would focus on payer accountability to ensure full parity compliance from all private insurers and the federal government; provider accountability, which meant developing the first set of quality standards and outcome standards for behavioral health; integration and coordination between the general medical and behavioral specialty systems; technology expansion, to build bridges between data and outcomes; and a new national focus on brain fitness and health, to drive funding into new translational neuroscience research into preventive and treatment interventions.

We discussed creating an ambitious online platform that would, for the first time, truly follow, measure, and help instigate parity implementation. It could start by helping individuals trying to file challenges when insurance companies refused to cover mental health care claims—allowing us to create a national database to analyze refusals of care. It would need to track parity progress on a state-by-state basis, looking at recent legislation and legal decisions that impact parity in coverage for mental illness and substance use disorder, and providing links so others could use the research. It would also track the parity implementation efforts of others—including advocacy groups and caregiver groups—who were doing their own work on everything from forcing disclosure of non-quantitative treatment limits to negotiating small technical glitches with big impacts (like the transition from DSM-IV to DSM-5 treatment codes) that could hurt people needing care. The platform (which we later called ParityTrack.org) would also offer everything from model state and federal legislation and rules to an easy way for anyone to email elected officials about mental health parity issues.

We also talked about how to make sure America's workplaces do a better job promoting mental health and wellness, making sure there is no discrimination in their health or disability coverage, in their company cultures, even in their advertising. We discussed how to bring together business leaders and thought leaders for a mental health leadership initiative modeled on the successful CEO Roundtable for Cancer, to focus on employer-sponsored mental healthcare and workplace wellness. Since a large percentage of healthcare is paid for by big self-insured companies, we felt a forum including them would not only help best practices in mental health coverage to proliferate but also spread the news of how their employee-assistance programs will help reduce absenteeism due to brain diseases and promote productivity.

After a three-hour session—parts of which were utterly exhilarating, other parts dispiriting, because there is so much to be done—we broke for dinner. We ate in the backyard, near the docks, with everyone at wooden tables under large fabric umbrellas. It was great to watch the lively conversations between people I had known my entire professional life—some of whom were fighting the stigma of mental illness before I even realized I had one—and people I had just recently met.

After dessert, the sun began to set over the bay, and everyone gravitated out to the wooden dock—not only all these thought leaders, but Amy and I and our kids. Harper and Owen were showing some of the world's experts on addiction facility management, insurance reimbursement, and healthcare program funding how the seagulls dropped clamshells from the sky onto the dock, and pieces got caught between the planks.

The kids started bending down and pulling the shell shards out of the dock and tossing them into the bay. And soon a handful of our guests were down on their hands and knees with them, helping with the effort.

I was standing on the end of the dock, talking to a healthcare accountant from PricewaterhouseCoopers. Amy was holding Nora. Harper and Owen and their new friends were having fun.

And I thought to myself: *For me, this is how the work will go on. Because I now have a chance to be healthy and happy enough to see it through.*

I do not kid myself. The diseases we have are chronic, not curable, and I am reminded of that all too often.

As we were finishing this book, we learned that one of our friends from that late summer day on the dock had completed suicide. He wasn't much older than me, he had two kids, and he had spent most of his adult life trying to help people get better healthcare. He knew so much and had helped so many, but in the end he was not able to save his own life.

His loss is one more reminder that I have to do everything in my power to keep up the common struggle—for Amy and our family, and everyone else who depends on me—to save every life I can, including my own.

Appendix I

WHAT YOU CAN DO

Now that you have read *A Common Struggle*, you might be wondering what you can do to improve care and coverage for mental illness and addiction, and end discrimination. I've been hearing this question for decades as a politician, and even longer as someone struggling with the illnesses and the stigma. We sometimes get too caught up in what we are hoping will happen in the future, with new discoveries, and forget just how many options and opportunities are available to us *right now*. So let's focus first on what you and I can do immediately, together.

First, don't be alone with your illness and your struggle. And don't be afraid to demand the best diagnosis, the best care, the best coverage, and the best way of staying current with the medicine and treatment. The illnesses are challenging enough, even when you do have all the information, caregivers you trust, and coverage that is equal to that for all other illnesses. You have to take the best possible care of yourself—or the person you are caring for—in order to be strong enough to advocate. If you or those close to you don't feel they understand the illnesses and treatments well enough, good basic resources include *Understanding Mental Disorders*, the consumer version of the *Diagnostic and Statistical Manual* used by all caregivers, the "Mental Health First Aid" training (www.mentalhealth-firstaid.org) offered nationwide by the National Council on Behavioral Health as well as the in-depth information on the websites from NAMI (https://www.nami.org/Find-Support), Mental Health America (which offers a help guide and very good basic online screening tools at http://www.mentalhealthamerica.net/mental-health-screening-tools), the National Council on Alcoholism and Drug Dependence (which offers an excellent guide on balancing medication-assisted treatment with abstinence and twelve-step peer support at https://ncadd.org/images/stories/PDF/Consumer-Guide-Medication-Assisted-Recovery.pdf) and the American Foundation for Suicide Prevention (http://afsp.org/find-support/). To make sure your treatment wishes are understood if your symptoms worsen, make an "advance directive" for your care choices with the help of the National Resource Center on Psychiatric Advance Directives (www.nrc-pad.org). If you and your caregiver feel your treatment is not being adequately covered by your insurance, explore your rights at ParityTrack.org, our online, state-by-state parity implementation watchdog, which we've created in partnership with the Thomas Scattergood Behavioral Health Foundation. There you can find our Parity Resource Guide (https://www.paritytrack.org/get-support/parity-resource-guide) and even register a complaint about denial of coverage at (www.parityquest.org). For a medical emergency with a mental illness or substance use disorder, dial 911 immediately; if it's an opiate overdose situation make sure you request naloxone. If you are having suicidal thoughts, call the National Suicide Hotline (800-273-8255).

Second, it is time to become educated about the political issues surrounding your illness, so you can vote and advocate effectively. The issues go far beyond just more funding for research for your individual disease—we also need to focus more strongly on larger goals that will help treat and cure all brain diseases. This is a big part of the reason why I wrote *A Common Struggle*—and created two nonprofits that are broadly inclusive of all mental illnesses and addictions (in the case of the Kennedy Forum www.thekennedyforum.org) and all brain diseases (in the case of One Mind www.onemind.org). I'm trying to provide and encourage leadership to bring together groups that sometimes compete for research dollars and public awareness in their own national and state lobbying. I'm also trying to help level some of the advocacy playing fields because, for a variety of reasons, the advocacy for some illnesses is heard above others—even if many more Americans suffer from illnesses with fewer or quieter advocates—and in some cases the advocacy for certain treatment approaches to illnesses are heard above others. For example, because of the historic anonymity in twelve-step recovery, there has not been as much public leadership for alcoholism and addiction advocacy as there has been for other mental illnesses. There is still an artificial divide in substance use disorders between those using medication-assisted treatment and some form of cognitive behavioral therapy (CBT) to detox and remain sober and those relying primarily on abstinence and twelve-step peer support—even though we know that the gold standard of treatment requires access to all of these together, based on your needs and symptoms at any given time. And with all these treatments, there are shortages of caregivers all around the country, as well as shortages of available appointments for in-network care. That is why we are working to create stronger advocacy on behalf of **all mental health**—including all mental illnesses and addictions, and all evidence-based treatments.

What I am trying to do is bring together as many stakeholders as possible—and their best ideas—to create an omnibus **National Behavioral Health Platform** which can offer an integrated and nonpartisan political agenda for the future of mental illness and substance use disorder care that is "secular" of guilds, political frictions and silos. It is also a platform that attempts to learn from the setbacks of the past, and takes advantage of the newest understandings of how to legally attack discrimination using state and federal parity acts, the protections inherent in the Affordable Care Act, and other laws in novel ways. It can help us get beyond assessing elected officials only on whether or not they voted for research funding for the exact illness we or our family members struggle with, and will help everyone see the big picture.

Starting on page 387, you can read through the entire National Behavioral Health Platform, which has been put together by the Kennedy Forum and the Scattergood Foundation—with input from many stakeholders—for use through the 2016 election and beyond, and will be periodically updated.

But, if you want to know what you should be demanding first—of your candidates and elected officials—**here is the lowest hanging fruit**:

1. **Every medical examination must include a mental illness and substance use disorder evaluation—one that is automatically connected, when indicated, to an aggressive plan of early diagnosis and intervention.** At every age, we need to be getting a simple "checkup from the neck up" every time we see a healthcare provider, starting with the depression screen that, though it is now fully covered under the Affordable Care Act, many doctors still aren't using. If you have any history of mental illness or addiction and your primary care physician isn't asking you, at each visit, the status of your illnesses, talk to them about it. To ensure our clinical workforce is better prepared to deliver these screenings, all healthcare providers should be required to take additional Continuing Medical Education classes on current brain health issues to keep their licenses to practice; similar continuing education is needed for attorneys, judges, and law enforcement officials. Further, the Centers for Medicare & Medicaid Services (CMS) and all private insurers should not only encourage these screenings through reimbursement but require that providers consistently use standardized outcomes measures to track patient progress. (Thanks to the Mood Disorders Association of Ontario, which coined "checkup from the neck up" and allows me to use it.)

2. **The Centers for Disease Control and Prevention (CDC) should establish a broad mental health surveillance system** so that we have accurate, regularly updated information and statistics on all aspects of the epidemics of mental illness and substance use disorder, including prevalence rates, types of treatment being used, availability of care, and comorbidities with other illnesses CDC already covers. The work that CDC already does on incidence of suicide and some other discreet areas of mental health and addiction, the National Survey on Drug Use and Health done by SAMHSA, and other smaller efforts are simply not sufficient for public officials, or the public, to understand and track the burdens of these diseases. Parity is about more than insurance; we also need parity in epidemiology.

3. **In order for research on brain diseases to catch up with basic science and medical research on the rest of the body, we call for a one-time five-year tripling of the budgets for the National Institutes of Health that**

cover the brain: NIMH, NIDA, NIAAA, and NINDS. Right now all the brain institutes combined receive less than 15 percent of the NIH's budget. This boost in funding should be used to integrate the institutes within a clinical research network that will study the brain and brain illnesses, develop new treatments, and conduct research on the dissemination of evidence-based therapies. The current segregation of the institutes into four separate bodies inhibits the ability of research at one institute from benefitting from findings produced at another. To make sure this extra funding is used to break down artificial barriers and silos between these medical areas, we propose an umbrella entity, the National Institutes of Brain and Behavior Disease, to coordinate the use of these extra funds, and the budget of SAMHSA. But this five-year period should also be used to slowly and logically phase out SAMHSA, because much of what it now accomplishes with grants—as part of an outdated "carve-out" way of approaching mental illness and substance use disorder—must be incorporated into a more structural approach to coverage that includes mental health along with all other health. Any areas in brain health requiring specialized grants and programs should be integrated into the appropriate section of HHS, including HRSA, AHRQ, CMS, and CDC.

4. **We must take immediate steps to dramatically increase our capacity for mental health and addiction care, which means aggressive action to increase the number of inpatient beds and coordinated outpatient stepdown services in this country, as well as incentivizing the training of more MDs, PhDs, MSWs, psychiatric nurses, and certified peers.** We support revising or further reinterpreting the IMD exclusion—a law from the 1960s meant to prevent dilapidated facilities from refilling their beds when Medicare/Medicaid was passed that has instead become the single largest impediment to quality inpatient mental health care, by preventing many facilities from getting Medicaid reimbursement for patients between the ages of twenty-two and sixty-four. While CMS recently changed the rule slightly, it still dramatically limits the number of inpatient beds available to anybody. Congress must also eliminate the arbitrary 190-day lifetime limit on inpatient psychiatric hospital care in Medicare—a

restriction that does not exist for any other inpatient Medicare service. To increase the number of caregivers, we must provide additional funding to the National Health Service Corps and create training grants for fellowships for mental health and addiction continuing education programs. These programs incentivize providers to enter into and stay in behavioral health care. We must also support the development of the Behavioral Health Minimum Data Set, a project sponsored by SAMHSA and HRSA, that tracks and studies the national mental health and addiction workforce.

5. **We must make an impact on the nation's rising suicide rate.** We support the important work of the JED Foundation in schools, the American Foundation for Suicide Prevention, the National Action Alliance for Suicide Prevention, and the Suicide Prevention Resource Center. The last two groups have also developed a unique effort called **Zero Suicide** (http://zero suicide.sprc.org) that brings the most modern tools and ideas to a special at-risk group: patients in hospital settings, whose suicides are considered the most clearly preventable of all. Zero Suicide began as an aspirational concept in the Air Force in the 1990s and was later used as an experimental benchmark in the Perfect Depression Care Initiative of the Henry Ford Health System. This new Zero Suicide for healthcare initiative employs a unique systems approach involving everyone who interacts with patients, and not just their clinicians, and a tool kit that allows much closer study of the processes leading to suicide attempts than previously possible. But it is time to make "zero suicide" our national standard of care, by accepting that most suicides represent a tragic course of illness for a brain disease and the only real way to prevent them is to improve brain health screening, diagnosis, and treatment. We need to better integrate means reduction, traditional hotlines and online media tools, and work to reduce the stigma associated with being open about suicidal ideation, suicide attempts, and completed suicides.

6. **Records for mental health and substance use disorder treatment must be integrated into electronic health-record systems so providers have the information needed to treat the whole person—while still protecting patient privacy.** HHS must finalize the update of federal regulation

"42 CFR part 2" so substance use disorder information can be incorporated into health records. Congress must amend the HITECH Act and CMS must update its final rule so that mental health professionals and facilities are eligible for financial incentives and reimbursement associated with electronic health records.

7. **Every county in the country should be implementing a system of diverting individuals with serious mental illnesses or co-occurring substance use disorders into community-based treatment and support services instead of putting them in jail.** The groundbreaking Eleventh Judicial Circuit Criminal Mental Health Project (CMHP) from Miami-Dade has been an incubator for programs, large and small, that can be emulated by counties nationwide. And for those already incarcerated with mental illnesses, states should adopt a version of the Mentally Ill Offender Community Transition Program in Washington State, a collaboration between the Department of Corrections and the Department of Mental Health that made a large impact on recidivism rates.

8. **We need to stop talking about "collaborative care" that is "outcomes driven" and actually start providing it.** There are programs around the country that are already doing this right, and can be replicated in every primary care setting. One is the Mental Health Integration Program (MHIP) in the state of Washington, sponsored by the Community Health Plan of Washington, and Seattle and King County Public Health. It provides excellent collaborative care for all mental illnesses and substance use disorders by bringing together primary care and community mental health centers; and it uses a unique payment system tied to quality improvement metrics, and a patient registry that tracks and measures patient goals and clinical outcomes, facilitating treatment adjustments if patients aren't improving. Another program is the chronic condition Healthcare Home initiative run by Missouri Healthnet, the state's Medicaid authority, for Medicaid recipients with severe mental illness. It combines many of the latest ideas about diverting "high utilizers" from emergency room care into more long-term coordinated care, but is among the first in the country to include a focus on high utilizers whose primary medical problem is

severe mental illness. Their cases are overseen by what are called "health homes" that combine aspects of primary care and community mental health, with cases actively overseen by nurse liaisons and case managers. For integration of care in emergency rooms and across socio-economic groups, an excellent model is the work done at Grady Health System in Atlanta with the Morehouse School of Medicine's Satcher Health Leadership Institute and the Georgia Department of Behavioral Health and Developmental Disabilities.

9. **Mental wellness programs should be required in all public and private schools.** Programs for social and emotional learning (SEL), executive function training, neurofeedback, mindfulness, and brain literacy help young people improve their traditional educations, but also allow development of better processing skills, promote emotional resilience, and help mitigate stress. They can also attack some of the underlying environmental triggers of mental illness—and the systems created by the interventions often help schools and parents identify at-risk students. These programs are easy to integrate into school curricula and don't take a lot of time every day. For SEL, we recommend the Responsive Classroom from the Center for Responsive Schools in northern Massachusetts (as does the Collaborative for Academic, Social, and Emotional Learning in Chicago, which has been evaluating these interventions for over twenty years); for executive function training, the ACTIVATE program from Yale's Dr. Bruce Wexler and C8 Sciences, which improves brain fitness with twenty-to-thirty-minute interactive game-like sessions several times a week, and also has healthcare applications for students with attention and autism spectrum disorders. One of the best combined interventions is Mind UP, developed with educators and neuroscientists by The Hawn Foundation.

10. **All American employers should reconsider their health insurance and employee assistance programs (EAPs) to see how they can improve diagnosis and treatment of mental illnesses and substance use disorders among their employees and executives—not only because it is the right thing to do and it is the law but because it is the single best way to save money on medical spending, absenteeism and presenteeism,**

and recruitment. It is crucial that companies and large organizations prioritize overall program quality over initial costs in improving their EAPs, which need to establish and maintain close contact with health insurance plans and available community resources, by following models like the Tufts Employee Assistance Program (http://hr.tufts.edu/benefits/employee-assistance-program). Since employees are often reluctant to seek help because of stigma, employers should implement evidence-based internal stigma-reduction programs, such as those featured in the Working Minds Project of the Mental Health Commission of Canada (http://www.mental healthcommission.ca/English/initiatives/11893/working-mind).

11. **We must respond to the epidemic of opioid addiction in a way that broadens diagnosis and treatment for all substance use disorders, and guarantee that insurers provide full coverage for these diseases. This must include a comprehensive range of evidence-based treatments such as residential care, intensive outpatient programs, cognitive behavioral therapy, and medication assisted treatment (MAT)— buprenorphine, methadone, and naltrexone.** Congress must amend the Drug Addiction Treatment Act of 2000 so that there is no longer any arbitrary limit to the number of patients to whom a specialty-trained physician can prescribe buprenorphine. State lawmakers should pass legislation that requires all pharmacies to carry naloxone, a life-saving drug that immediately reverses the effects of an opioid overdose. To address prevention, all physicians, nurse practitioners and physician assistants that prescribe opioid medications should follow the CDC Guideline for Prescribing Opioids for Chronic Pain.

12. **It is time for the Department of Health and Human Services, the Department of Labor, and state regulatory agencies to end the managed care secrecy that allows all American medical insurers (including the federal government) to discriminate against those with mental illness and addictions.** These departments must use the legal power they *already have* to demand detailed disclosures of how insurers make their decisions to approve or deny coverage for all medical, surgical, and mental health care. The departments have issued guidance about

disclosure, but it is still not sufficient. Making this information transparent is the only way to assure that the standards used for decisions on medical/surgical cases and mental health cases can be properly compared. The law has required this disclosure since the parity act was passed in 2008 and insurers still haven't complied (although some state agencies have begun to audit and fine health plans not in compliance). And we're not singling out the private insurance companies. We also call on the major public insurers—the Centers for Medicare and Medicaid Services (CMS) and its various entities, as well as the Office of Personnel Management (OPM), which oversees medical benefits for federal employees, the Departments of Defense (DOD) and Veterans Affairs (VA), the Indian Health Service (IHS) and others—to disclose the same criteria and protocols for their coverage decisions. This could be done in the form of blinded real-life scenarios and court decisions that can be used to guide decisions and clarify what violates the law, the way that the Internal Revenue Service often explains the ramifications of new tax regulations. Once these criteria and protocols have been shared, it would be essential for DOL and HHS to begin detailed random audits of health plans to determine compliance. We also call on the Department of Justice (and state Attorneys General) to get involved in enforcing such disclosures and transparency, since their investigations and consent decrees now often take the place of traditional regulation.

In the meantime, here is what you can do to immediately help the parity cause. Go to www.paritytrack.org. Do the quick online registration, and make your voice heard with the political outreach app and the national appeal/denial registry. From the site you can send an email directly to your state insurance commissioner and regional office of the Department of Labor, urging them to conduct random audits of health insurers practices concerning behavioral health, and to check all healthcare complaints for evidence of non-compliance with parity laws. (Many complaints are filed that don't mention the actual word "parity" so regulators need to look harder at whether feedback from consumers and caregivers represent non-compliance with parity laws.) You can also **email your state legislators and members of Congress to urge them to pass even stronger laws to protect you from discriminatory insurance practices**. And, if your doctor has ordered behavioral health care which your insurance company has denied, **you can immediately file an appeal** (and, if it's an emergency, an expedited appeal.)

This is just the beginning. There is a lot of work to do and, frankly, it is going to take contributions from everyone. The good news is that we already have many evidence-based programs ready to implement across our country, and smart public policies awaiting approval, passage or, in some cases, refunding. And I'm pleased to say there has been some notable progress since we put this kind of political agenda together for the hardcover edition of *A Common Struggle* in 2015. The President announced a large proposed budget increase in the fight against the rising epidemic of opiate addiction, overdose and suicide. He also finally created an interagency Mental Health and Substance Use Disorder Parity Task Force, which is scheduled to make its first recommendations just before the 2016 election.

The Centers for Medicare and Medicaid Services announced a new final rule that will strengthen access to mental health and substance use disorder services for children in the CHIP program and those with low incomes receiving Medicaid. The US Preventive Services Task Force made new recommendations that doubled down on screenings for depression, especially for pregnant women. But there is still so much to do.

On the pages that follow, you'll find our National Behavioral Health Platform, as well as more information on how to connect with our organizations, including the Kennedy Forum, ParityTrack, and One Mind.

Thank you for joining me in the common struggle.

Patrick J Kennedy

THE NATIONAL BEHAVIORAL
HEALTH PLATFORM
A NONPARTISAN APPROACH
TO MENTAL ILLNESS
AND SUBSTANCE USE DISORDERS

Since I left Congress in 2010 and starting working more broadly on the politics of mental health and addiction, my staff and I have been gathering, deconstructing, editing, and re-editing lists of programs and policies that we know already work—yet they haven't been fully adopted across the country. Below you'll find our expanded working list of these programs and policy needs in a variety of areas. It is meant to be understandable and useful to everyday medical consumers and their families, as well as to caregivers and policymakers. And I hope it serves as a reminder that even though we have much to learn about the brain, how it works, and what to do when it doesn't work as well as we like, we really have not yet tried, on a national scale, much of what we already have proven can be successful.

For the 2016 elections and beyond, we hope this platform will prove useful in helping you decide which candidates and causes to support, and what specific bills and programs to advocate for in your area of strongest personal interest and commitment.

The goal of our ongoing platform project is to use an interdisciplinary public health approach to target six key areas: **access to services, prevention and early intervention, vulnerable populations, the behavioral health workforce, social determinants, and research**.

I. Access to services for behavioral health care is woefully inadequate, there is little continuum of care, and treatment for mental illness and substance use disorders remains medically and economically segregated from general health care. Furthermore, mental health care is often left out of programs targeting the rapid raise in opioid use and suicide. The recommendations below address this lack of access to behavioral health services and unfair medical management.

PARITY
- HHS and DOL should strongly enforce the federal parity law by conducting no fewer than twelve random audits of health plans on an annual basis for compliance
- Federal and state regulators, and accreditation agencies, must require all health plans to disclose medical management criteria and protocols and how they are applied for both behavioral health care and medical/surgical care
- DOL, state insurance departments, and other applicable regulatory agencies should conduct audits or market conduct exams of any plan with three or more behavioral health complaints of the same type
- Congress must extend the federal parity law to Medicare and Medicaid fee-for-service
- Congress must amend the federal parity law so that it clearly states that mental health and substance use disorder benefits include residential treatment and that residential treatment is comparable to sub-acute inpatient medical/surgical treatment such as hospice care or care in a skilled nursing facility
- Congress must amend the federal parity law so that mental health conditions and substance use disorders are defined as any listed in the ICD-10 or found in the DSM-5.

- The federal government should release further regulations on non-quantitative treatment limitation compliance with examples of appropriate and inappropriate use. These regulations must clearly define the terms processes, strategies, evidentiary standards, or other factors.
- State insurance departments and other applicable state agencies should develop, implement and enforce strong requirements that health plans have an adequate number of behavioral health providers in their networks.
- DOL and state insurance departments should scrutinize all consumer complaints regarding prior authorization, fail first protocols, and concurrent medical necessity reviews for non-quantitative treatment limitation compliance under the federal parity law
- An online resource for consumer and provider reports of potential non-compliance with the federal parity law should be developed (this tool can consolidate complaints from other registries, such as www.parityquest.org)
- State legislatures throughout the country should introduce and pass legislation that increases parity protections, requires insurer transparency, and demands regulatory agency accountability (a model legislation is available at www.paritytrack.org/model-legislation)
- Attorney Generals with jurisdiction should investigate the actions of insurance plans if they receive numerous complaints regarding inadequate compliance with state or federal parity laws
- Insurers must approve of in-plan exceptions when the insurer's network does not have any provider accessible, available, or qualified capable of providing a medically necessary service. This information must be made publically accessible on the website that lists network providers and be communicated when a beneficiary calls to inquire about network providers
- Medical necessity determinations for eating disorder treatment should be based upon the overall medical and mental health needs of the patient—and not solely on body weight or body mass index. States should consider legislation similar to the recent Missouri law guaranteeing this: http://www.senate.mo.gov/15info/pdf-bill/tat/SB145.pdf

INTEGRATED CARE

- CMS should remove payment obstacles to facilitate the integration of behavioral health care into all other medical settings, including primary care, emergency rooms, and Federally Qualified Health Centers
- States should revise their Medicaid payment policies to allow for the billing of behavioral health and primary care services provided the same day
- States should implement integrated managed care programs for dual eligible enrollees in Medicare and Medicaid
- Congress should extend Medicare and Medicaid reimbursement for electronic health care use to mental health professionals and facilities
- Behavioral health providers must take advantage of incentives in the Physical Quality Reporting System program
- Federal and state governments, the National Quality Forum, accreditation agencies, purchasers of insurance and other stakeholders should continue to integrate behavioral health metrics into their core set of health care quality measures
- All health care plans should adopt value-based payment models based on measurement systems that integrate behavioral and physical health metrics
- Research on behavioral health integration through collaborative care, such as studies conducted by the Advancing Integrated Mental Health Solutions Center at the University of Washington, should be disseminated nation-wide

SUBSTANCE USE DISORDER SPECIAL ISSUES

- Insurers must cover residential treatment for substance use disorders as a first course of treatment rather than requiring patients to fail first at outpatient treatment
- Insurers should develop a reimbursement system for certified peer specialists in alcoholism and addiction treatment
- Congress should strengthen prescription drug monitoring programs, encourage training of family and first responders in naloxone, and incentivize the use of medication assisted treatment in all healthcare settings through additional funding and supports
- Needle exchange programs should incorporate treatment motivation and

incentive programs, such as those pioneered by the Baltimore Syringe Exchanged Program (http://health.baltimorecity.gov/hiv-std-services/com-
munity-risk-reduction)

- Communities should establish Family Treatment Drug Courts, an alternative to regular dependency courts, which aim to improve the safety and
well-being of children in the welfare system by providing parents access to
drug and alcohol treatment, judicial monitoring, and individualized services that integrate the needs of the entire family
- Policymakers and health care providers should rely on resources produced
by the National Center on Addiction and Substance Abuse, a national
nonprofit research and policy organization, in developing policies and
programs addressing addiction (http://www.centeronaddiction.org/about)
- Federally funded pain research studies should incorporate recommendations made by the Interagency Pain Research Coordinating Committee
so that pain management is less reliant upon the use of prescription opioids
- States should allow partial fills of schedule II controlled substances so
long as the total quantity for all partial fillings does not exceed the total
quantity prescribed
- The FDA should issue guidance as to how approved labeling on opioid
prescriptions may include statements that deter misuse
- States should revise their Essential Health Benefit benchmark plans to
comply with the ACA regarding SUD coverage so that addiction treatment is accessible and affordable
- Congress should amend the Drug Addiction Treatment Act of 2000 and
the Controlled Substances Act so that nurse practitioners and physician
assistants are allowed to be certified to prescribe medication-assisted
treatment
- HHS must expand access to medication assisted treatment by increasing
the highest limit on the number of patients eligible providers can treat
from 100 to 500

INTERNATIONAL RECOMMENDATIONS

- All countries should use tools developed through the WHO Mental
Health Gap Action Program to address the severe lack of resources for

mental, neurological, and substance use disorders and help implement evidence-based and low cost interventions

- Countries that recently created or are in the process of implementing universal health coverage must incorporate mental health care into their national benefits plans upon initiation of the program in order to avoid the siloing of mental health and addiction from other health disorders
- Non-profits and international organizations must support programs that train community health workers in how to treat individuals with mental health and substance use disorders, such as Partners In Health MESH-Mental Health program
- All countries should develop and maintain a National Mental Health Plan with clear indicators that align with the WHO mental health action plan 2013-2020
- All countries should release data to and support the International Association for Suicide Prevention's efforts to conduct cross-national comparisons of suicide aimed at providing insight into the growing clustering and contagion of suicidal behavior
- All national disaster and emergency response initiatives must include a mental health component based on the WHO mental health and emergency resources (http://www.who.int/mediacentre/factsheets/fs383/en/)
- The International Narcotics Control Board should make fentanyl a regulated substance

II. Prevention and Early Intervention can decrease the chronic and debilitating outcomes associated with mental illness and addiction. Yet the United States' health system continues to rely on expensive interventions implemented only long after the onset of disease. The following recommendations prioritize prevention in an attempt to avoid adverse health outcomes and curb costs.

COMMUNITY-BASED SERVICES
- Congress should expand the Medicaid home and community-based services waiver to include youth who are in need of services provided in a psychiatric residential facility, including Coordinated Specialty Care for First Episode Psychosis

- Congress should extend Section 223 of the Protecting Access to Medicare Act to facilitate the development of certified community behavioral health clinics
- Congress should pass the Expand Excellence in Mental Health Act and implement alternative payment models that incentivize coordination between community-based services
- States should take advantage of the Medicaid home and community based services HCBS waiver
- State insurance commissioners should require healthcare plans cover evidence-based home visiting programs, such as the Nurse Family Partnership, and encourage their integration into managed care plans and integrated care models
- The SAMHSA Substance Abuse Prevention and Treatment and the Community Mental Health Services Block Grants should be integrated into funding structures used to deliver grants for other medical care to eliminate the siloing of behavioral health from other medical grants
- All programs operated or supported by SAMHSA should incorporate the best available science, use evidence-based practices, and measure their effectiveness and efficiency through the adherence to clearly identified goals

LAW ENFORCEMENT
- All law enforcement personnel should complete a 40-hour Crisis Intervention Team program based on the Memphis Model, an internationally-recognized best practice for pre-arrest jail diversion for those in a mental illness crisis, which can be accessed at www.cit.memphis.edu
- All law enforcement agencies and first responders should be required to carry naloxone in either the injection or intranasal form
- All states should enact Good Samaritan or 911 drug immunity laws that provide immunity from supervision violations, low-level drug possession, and use offenses when an individual experiencing or witnessing an opiate-related overdose calls 911 for assistance or seeks medical attention

SCHOOLS AND UNIVERSITIES
- All colleges and universities must increase behavioral health resources to be sufficient to address the long wait times frequent on campuses

- The Department of Education, in collaboration with the HHS and other agencies, should develop social and emotional learning standards for elementary and secondary schools aimed at improving mental wellness
- The Department of Education, in coordination with the NIMH, should develop and disseminate evidence based brain-building interventions for schools
- The Department of Education should develop and disseminate guidance on the implementation of multitier systems of supports for behavioral health services in school systems
- Colleges and universities should create and implement strategic plans for mental illness and substance use disorder prevention based on The Jed Foundation's Campus Program Framework (https://www.jedfoundation.org/professionals/programs-and-research/CampusProgram)

SCREENING

- All disciplinary actions in schools should be accompanied by a mental health screening
- The Department of Education should require mental health screening as a component of annual school physicals that include recommendations for considering family member mental health when necessary
- State health insurance commissioners should require healthcare plans reimburse for Screening, Brief Intervention, and Referral to Treatment, an approach where primary care staff assess patients' substance use risk and refer to appropriate treatment
- Screening pregnant women for perinatal mood disorders, anxiety disorders, and substance use disorders should become the standard of care
- Congress should enact legislation requiring all health plans to reimburse for evidence-based mental health screening during annual well-child exams and adult annual physical exams. They should include an adverse childhood experience (ACE) component, as higher ACE scores are associated with a greater likelihood of numerous medical and behavioral conditions
- CMS should enforce the federal Medicaid law requiring states provide early and periodic screening, diagnosis, and treatment for Medicaid eligible children and adolescents

Suicide

- States should increase funding for and assist in the implementation and evaluation of state suicide prevention plans that focus on suicides across the lifespan
- Congress should pass the Garrett Lee Smith Memorial Act Reauthorization of 2015, which funds several research, training, prevention, and technical assistance programs aimed at decreasing suicide, including the Youth Suicide Early Intervention and Prevention Strategies, and Mental Health and Substance Use Disorder Services on Campuses programs
- All colleges and universities should develop evidence-based suicide prevention plans to respond to the high incidence of suicide in young adults
- All secondary schools, and even elementary schools, should also have evidence-based suicide awareness plans, based on the Model School District Policy on Suicide Prevention (https://afsp.org/wp-content/uploads/2016/01/Model-Policy_FINAL.pdf), to respond to the growing problem of suicide in younger children

Emergency Response

- All hospitals should create behavioral emergency response teams (BERT) to assist staff in non-behavioral health units treating patients with acute psychiatric disorders experiencing violent behaviors
- All offices of emergency management should develop a comprehensive mental health disaster plan using PsySTART Rapid Mental Health Triage and Incident Management System (http://www.cdms.uci.edu/PDF/PsySTART-cdms02142012.pdf)
- All states should pass legislation requiring school districts to develop evidence-based plans detailing how they will handle emotional and behavioral distress, including suicidal thinking and behavior, and threats of violence, during the school year

III. Vulnerable Populations are more severely impacted by behavioral health disorders than the general population. Individuals in the criminal justice system, veterans and active members of the military, marginalized populations, and pregnant women are among the groups that will benefit from targeted efforts to achieve health equity and improve health outcomes.

- Congress should require that all programs and treatments receiving federal funding are culturally and linguistically sensitive, age appropriate and trauma-informed
- HHS should create the Inter-Departmental Serious Mental Illness Coordinating Committee, which will evaluate the effect on public health of federal programs related to serious mental illness that includes data about health outcomes and other social outcomes such as employment, homelessness, and incarceration rates

CRIMINAL JUSTICE SYSTEM

- States and counties should implement evidence-based pre-arrest, pre- and post-booking, pretrial, and presenting diversion programs for offenders with a serious mental illness or substance use disorder and connect individuals with appropriate services
- Federal and state legislatures should provide financial incentives for prosecutors and attorney generals who demonstrate a commitment to evidence-based alternatives to incarceration
- Federal, state and other correctional authorities should replace solitary confinement with evidence-based and cost-saving mental health care, such as crisis intervention training for correctional officers and mental health step-down units
- States should increase enrollment of the criminal justice population in Medicaid or private insurance to ensure that individuals with mental health and substance use disorders receive appropriate treatment and support services while incarcerated and are connected with appropriate community services upon release
- Congress should appropriate full funding for the Justice and Mental Health Collaboration Act
- Post-secondary educational institutions should adopt admissions policies that do not unfairly discriminate against individuals with a criminal record

VETERANS AND ACTIVE MEMBERS OF THE MILITARY

- In cases where the VA is incapable of meeting care demands, reimbursement for licensed mental health providers external to the agency should be made available

- Congress should appropriate additional funding to the Department of Veterans Affairs to increase the number of behavioral health professionals in the Veterans Health Administration available to veterans and their family members
- Congress should consider extending the National Health Service Corps to include Veteran's Administration Hospitals
- States and counties must collect and publish data on the number of veterans incarcerated in the criminal justice system

INDIVIDUALS WITH DEVELOPMENTAL DISABILITY COMORBID WITH MENTAL ILLNESS OR SUBSTANCE USE DISORDER

- States must prioritize mental health diagnosis and treatment for individuals with co-occurring developmental disability, mental illness, and substance use disorder by taking advantage of federal programs, such as Medicaid waivers, Money Follows the Person, and the Balancing Incentive Payment program
- Insurers should reimburse for day rehabilitation treatment programs for adults with dual diagnoses of intellectual disabilities and mental illness that promote independence and focus on transitional planning, similar to the Harris County ADAPT program, www.mhmraharris.org/idd/Brochure%20ADAPT.pdf
- Individuals and facilities treating children and adults with co-occurring disabilities must meet qualifications standards, such as the NADD Accreditation and Staffing Certification Guidelines (http://thenadd.org/products/accreditation-and-certification-programs/)
- State legislatures should amend their laws about insurance coverage of pervasive developmental disorder so that all developmental disabilities are included

MARGINALIZED POPULATIONS

- Training and continuing-education programs must incorporate cultural competency elements focused on under-served populations, including racial, ethnic, and sexual minorities, and be based on evidence-based standards
- The Indian Health Services, a division of the HHS, must develop a strategy to address the high incidence of suicide and untreated substance use disorders in Native American communities

- The Model Adolescent Suicide Prevention Program, originally developed for a small tribe in New Mexico, should be disseminated to other Native American tribes (http://legacy.nreppadmin.net/ViewIntervention.aspx?id=251)

PREGNANT WOMEN
- Pregnant women with opioid use disorder should be connected with appropriate medication assisted treatment during pregnancy and remain in treatment after they have given birth
- Congress should appropriate federal funding to the Centers for Disease Control and Prevention to sponsor fetal alcohol syndrome disorder practice and implementation centers in every region

IV. **The Behavioral Health Workforce** is unable to meet the needs of the growing population requiring mental health and addiction services. Mental health professional shortage areas exist throughout the country. Training programs do not reflect the diverse needs of patients. Many facilities offering behavioral health treatments do not meet accreditation standards. The following recommendations combat the growing workforce crisis in mental health and addiction care.

- Congress should increase funding for the National Health Service Corps scholarship and loan repayments program to increase the supply of behavioral health professionals
- Federal and state governments should create training grants for fellowships and stipends for advanced education programs in behavioral health care
- Medical training programs must include discussions of safe-prescribing practices, including the use of opioid treatment alternatives when appropriate
- Behavioral health provider organizations should conduct annual cultural competence self-assessments
- Congress should create a Minority Fellowship Program designed to increase providers' knowledge of issues related to prevention, treatment, and recovery support for mental and substance use disorders among racial and ethnic minority populations (http://www.samhsa.gov/minority-fellowship-program)

- Public and private health systems should incentivize the effective use of telehealth
- Continuing Medical Education for state medical licensure should include training in evidence-based care coordination and valued-based payment systems
- All health care plans that offer behavioral health benefits must meet accreditation standards developed by URAC or the National Committee for Quality Assurance
- National peer credentialing standards for individuals in clinical settings must be developed to encourage peer specialist reimbursement
- All facilities and programs serving persons with mental illness, including, hospitals, community mental health centers, clinics, nursing homes, rehabilitation programs, correctional institutions, and networks, should seek accreditation

V. Social Determinants which are known to trigger and exacerbate mental illness and substance use disorders must be addressed in combination with policies aimed at service access.

EDUCATION
- Congress should amend the Elementary and Secondary Education Act to fund teacher and principal training and professional development in mental wellness programs, such as social and emotional learning, early warning sign identification, and trauma-informed approaches
- Federal Title I education funds and other congressional funds should be used to replace zero tolerance policies with programs that consider behavioral health, such as trauma-informed programs and positive behavioral support
- Congress should amend the Head Start Act to require that in providing and allocating resources for training and technical assistance the Department of Health and Human Services must give priority to the implementation of evidence-based trauma-informed programs, age-appropriate positive behavioral interventions and supports, early childhood mental health consultation, and prevention of suspension and expulsion

WORKPLACE

- Employers should ensure that they are fully compliant with the Americans with Disabilities Act regarding current and prospective employees with mental illnesses and substance use disorders. They must offer them the same accommodation they would any other medically disabled person.
- The Occupational Safety and Health Administration should develop a national psychological health and safety in the workplace standard—similar to physical health and safety standards—to help organizations achieve measurable improvement in the psychological health of employees
- Employers should ask employees to complete health risk appraisals that include questions relating to behavioral health. Individuals who screen positive should be connected with relevant employee assistant programs
- Employers should design their health insurance benefits in accordance with the Employer Guide for Compliance with the Mental Health Parity and Addiction Equity Act (http://www.workplacementalhealth.org/ParityGuide15) published by Milliman, Inc. and the Partnership for Workplace Mental Health
- Employers should adhere to the guidelines of Employee Assistance Professionals Association (http://www.eapassn.org/Portals/11/Docs/EAPAStandards10.pdf) and measure the performance of EAPs with validated tools, such as those provided within the Workplace Office Suite (http://chestnutglobalpartners.org/wos)
- Employers should create an easily accessible summary of behavioral health benefits to help consumers navigate the healthcare system
- Employers should implement workplace wellness programs similar to Wellness Works, a California workplace education and training program (http://www.wellnessworksmentalhealth.org/)
- Employers should pledge to avoid using language in advertisements and organizational documents that perpetuates negative and inaccurate stereotypes about people with mental illnesses and substance use disorders

EMPLOYMENT

- CMS should revise Medicaid regulations to extend the Medicaid Rehabilitation Option to cover vocational and employment support services

- Federal and state entities should track unemployment rates among individuals identified as living with a behavioral health disorder
- Titles I and II of the Americans with Disabilities Act must be interpreted and enforced in ways that limit discrimination and maximize employment opportunities for individuals with mental illness
- Expand eligibility for supplemental security income and supplemental security disability income to include people with substance use disorders
- The VA should have authority to provide supportive-employment services to veterans

HOUSING
- States should increase funding and fully implement evidence-based housing programs, such as Housing First (http://legacy.nreppadmin.net/ ViewIntervention.aspx?id=365), to reduce homelessness among individuals with mental illness and addiction
- CMS should revise Medicaid regulations to extend the Medicaid Rehabilitation Option to cover housing support services
- Federal and state entities should track homelessness rates among people identified as living with a behavioral health disorder

VI. Research is needed to better understand the etiology of brain diseases and to create a proper evidence base for treatment development and implementation. The recommendations below encourage sustained and sufficient funding for both public and private mental health and addiction research.

- No brain health research should be funded unless it employs the open science principles required to make its results shareable across disciplines and around the world. All funders and researchers should incorporate the One Mind Open Science Principles into their protocols, so that informed consents for medical information collection allow de-identified data to be shared to study a broad range of conditions, research employs the most widely accepted common data elements, and data can be made available to the research community as early as possible (http://onemind.org/Our-Solutions/Open-Science)

- The NIH should appropriate equitable funding to the NIMH, NIDA, and NIAA that is comparable to funding for the other institutes. This funding would support research on the etiology of brain diseases, treatment development, the evaluation of clinical practices, and outcomes monitoring
- Congress should continue to appropriate funding to the NIMH Research Domain Criteria (RDoC) initiative
- Research institutes focused on mental illness and substance use disorders should follow the model of the National Network of Depression Centers, based off of the National Comprehensive Cancer Network, which facilitates collaboration between different centers to reach the critical mass necessary for large clinical trials and data registries
- Congress should appropriate funding to the NIMH for research on the determinants of self-directed violence
- State should amend existing state laws to include brain donation within existing organ donation policies
- Congress should incentivize pharmaceutical companies in the development of new medications targeting the central nervous system by creating a regulatory pathway to hasten the conditional approval of beneficial CNS drugs
- Federal research grants for behavioral health treatments should include a translational research component on the financial, ethical, logistic, and regulatory aspects impacting dissemination of therapies into clinical and community settings
- Congress should increase funding to the CMS to expand the National Violent Death Reporting System nationally and to facilitate coordination between the states
- National and/or state standards protecting psychiatric research participants must include stronger provisions on informed consent, advanced directives, and right to withdraw

FOR MORE INFORMATION
ABOUT OUR PROGRAMS

THE KENNEDY FORUM

- Policy incubator and convener for the entire community of mental health and addiction
- Gathers experts from across the spectrum of behavioral health to discuss and promote best practices and policy solutions in areas requiring collaborative leadership, including parity implementation, outcomes-based care, integration, technology, and mental wellness
- Launching a global brain health leadership enterprise with One Mind and Johnson & Johnson—One Mind Initiative at Work—which will provide a forum for select visionary corporate leaders and thought leaders committed to improving behavioral health through the workplace
- Holds conferences and meetings, including the annual "State of the Union in Mental Health and Addiction"
- Works closely with the Kennedy Center for Mental Health Policy and Research, Satcher Health Leadership Institute, Morehouse School of Medicine and the Kennedy Forum Illinois
- To join the Kennedy Forum and get regular updates on legal, medical and scientific news, go to www.thekennedyforum.org

ParityTrack.org O

- Collaboration between the Kennedy Forum and the Thomas Scattergood Behavioral Health Foundation that provides live, interactive resources, on a state-by-state basis, to improve implementation and enforcement of the Mental Health Parity and Addiction Equity Act of 2008, the additional behavioral health protections of the Affordable Care Act, and any new legislation or regulations.
- Provides technical assistance to legislators, regulatory agencies and advocates, develops model state parity legislation, and aggressively aggregates legal cases and decisions that impact implementation and enforcement of parity laws.
- For consumers, family members and caregivers, ParityTrack also provides critical information, on a state-by-state basis, to explain relevant legislation, regulations, and litigation so everyone understands their rights under the law. Explains common parity violations, to help better educate consumers on a host of issues that might arise when seeking or accessing treatment.
- Provides contact information for consumers and family members to reach out to state insurance commissioners, insurance companies and other local resources.
- ParityTrack also has debuted an app that allows any complaints you file concerning denials of care to become part of a national database at www .parityquest.org.
- For more information, visit www.paritytrack.org.

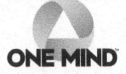

ONE MIND

- International forum for open science, sharing of big data, and advanced collaboration in brain research, which will accelerate replication and validation of results, allow increased data integration and power for statistical analysis, and accelerate the translation of basic research to clinical use so patients receive improved diagnostics and treatments

- Built open data portal with open science principles that will greatly accelerate the discovery of better diagnostics, treatments and, some- day, cures for diseases and injuries of the brain
- Creates global public-private partnerships among governmental, corporate, scientific, and philanthropic communities
- Holds annual summit of international brain research community to share innovation and best practices, and take on new research challenges that will benefit a broad range of brain diseases
- To join the One Mind effort and get regular updates on its brain science efforts, go to www.onemind.org.

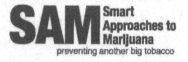

- Champions smart policies that promote getting the science out to the public about today's high-potency marijuana and encourage decreasing marijuana use—without harming marijuana users with arrest records that stigmatize them for life
- Works to stop the commercialization of marijuana and marijuana-edible products by fighting Big Marijuana—the Big Tobacco of our time
- Promotes research on marijuana's medical potential and helps to assure that medicines made from marijuana's active ingredients can be dispensed by board-certified physicians to appropriate patients in pharmacies like any other medicine
- For more information, visit www.learnaboutsam.org.

AFTERWORD AND
ACKNOWLEDGMENTS

From Patrick Kennedy

The biggest challenge of working on this book has been keeping it scrupulously honest about my illnesses and how they affected my relationships, even if it reminded me again and again how much time and love and productivity I have lost to being sick. That has been especially true when going back over my relationship with my father. I did this to show the generational differences between approaches to mental illness and addiction—and to help personalize the challenges of mental health parity as they exist in all families. But in rereading parts of the book, I am constantly reminded of how much I miss my father and, perhaps more importantly, how I missed the chance for him to see me in recovery, with a wife and family, carrying on my work in a healthier way. I hope the book captures both the wonderful times we shared, as well as the missed opportunities. I hope it serves as a reminder to me and to others how these illnesses affect families and, if not treated properly and chronically, can rob us of our chance to connect, to love, and to process conflict in the relationships that matter most.

I wanted to make one point about all the political processes described in this book. While I have tried to describe some of my recollections of what I was doing, or trying to do, during various efforts as an elected official—and now as an advocate—nobody in Washington does anything by themselves. There are hardworking colleagues and cosponsors and staffers and lobbyists and advocates involved in every move we make—but listing and thanking everyone involved turns narrative into the Congressional Record. I am eternally grateful to my colleagues in politics, business, and advocacy, and want to thank everyone who supported me as a state rep in Rhode Island and during my years as a Congressman from Rhode Island's First District. And I learned the true value of their friendship after I no longer sat on an appropriations committee that mattered to them, or could cast a vote—and they still were there for me, in so many ways, and support what we are trying to do now. The same is true for many of my father's best and brightest, who have been there for me during this journey as a constant reaffirmation of how the work goes on and the cause endures.

I should also note that while we did our best to navigate the various rules for properly identifying the various brain disorders and those who have them, there is no perfect way to conform to everyone's idea of what is correct—especially in a long narrative where there simply must be synonyms to avoid endless word repetitions. Beyond making sure that nobody in the book is described as "being" their illness unless they actually preferred it (some with alcoholism would rather be referred to as alcoholic), we did use disease, disorder, and illness interchangeably, as we did addiction, dependence, and substance use disorder; intellectual disability and developmental disability; and quite a few other terms. While we had many discussions about the best way to do the right thing in these usages, I'm sure there are instances where, no matter how good our intentions, some readers might be upset by some word choices.

If I started making a really inclusive list of those who deserve recognition, it might never end. But I especially want to thank my family and friends, as well as all of those who have been with me since I left Congress. These include the staff at One Mind and the Kennedy Forum, our ParityTrack partners at the Thomas Scattergood Behavioral Health Foundation, our partners at the Satcher Health Leadership Institute at Morehouse University and the Kennedy Center for Mental Health Policy and Research, and the team at Kennedy

Forum Illinois: Garen and Shari Staglin; Allan Fox; Bill Emmet, Dr. Henry Harbin, Garry Carneal, and Lauren Alfred; Joe Pyle, Alyson Ferguson, Timothy Clement, Amanda Mauri, and Luke Butler; Dr. David Satcher and Dr. Glenda Wrenn; Peter and Mimi O'Brien; and Jeff Valliere of Cura Strategies. I'd also like to thank my personal team: Keith Lowey, Kara Kukfa, Brendan Fairfield, Nicole Steed, and Kate Borchers.

And I want to acknowledge all those within the anonymous twelve-step recovery community, who are always there wherever I go and whenever I need them, and my closest and most supportive family member in that community Chris Lawford.

I want to thank my co-author, Stephen Fried, who has been my navigator in this venture. We often described this book as some kind of Lewis and Clark journey across many Americas, without my realizing that by the end, after traversing so much challenging political and personal terrain, it would feel like he had become my Clark. The path to this book wasn't always easy or direct, and there were times when I wondered if we were going to land in a new place or fall off the end of the earth. But with Stephen as navigator, we knew when to take chances and how to remain fixed on our ultimate destination.

Thanks to my publishers David Rosenthal and Aileen Boyle at Blue Rider Press, to our agent on the book, David Black, and to my attorney, Ike Williams.

Ultimately, the only reason I was able to write this book—in fact, the only reason I am still alive to tell this story—is because of my wife Amy and our kids, Harper, Owen, Nora, and Nell. Amy saw something in me that I had not been able to find in myself, and instead of running away from me she ran toward us. Her belief in me and in our love has been so inspiring but also so steadying; I can only wish that everyone involved in the common struggle finds this kind of closeness and partnership with someone so grounded and so hopeful. She and our children inspire, amuse, and emotionally support me every day of my life. Thank God for them.

From Stephen Fried

In late March of 2011, Patrick Kennedy and I were introduced via e-mail by a mutual friend in Tucson, Dr. Raymond Woosley, who thought we might have a lot to talk about. A week later we were having lunch in New York, where neither of us lived: I was commuting there on Thursdays from Philadelphia to teach at Columbia Journalism School, and Patrick was commuting there (and to DC, Boston, Philadelphia, and other locations) from Absecon, New Jersey, where he and his then-girlfriend Amy, and her daughter Harper, were living with Amy's parents.

It was an intriguing and energizing lunch, and it reminded me how much I missed writing about mental health, addiction, and brain science. These subjects had fascinated me during the first twenty years of my journalism career in magazines and nonfiction books, but it was getting harder to find editors interested in assigning ambitious stories in these areas, so I had been focusing more on writing narrative history books, teaching narrative journalism, and lecturing.

It turned out Patrick and I knew a lot of the same people in the world of brain science and politics, but from different perspectives. I had covered many veterans of the "Decade of the Brain" who had lived through that cycle of great bravery and hope and the failed 1996 mental health parity bill. Much of this journalism had been inspired by my wife, author Diane Ayres, and her medical issues after one pill of a new antibiotic triggered a seizure and a mood disorder—leaving her, and us, in an area where neurology and psychiatry have always crossed over, even though neurologists and psychiatrists often want patients to pick sides. Because I wrote about her illness and pharmaceutical safety, my wife and I became friendly with some of my sources, especially Dr. Kay Redfield Jamison—who first "came out" with her manic-depressive illness in a piece I wrote for the *Washington Post Magazine* in 1995—and her late husband, schizophrenia researcher Dr. Richard Wyatt. I covered the rise of NAMI in Washington for *The New Yorker* (don't look for the piece, they killed it—but left me with many exclusive interviews, including one with the late Paul Wellstone, that were helpful for this book), I spent a year covering the internal life of the nation's first psychiatric hospital in Philadelphia, I covered the family who invented the "false memory" controversy, I covered the sexual side effects of some psychiatric drugs and the difficulties of titrating down off others.

When I heard Patrick describe what he wanted to accomplish in his post-congressional advocacy, it made me want to watch and perhaps participate. Especially since one of his major goals was to break down the barriers between the medical professions interested in the brain. As I explained at our lunch, after many years of having my wife's case handled by a mental health professional—with all the discrimination, unfair deductibles, and managed care challenges—she had several more seizures and was now being treated primarily by a neurologist. And as soon as that switch took place, our healthcare provider started calling us all the time, asking how they could help her manage her epilepsy. Family members were suddenly more supportive of her care; nobody asked anymore if she "really" needed those medications, the way they did when her primary diagnosis was bipolar disorder (even though she was still taking the same anticonvulsant meds, which are used for both illnesses).

At our first meeting, Patrick didn't tell me much about his own personal situation; we were there to talk about the upcoming One Mind debut. So I didn't understand at the time just how recently his life had changed, and how new his new perspective really was: it was only years later, when we were deep into this book, that I realized that on the day we had met Patrick considered himself just a couple months sober.

We talked and e-mailed before, during, and after One Mind, but never actually decided to work together. Months later, *Philadelphia* magazine asked if I wanted to write about Patrick and his new life in South Jersey with Amy. I asked if they were up for this, because everything I had seen and heard during our conversations and at One Mind would be on the record. They bravely said okay, and we started, right away, doing some incredibly personal and moving interviews. After the piece came out, I was asked if I would consider doing a book project with him.

Patrick had been teaching a course on mental health policy at Brown after leaving Congress, with his friend Dr. Judith Bentkover, and thought the lectures might make an interesting book. I said I'd be happy to help him find someone else to write it, but would only be interested in collaborating if the book was something much bolder, something that could make a bigger impact. I thought it would be great if Patrick wanted to co-write a book that told the true, behind-the-scenes story of mental health and addiction politics and science, and included a lot of his own experiences with the challenges of these illnesses in his own family—as a mirror onto all the families similarly affected. Patrick liked the idea and his lawyer, Ike Williams, came up with the title, *A Common Struggle*.

For the next two years, we did periodic, long interviews—each one usually two and a half to three hours—that moved effortlessly from public policy, really private stuff about Patrick's illnesses past and present, discrimination against brain diseases, the challenge of building two nonprofits from scratch, and his family. When we started, Patrick's stepdaughter, Harper, was four and Amy was pregnant with Owen. I was often there when Harper got home from day care and later from school, and we always stopped the interviews so she could regale us with what happened that day. After Owen was born, we did many interviews when Patrick was in charge of watching him, and so it was not uncommon for our discussions to go to a whisper as he rocked Owen to sleep in his arms. Later, Owen would sometimes crawl up, and then march up to Patrick's third-floor office during a session and demand that his dad read him a book. Patrick always stopped, read him one, and then convinced him to go back downstairs and take a nap. When we were finishing the book, Nora was just getting old enough to start coming up with her brother to double-team their dad.

Besides these sessions—we did over forty of them—Patrick gave me access to all of his medical records, including all the notes from his psychiatrists and psychologists, inpatient and outpatient (none of which he had ever read), and his handwritten worksheets from rehabs. He also gave me all his office political files on mental health parity and other healthcare bills, and I attended several years' worth of conferences and symposia where Patrick spoke. I also interviewed Amy at length several times; Amy and I did an interview session with Patrick's mother; and Patrick and I interviewed a small number of very important people in his life. The process was often surreal, since this was, in many cases, the first time Patrick and people close to him were admitting out loud just how ill he had been at various times, and how much about his health had gone unspoken. The process was like psychotherapy or twelve-step sharing, with an investigative reporter involved.

After I wrote a draft of the book, Amy very actively joined the process of editing. The three of us spent several months—in long sessions on the phone, in person in Patrick's study, in limos, and when Amy was pregnant with Nell and not feeling so great, we worked together while she was lying on the couch in the living room, buried in manuscript pages. It was intense, fascinating, and really, really personal.

I'm not sure anybody has ever trusted me with this level of private detail and revelation before. Patrick and Amy are really brave, and committed to what they want to accomplish, and I thank them for letting me be part of it.

I also want to thank those who taught me how to write about mental illness, addiction, and healthcare, Dr. Sandy Bloom and Ruth Anne Ryan; Dr. Kay Redfield Jamison and Dr. Richard Jed Wyatt; Dr. David Flockhart and Dr. Raymond Woosley; Dr. Ray DePaulo, Laurie Flynn, Dr. Martin Orne, Dr. Jennifer Freyd, Dr. Jody Foster, Dr. Michael Miller, Dr. Bradley Fenton, Dr. Michael Sperling, Dr. Steven Galetta, Dr. Jeffrey Lieberman, and all the consumers and families, living and dead, whose lives have been shared with me.

My thanks to my assistant on this book, Amanda Mauri—an MPH grad student at Penn who got quite an education in the politics of public health—and to the Penn undergrads who helped with political and archival research: Jessica Goodman, Debby Chiang, Melanie Bavaria, Maxwell McAdams, Rebecca Heilweil, and Laine Higgins.

Thanks to my unstoppable agent, David Black, and to our publishers, David Rosenthal and Aileen Boyle at Blue Rider.

And, mostly, thanks to my wife and editor, Diane Ayres, who is responsible—personally and professionally, as if they can be separated— for most of the insights I brought to this book, and most of my abilities to write and finish it.

INDEX

ABOUT THE AUTHORS

The Honorable **Patrick J. Kennedy** is a former member of the U.S. House of Representatives and the nation's leading political voice on mental illness, addiction, and other brain diseases. During his sixteen-year career representing Rhode Island in Congress, he fought a national battle to end medical and societal discrimination against these illnesses, highlighted by his lead sponsorship of the Mental Health Parity and Addictions Equity Act of 2008—and his brave openness about his own health challenges. The son of Senator Edward "Ted" Kennedy, he decided to leave Congress not long after his father's death to devote his career to advocacy for brain diseases and to create a new, healthier life and start a family. He has since founded the Kennedy Forum, which unites the community of mental health, and co-founded One Mind, a global leader in open science collaboration in brain research. He lives in New Jersey with his wife, Amy, and their four children.

www.patrickjkennedy.net

Stephen Fried is an award-winning magazine journalist, a bestselling author, an adjunct professor at Columbia University Graduate School of Journalism, and a lecturer at the University of Pennsylvania. He is the author of two books on healthcare, mental health, and addiction—*Bitter Pills: Inside the Hazardous World of Legal Drugs,* and *Thing of Beauty: The Tragedy of Supermodel Gia*—as well as *The New Rabbi, Husbandry,* and his recent historical biography *Appetite for America: Fred Harvey and the Business of Civilizing the Wild West—One Meal at a Time,* which was a *New York Times* bestseller. Fried lives in Philadelphia with his wife, author Diane Ayres.

www.stephenfried.com